Practical Management of Pediatric Cardiac Arrhythmias

Edited by

Vicki L. Zeigler, RN, MSN

Pediatric Arrhythmia Nurse Specialist
Certified Legal Nurse Consultant
Azle, Texas

and

Paul C. Gillette, MD

Medical Director of Cardiology
Cook Children's Heart Center
Fort Worth, Texas

Futura Publishing Company, Inc.
Armonk, NY

Library of Congress Cataloging-in-Publication Data

Practical management of pediatric cardiac arrhythmias / edited by
Vicki L. Zeigler and Paul C. Gillette.
      p. ; cm.
      Includes bibliographical references and index.
      ISBN 0-87993-466-2 (alk. paper)
      1. Arrhythmia in children.   I. Zeigler, Vicki L.   II. Gillette,
Paul C.
      [DNLM: 1. Arrhythmia—diagnosis—Child.   2. Arrhythmia—
therapy—Child. WG 330 P3713 2001]
      RJ426.A7 P394 2001
      618.92'128—dc21   2001023867

Published by
Futura Publishing Company
135 Bedford Road
Armonk, New York 10504

LC#: 2001023867
ISBN#: 0-87993-466-2

Every effort has been made to ensure that the information in this book is
as up to date and accurate as possible at the time of publication. However,
due to the constant developments in medicine, neither the author, nor the
editors, nor the publisher can accept any legal or any other responsibility
for any errors or omissions that may occur.

Printed in the United States of America on acid-free paper.

Dedication

This book is dedicated to our friends:

Scott and Carol Elkins, whose hearts are as big as Texas
AND
Craig and Melodie Greene, whose faith and devotion are an
inspiration to us all.

Acknowledgments

We would like to thank Laurie Browning for her secretarial assistance in preparing parts of this manuscript. We would also like the thank the following manuscript reviewers for taking time out of their busy schedules to review specific chapters for us: Jack Chapin, Linda Herrell, Chris Hickman, Patty Hussey, and our honorary co-editor, Dianne Marlow. Last, we would like to thank Steven Korn for his encouraging words and patience during this manuscript preparation and Joanna Levine for her expert editorial skills. We could not have completed this project without all of you. Thanks.

Foreword

The management of cardiac arrhythmias in children has become a more important and complex problem than in past years. Over the last several decades, our understanding of the mechanisms and etiologies of arrhythmias has improved drastically. As more and more patients with both simple and particularly complex congenital heart disease survive operations, there is an increasing population of patients with simple and complex cardiac arrhythmias. Coupled with this increasing need for management of complex arrhythmias has been the introduction of new antiarrhythmic medications, mapping and ablation techniques, and enhanced device therapy with improved leads and improved functional characteristics. Although the most complex problems must be dealt with by those sub-subspecialists in cardiac arrhythmia management, many other health care professionals, including pediatricians, pediatric cardiologists, and pediatric cardiac nurses without specific advanced training in arrhythmia management, also participate in their care. This care requires not only highly technical components, but holistic patient and family-focused aspects as well.

This book serves as a very useful source of current information and practical data about the diagnosis and management of all aspects of care for all caregivers, from novice to expert, who care for children, adolescents, and young adults with arrhythmias. This text includes succinct information on implications for clinicians and patient and family considerations, with precise "how to" information regarding specific treatment modalities and management techniques. The editors and authors are all nationally recognized experts in the field and have provided a very useful text for all, which can be a valuable asset to all of us practitioners who deal with this increasing population of pediatric, adolescent, and young adult patients.

Thomas P. Graham, Jr., MD
Ann & Monroe Carell Family Professor of Pediatrics
Director, Pediatric Cardiology
Vanderbilt University Medical Center

Contributors

John M. Clark, MD   Director of Electrophysiology, Children's Hospital Medical Center of Akron, Akron, Ohio

Karen Corbett, PhD, RN   Assistant Professor, College of Nursing, Medical University of South Carolina, Charleston, South Carolina

Macdonald Dick II, MD   Professor, Department of Pediatrics and Communicable Diseases, University of Michigan; Director, Pediatric Electrophysiology, Division of Pediatric Cardiology, University of Michigan Hospitals, Ann Arbor, Michigan

Paul C. Gillette, MD   Medical Director of Cardiology, Cook Children's Heart Center, Fort Worth, Texas

Debra G. Hanisch, RN, MSN, CPNP   Nurse Practitioner, Pediatric Cardiology, Lucile Packard Children's Hospital at Stanford University Medical Center, Palo Alto, California

Barbara J. Knick, RN, CVT   Electrophysiology Coordinator, Pediatric Cardiac Catheterization Laboratory, Division of Pediatric Cardiology, The Children's Heart Center of South Carolina, Medical University of South Carolina, Charleston, South Carolina

Sarah S. LeRoy, RN, MSN, CPNP   Pediatric Nurse Practitioner, Division of Pediatric Cardiology, University of Michigan Hospitals, Ann Arbor, Michigan

Ann Lewis, RN, BSN   Pacing Sales Representative, Medtronic, Incorporated, Raleigh, North Carolina

Dianne Marlow, RN, BSN, CLNC   Certified Legal Nurse Consultant; Clinical Nurse Coordinator, Cardiology Department, Texas Children's Hospital, Houston, Texas

J. Phillip Saul, MD   Professor of Pediatrics, Chief, Division of Pediatric Cardiology, The Children's Heart Center of South Carolina, Medical University of South Carolina, Charleston, South Carolina

Sherry J. Taylor, RN, BSN   Cardiology Nurse Clinician, Children's Hospital Medical Center of Akron, Akron, Ohio

George F. Van Hare, MD   Associate Professor of Pediatrics, Stanford University School of Medicine; Director, Pediatric Arrhythmia Center, University of California, San Francisco and Stanford University Medical Center, Palo Alto, California

Vicki L. Zeigler, RN, MSN   Pediatric Arrhythmia Nurse Specialist, Certified Legal Nurse Consultant, Azle, Texas

Contents

Chapter 1

Mechanisms, Diagnostic Tools, and Patient and Family Education

Vicki L. Zeigler, RN, MSN, Dianne Marlow, RN, BSN, and Paul C. Gillette, MD

Cardiac arrhythmias in children are similar in many ways to those found in the adult population. Due to an increased understanding of arrhythmia mechanisms in children as well as better diagnostic tools, clinicians are able to diagnose and treat arrhythmias in children earlier and in a more organized manner. In order for a clinician to understand arrhythmogenesis in children, he or she must possess basic knowledge of the mechanisms and substrates of these arrhythmias. With a rudimentary understanding of these mechanisms and the diagnostic tools necessary to perform a complete clinical evaluation of the child with an arrhythmia, the clinician becomes much better equipped to deal with the various substrates as well as the various arrhythmia treatment options.

This chapter is intended to familiarize the clinician with the mechanisms of arrhythmias in children and the diagnostic tools that are used in their clinical evaluation, whether in assessing a new-onset arrhythmia or a chronic rhythm disturbance that requires intermittent follow-up. The diagnostic tools included in the following discussion are: history and physical examination, 12-lead electrocardiogram (ECG), signal-averaged ECG (SAECG), 24-hour ambulatory monitoring, transtelephonic monitoring (TTM), exercise stress testing (EST), hospital-based telemetry monitoring, and intracardiac electrophysiology studies (IEPS). Last, this chapter reviews the principles of educating children and their families, with an emphasis on family-centered care and children's understanding of illness.

From Zeigler VL, Gillette PC: *Practical Management of Pediatric Cardiac Arrhythmias.* Armonk, NY: Futura Publishing Co., Inc.; ©2001.

Mechanisms

The mechanisms of cardiac arrhythmias in children are similar to those seen in adults, and consist of reentry, abnormal automaticity, and triggered activity. Cardiac arrhythmias can begin at the cellular level due to abnormal ionic flux with mechanisms associated with ions, channels, or other electrophysiologic features such as gross anatomic abnormalities. This section of the chapter provides a definition of the aforementioned mechanisms, followed by a discussion of their application to the tachyarrhythmia and bradyarrhythmia substrates commonly seen in the pediatric population.

Reentry as an arrhythmia mechanism was first described in 1914 by Mines.[1] In order for reentry to occur, there must always be an anatomic or functional circuit, an area of slow conduction, and a zone of unidirectional block. Reentry occurs as a result of a circuit that is created when an impulse continues to circulate in a portion of myocardial tissue after the remainder of the heart completely repolarizes. If this residual impulse exists long enough to allow recovery of other cardiac tissue from its refractoriness, a new depolarization can occur. If this scenario is repeated on a continuing basis, a tachycardia will ensue. Reentry can occur around an anatomic (e.g., accessory pathway) and/or functional (e.g., atrial flutter) barrier or result from intramyocardial microreentrant circuits, the latter of which is seen with atrial fibrillation and some atrial flutter. Reentrant tachyarrhythmias can be induced and terminated by premature stimulation or rapid pacing.

Abnormal automaticity is characterized by nonautomatic cells that acquire diastolic depolarization.[2] Automaticity is the ability of a cell to depolarize spontaneously,[3] and is found in sinus node, atrial, atrioventricular (AV) nodal, and His-Purkinje cells. The cellular mechanism involved in abnormal automaticity is similar to that which underlies the automaticity of the heart's natural pacemaker cells, with calcium and delayed potassium currents playing a major role. Cardiac arrhythmias resulting from altered or abnormal automaticity include atrial and junctional ectopic tachycardias and some ventricular tachycardias (VTs) as well. Arrhythmias resulting from abnormal automaticity cannot be induced or terminated by underdrive or overdrive pacing or by premature stimuli.

Triggered activity requires a preceding stimulus in order to initiate a depolarization,[4–6] and consists of early afterdepolarizations (EADs) and delayed afterdepolarizations (DADs). Both types of afterdepolarizations are triggered by cell activation, but they generally occur under (or in) different circumstances. EADs occur when repolarization is prolonged disturbing the spread of normal impulses producing rate-related block; this rate-related block in turn can encourage reentry circuits or produce entrance block that can protect an automatic focus. In addition to prolonged repolarization, EADs are often bradycardia dependent[6] and may account for the arrhythmias associated with specific electrolyte imbalances, long QT syndrome (LQTS), premature ventricular contractions (PVCs), and some postoperative ventricular arrhythmias associated with cell injury or damage. DADs, on the other hand, occur after repolarization has been completed and are more tachycardia dependent. The postdrive facilitation seen in DADs may be involved in the spontaneous acceleration (or warm-up) of some clinical tachycardias, as well as playing a role in "catecholamine-dependent" ventricular arrhythmias. A summary of the mechanisms associated with tachyarrhythmias in children can be found in Table 1.

Tachyarrhythmias

Tachyarrhythmias in children are generally due to reentry or abnormal automaticity. Reentry is responsible for 90% of all tachyarrhythmias in children and may involve abnormal structures, normal structures, or both. The following discussion is subdivided into supraventricular and ventricular tachyarrhythmias, with an emphasis on the underlying substrates specific to children.

Table 1
Mechanisms of Tachyarrhythmias in Children

Reentry
   Sinus node reentry tachycardia
   Atrioventricular reentry tachycardia (with and without WPW)
   Atrioventricular nodal reentry tachycardia
   Intraatrial reentry tachycardia
   Atrial flutter
   Atrial fibrillation
   Atriofascicular tachycardia
   Nodofascicular tachycardia
   Nodoventricular tachycardia
   Bundle branch reentry tachycardia
   Ventricular tachycardia (reentrant)
   Ventricular flutter
   Ventricular fibrillation

Abnormal/altered automaticity
   Atrial ectopic tachycardia
   Junctional ectopic tachycardia
   Accelerated idioventricular rhythm
   Ventricular tachycardia (automatic)

Triggered activity
   Pause-dependent torsades de pointes (EADs)
   Arrhythmias secondary to digoxin toxicity (DADs)
   Ventricular tachycardia (DADs)

DAD = delayed afterdepolarization; EAD = early afterdepolarization; WPW = Wolff-Parkinson-White.

Supraventricular Arrhythmias

The most common supraventricular reentrant tachyarrhythmia seen in children involves antegrade conduction over the AV node and retrograde conduction over an accessory pathway (also known as AV reentry tachycardia) with the atria and ventricles completing the tachycardia circuit. In most cases, the structure with unidirectional block is the accessory pathway, while the AV node possesses the characteristic of slow conduction. Temporary interruption of the reentry circuit may be accomplished by creating block in one pathway, by premature depolarizations, or by capturing the circuit (i.e., entrainment). Entrainment occurs when a premature stimulus or train of premature stimuli capture the reentry circuit and increase the rate to that of the pacing rate. At the cessation of pacing, the reentry circuit can continue at the pacing rate, return to the original rate, or terminate depending on the properties of the pathway and its response to pacing. Interruption of reentry circuits due to an accessory pathway can be accomplished using acute management strategies such as adenosine administration, vagal maneuvers, and cardioversion.

Gillette[7] studied 35 patients, aged 1 week to 18 years, using IEPS and found 33% to have AV reentry tachycardia secondary to an accessory connection. Ko and colleagues[8] performed transesophageal electrophysiology studies on 135 children, of which 73% had supraventricular tachycardia (SVT) due to an accessory connection. The specific substrates of reentrant SVT seen in children include both orthodromic and antidromic SVT with manifest or concealed Wolff-Parkinson-White (WPW) and the permanent form of junctional reciprocating tachycardia (PJRT).

The second most common reentrant SVT in children is AV nodal reentry tachycardia (AVNRT), which typically appears between the ages of 5 and 10 years.[9] This reentrant rhythm involves two distinct functional and probably anatomic pathways[10,11]; the tachycardia circuit involves one limb within the AV node and the other in fibers adjacent to the AV node.[12] These pathways allow dissociation of conduction within the AV node allowing impulses to reenter the AV node in a retrograde fashion as depolarization spontaneously proceeds to the ventricles. In Gillette's early series of 35 patients[7] (with almost half with concomitant congenital heart disease [CHD] or cardiomyopathy), 24% had AVNRT. In Ko's series of 135 patients[8] (which excluded patients with concomitant CHD and cardiomyopathy), the incidence was 13%. In the series of 30 fetuses studied by Naheed and colleagues,[13] none had AVNRT, supporting the hypothesis of an age-related incidence of the various types of SVT seen in children.

The remainder of reentrant SVTs seen in children includes atrial flutter, intraatrial reentry tachycardia (IART) after repair of CHD, and, rarely, atrial fibrillation. With classic forms of atrial flutter (which pediatric patients rarely exhibit), the tachycardia circuit consists of fixed anatomic obstacles, particularly the orifice of the inferior vena cava and the coronary sinus (CS) os, in addition to the functional slowing of conduction around incisions. The circuit is dependent on a critical-length macroreentrant pathway that is confined primarily to the right atrium. IART, most commonly seen in patients after surgery for CHD, is probably more common in children than classic atrial flutter.[14–16] This reentrant supraventricular arrhythmia is thought to be localized to atrial tissue, specifically due to scar formation at the atriotomy site. Recent investigations into these reentry mechanisms have allowed more precise mapping of the arrhythmia substrate with successful radiofrequency ablation in 5 of 7 patients.[17]

Atrial fibrillation is an uncommon arrhythmia in children that is thought to result from multiple, partially independent reentry wavelets that circulate concurrently.[18] It is generally perpetuated by dilated atria, shortened atrial refractoriness, and inhomogeneous conduction. These conduction and refractory properties of the involved atrial tissue define the functional obstacles of the multiple reentry circuits responsible for atrial fibrillation.[19]

Supraventricular arrhythmias resulting from enhanced automaticity include both atrial and junctional ectopic tachycardias. Atrial ectopic tachycardia (AET) accounts for approximately 4% to 6% of all SVTs in children[9] and occurs when cells other than the normal pacemaker cells have a higher spontaneous rate.[20,21] This higher rate occurs because of more rapid phase 4 depolarization or reduced threshold for initiating an all-or-none action potential. Junctional ectopic tachycardia, although it can be congenital, most commonly occurs after surgery for CHD. The enhanced automaticity is due to irritation of the His bundle during surgery. This particular postoperative supraventricular arrhythmia is usually self-limiting, but can contribute to morbidity and mortality in these patients if not promptly identified and managed. Supraventricular arrhythmias that are secondary to triggered activity are rare in children. Although the precise mechanism of multifocal or chaotic atrial tachycardia is unknown, there is some evidence pointing toward triggered activity.[22]

Ventricular Arrhythmias

The mechanisms of ventricular arrhythmias are similar to those of supraventricular arrhythmias and include reentry, enhanced or abnormal automaticity, and triggered activity.[23–26] VT, due to abnormal ventricular impulse generation and/or conduction, arises primarily within the peripheral Purkinje system but may also arise within the His bundle and bundle branches or in the ventricle.[27,28] Vetter and colleagues[29] report that 60% of VTs are due to reentry and the remaining 40% are due to abnormal automaticity. Specific reentrant ventricular tachyarrhythmias include VT after surgery for CHD, right ventricular outflow tract (RVOT) tachycardia, and left ventricular or fascicular tachycardia.

In most pediatric patients, ventricular tachyarrhythmias are a result of surgery for CHD.[30] The most studied of these patients are those with tetralogy of Fallot whose ventricular arrhythmias have been mapped to the ventriculotomy site.[31,32] The presence of fractionated and delayed local electrograms seen postoperatively provides evidence of the potential area of slow conduction which is a required part of the reentrant circuit.[33]

According to Vetter and colleagues,[29] enhanced or altered automaticity accounts for 40% of ventricular arrhythmias in children. These arrhythmias are more likely to occur under abnormal myocardial conditions such as hypoxia, variances in the concentration of extracellular ions critical for excitation (e.g., potassium), various membrane active drugs (e.g., antiarrhythmic drugs), or structural changes in ion channels.[34]

Ventricular tachyarrhythmias associated with digoxin toxicity as well as torsades de pointes are thought to result from triggered activity. Triggered activity, specifically EADs, has been recorded in patients with LQTS[35,36] and may be the mechanism for torsades de pointes and/or VT in this subgroup of patients.

Bradyarrhythmias

The bradyarrhythmias seen in the pediatric population consist of sinus bradycardia, sick sinus syndrome, acquired second- or third-degree AV block, and congenital complete AV block. Abnormal sinus node function may be due to inadequate intrinsic control, especially excessive vagal tone, or to anomalous intrinsic activity, i.e., abnormal automaticity or sinoatrial (SA) conduction.[37] Sinus bradycardia is relatively rare in the child with an anatomically normal heart, and rarely occurs without concomitant atrial reentrant tachycardia in children who have undergone surgery for CHD.

Sick sinus syndrome is an electrocardiographic diagnosis consisting of bradycardia, reentrant atrial tachycardia, and a blunted heart rate response to exercise. The abnormal impulse formation of the sinus node is probably due to trauma to the sinus node, its approaches, or the sinus node artery, occurring as a result of the CHD surgery. The underlying abnormality of the reentrant tachycardia seen in these patients is probably not related to the sinus node itself, but involves zones of the electrically impaired atria with abnormal conduction and refractory characteristics.[38,39]

Surgically acquired AV block is the most common mechanism of bradycardia in children, and occasionally may be due to injury to a coronary artery during surgery. Congenital malformations of the cardiac conduction system are an important cause of bradyarrhythmias as well. The conduction system may fail to develop in any area or it may be destroyed after its development but before birth. Abnormal development is responsible for congenital complete AV block in patients with major cardiac malformations such as asplenia. Developmental abnormalities may also predispose to the later development of AV block in congenitally corrected transposition of the great arteries. In patients with anatomically normal hearts, complete AV block is usually caused by an antibody response that results in fatty replacement of the AV node.

The understanding of the mechanisms of arrhythmias is important because it can aid the clinician in determining if treatment is indicated and what type of treatment will be most beneficial to the child with a specific cardiac rhythm disturbance. Once the mechanism is identified and the specific substrate elucidated, a comprehensive plan of care can be developed with the patient and family.

Diagnostic Tools

There are a multitude of tools that can be used by clinicians in the initial and ongoing evaluation of children with cardiac arrhythmias. There are several adjunct diagnostic tools that are not discussed in depth in this chapter, but warrant some discussion because they may aid the clinician in determining or confirming an etiology for specific cardiac arrhythmias. One of those tools, the echocardiogram, can provide the clinician with a great deal of information. In the postoperative arrhythmia patient, the clinician should note any anatomic and/or structural findings that may propagate the arrhythmia. The effect of the arrhythmia on overall hemodynamics may be evidenced by chamber enlargement and/or dysfunction. In patients scheduled for transvenous device placement, the echocardiogram should be used to identify the presence of intracardiac shunts and can be performed with contrast if necessary.

The transesophageal echocardiogram may aid the clinician in identifying problems that the transthoracic echocardiogram cannot, e.g., thrombus identification in patients prior to elective cardioversion.[40] Magnetic resonance imaging can be helpful in identifying and assessing some myocardial tumors that cause ventricular arrhythmias.[41] Cardiac catheterization is a helpful tool, especially for patients with VT, since the use of angiography is helpful in identifying arrhythmogenic right ventricular dysplasia.[42] For a more definitive diagnosis of arrhythmogenic right ventricular dysplasia, viral myocarditis, or cardiomyopathy, an endomyocardial biopsy can be extremely useful.[43,44]

The diagnostic tools included in the following discussion are: history and physical examination, 12-lead ECG, SAECG, 24-hour ambulatory electrocardiography, transtelephonic electrocardiography, EST, telemetry monitoring, and, finally, IEPS. The discussion regarding these diagnostic tools includes their specific and various uses, the advantages and disadvantages of each, the specific implications for clinicians, and, finally, the patient and family considerations.

History and Physical Examination

The history and physical examination of children with cardiac rhythm disturbances are important diagnostic tools for the cardiovascular clinician, and interview strategies must take the child's developmental age into account.[45] The clinical evaluation of the child with a cardiac arrhythmia is generally prompted by the frequency and severity of the episodes, with the type of symptoms being dependent on the following variables: the child's heart rate during the arrhythmia episode, the child's age, the activity being pursued when the arrhythmia occurs, and the presence of associated structural or congenital heart disease.[46] The history generally starts with the child's chief complaint, and is followed by a history of the present illness, past history of any illnesses, current health status, and, importantly, a family history. The presenting symptoms associated with cardiac arrhythmias include palpitations (most common), irregular heart rate, heart failure (occasionally), syncope, cardiac arrest (rare), and sudden death (rare).

Uses

The *history* is performed in order to: 1) gather information (in order to form an initial, tentative diagnosis); 2) initiate a relationship with the patient and family; and 3) initiate a definition of the clinician's therapeutic goals.[47] A detailed family history, especially cardiovascular, is important to obtain, as it may form a basis for any familial or genetic etiologies behind the cardiac rhythm disturbance.

The *physical examination* of the child with a cardiac arrhythmia may or may not provide information pertinent to the child's clinical condition and is probably most helpful in children who present with their clinical arrhythmia or experience an episode in the presence of the cardiovascular clinician. The physical examination can allow the clinician to make an objective assessment of the child's hemodynamic status during the arrhythmia episode.

Advantages/Disadvantages

The major advantage of a history is that it may provide a wealth of information regarding the child's symptoms relative to an arrhythmic event. The description of symptoms and/or episodes by the parent and/or child can provide clues to the clinician that are often needed to delineate how best to proceed in the arrhythmia evaluation. A history is generally cost effective and the family history component is often very helpful in identifying familial and/or genetic disorders and/or risk factors for sudden cardiac death. A disadvantage of obtaining a history is that some individuals are poor historians and may even provide irrelevant information.

The advantages of a physical examination can also be the disadvantages for patients with anatomically normal hearts and intermittent symptoms. In patients with frequent ectopy, cardiac auscultation may provide clues regarding the arrhythmia, specifically irregular heartbeats. One major advantage of the physical examination if the patient is experiencing an arrhythmic event in the presence of the clinician is the ability to perform an assessment of the hemodynamics of that arrhythmia. The clinician can assess the child's respiratory status, color, and peripheral pulses in order to make a determination regarding potential treatment options. In patients with implanted devices, the physical examination can be used to assess the device pocket as well as the incision for any signs of erosion or infection, respectively. The disadvantages include the inability to detect any physical abnormalities in patients with cardiac arrhythmias and limited information in uncooperative and irritable children.

Implications for Clinicians

During the interview regarding the child's history, it is critical that the cardiovascular clinician convey to the child's parent(s) that he or she is interested in the child as well as the arrhythmia.[48] The parent should be allowed to talk freely in the beginning in order to express concerns in his or her own words. The clinician should look directly at the parent and child intermittently throughout the interview.

The symptoms associated with cardiac arrhythmias in children are varied and are described differently depending on the child's age. The older child and/or adolescent may be able to describe a history of palpitations, while the younger child may complain of a stomachache or their heart "beeping." Children less than 5 years of age generally are unable to provide any relevant data, so the clinician must rely on the child's parent or caregiver for this information. During the interview, the child should remain dressed in order to decrease anxiety and apprehension.[47] The parent and child should be referred to by name and should not be "talked down to," since the sympathetic listener frequently obtains more accurate information than does the harried, distracted interviewer.[48] Specific questions that can be used by clinicians to elicit information regarding cardiac arrhythmias in children can be found in Table 2.

The questions asked by the clinician regarding family history should focus on the presence of any known cardiac arrhythmias in family members, any sudden death (especially at an early age) episodes, and whether anyone has had syncope or "seizurelike" activity. It is also important to elicit whether the child has been previously diagnosed with seizures, since many patients with LQTS are often initially diagnosed with seizures.[49] Since more and more medications, herbs, and dietary supplements can result in QT prolongation, the clinician should inquire about any medications that the child

Table 2
Questions Used to Obtain Information Regarding Cardiac Arrhythmias

1. How many times have the episodes occurred?
2. How frequent are the episodes?
3. How long do the episodes last?
4. What initiates an episode?
5. How does the child look during an episode?
6. Where does the episode make it feel "funny"?
7. What makes the episode stop?

may be taking at the time or may have been taking during the occurrence of an episode. Information regarding hospitalizations and/or surgeries should be elicited with an emphasis on those related to the arrhythmia episodes.

The physical examination should include the traditional inspection, palpation, percussion, and auscultation. With younger children, the clinician should take any available opportunity when the child is quiet to auscultate the heart. Distracting the child and/or allowing him or her to handle the stethoscope can provide reassurance and decrease anxiety. In many instances, the child may be more comfortable in the parent's lap, and if possible the clinician should proceed with the physical examination in this manner. Since removing the child's clothing promotes fear and anxiety, the child should remain clothed for the majority of the examination when feasible. A hospital gown placed backwards, with the ties in front, provides privacy for the school-aged to adolescent female patient and ease of auscultation for the clinician.

Patient and Family Considerations

The history and physical examination can be used to establish rapport with the patient and family. The clinician should introduce himself/herself to the patient and family and then provide an explanation of the events to follow. If the child is old enough to participate, he or she should be encouraged to do so and should be told exactly what to expect during the physical examination. This will hopefully decrease patient/family anxiety while also allowing the clinician to gather information regarding the child's symptomatology.

12-Lead Electrocardiography

The 12-lead ECG, long thought to be the hallmark of noninvasive cardiac arrhythmia diagnosis, is a graphic depiction of the heart's electrical activity. The standard 12-lead ECG uses 10 surface electrodes/leads with a frontal plane view consisting of 3 bipolar limb leads (I, II, and III),[50] augmented limb leads consisting of 3 unipolar leads (aVR, aVF, and aVL),[51] and a horizontal plane consisting of 6 unipolar chest leads (V_1 through V_6).[52] Routine recordings are obtained at 25- or 50-mm/s paper speed with an amplitude of 1 mV/cm. A 10-second rhythm strip can serve as a useful adjunct in many patients. The 15-lead ECG includes the additional leads of V_3R, V_4R, and V_7, also known as the "right chest leads." These additional leads may be helpful in identifying the presence of right ventricular hypertrophy (V_3R and V_4R) or left ventricular hypertrophy (V_7).[53]

Uses

The 12-lead ECG can be used to assess heart rate and rhythm, QRS duration and morphology, P wave morphology and relationship to the QRS complex, intervals, axis, and hypertrophy. With regard to cardiac arrhythmia assessment, in many cases, a 12-lead ECG that does not show abnormalities is not nearly as helpful as one with abnormalities. Specific abnormalities that can be found on the resting 12-lead ECG include ventricular preexcitation (e.g., WPW), prolonged QT interval, ventricular hypertrophy, diffuse ST-T wave changes, and AV block. The 12-lead ECG can also be used to assess and document premature ectopy (atrial, junctional, and ventricular), narrow and wide QRS tachycardias (with and without AV block), bradycardia (sinus and junctional), bundle branch block, intraventricular conduction delay, and pacemaker function (or malfunction). It has also been used to determine pathway location in patients with accessory connections.[54]

Advantages/Disadvantages

The biggest advantage of the 12-lead ECG is the wealth of information that can be gleaned from it, especially if the child is experiencing an arrhythmia during its acquisition. Once all of the electrodes and leads have been placed, the data can be quickly acquired. If the arrhythmia occurs during ECG acquisition, the arrhythmia can be documented in multiple leads, making some substrates easier to identify. The ability to transmit ECGs by modem to a computerized data station provides the additional advantages of storage and retrieval.

The disadvantages of the 12-lead ECG is that it requires multiple electrodes and leads that can be upsetting to some children. The child must be still during data acquisition; this can be quite a feat in specific age groups. Additionally, if symptoms do not occur during ECG performance, additional diagnostic tools may be necessary for arrhythmia documentation.

Implications for Clinicians

The quality of a 12-lead ECG is extremely dependent on the skill and expertise of the individual performing it. It is critical for clinicians to remember that the assessment of heart rate, conduction intervals, axis, and hypertrophy are all age specific,[55] so it is extremely important that the child's age be included somewhere on the ECG report. The clinician must be aware of various factors that affect the quality of the 12-lead ECG, including patient movement, incorrectly placed electrodes, lack of correct skin preparation, static/alternating current, poor signal quality, broken lead wires, and improper grounding.

Clinicians performing 12-lead ECGs have a large responsibility because it is best if the child is still and quiet when the ECG is being obtained. This requires some ingenuity at best, but can be accomplished with skill and patience. In small children who are extremely agitated, it may be helpful to allow the child to be held by the parent rather than being placed on an impersonal examination table. To the older child, an explanation regarding the importance of being still and quiet can be given, and will be met with cooperation in most cases. The clinician should allow the child to participate as much as possible to gain trust and decrease anxiety.

Lead placement is extremely important for accurate ECG assessment. The most common mistake that individuals make when placing ECG leads is reversing the limb leads, specifically the right and left arm (Figs. 1 and 2). Most cardiologists can immediately detect this, but it can result in false-positive readings on the ECG if not recognized. It is important that the skin be free of oils and lotions prior to electrode placement. The clinician should ensure that all equipment is in proper working order prior to obtaining the ECG, including the machine itself and the lead wires. In most centers, the biomedical engineering department performs quality controls on all patient care equipment.

Once the ECG is obtained, and prior to removal of the leads and electrodes, the clinician should evaluate the ECG for quality. If the quality is poor, the ECG should be repeated. The reasons for poor quality should be assessed by the clinician with efforts to correct any noted problems. The ECG should always first be recorded at full calibration. Half calibration can be included as well if too much overlap of QRS complexes occurs. Making the initial recording at half calibration may reduce apparent motion artifact, but also reduces accuracy of interpretation.

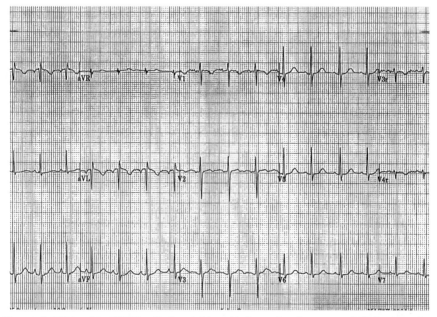

Figure 1. Fifteen-lead ECG with the right and left arm leads reversed. This gives the appearance of dextrocardia on the six limb leads, but not in the chest leads. The rhythm, which appears to originate in the left atrium as evidenced by the negative P waves in leads I and aVL, is clearly normal in lead V_6 with positive P waves.

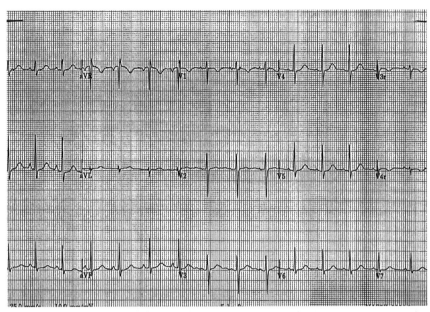

Figure 2. The same patient as in Figure 1, with the arm leads in their proper position.

Patient and Family Considerations

In order to gain the trust and cooperation of the patient and family, it is important to explain to them the importance of this particular diagnostic tool. If the child is old enough, an age-appropriate explanation should be given prior to electrode placement. Once a satisfactory ECG has been obtained, most children want to remove the "stickers" themselves and often want to take them home as souvenirs.

Signal-Averaged Electrocardiography

The SAECG is a method for recording high-resolution ECGs in which multiple PQRS complexes are recorded from three sets of orthogonal electrodes in the X, Y, and Z axes. The signals obtained are then digitized, summed, and filtered.[56] The three parameters measured by the SAECG include: 1) a filtered QRS duration; 2) the amplitude of the terminal 40 ms of the filtered ECG complex; and 3) the root mean square of the terminal 40 ms of the QRS complex.[57] A total of 256 beats are averaged and the presence of low-amplitude, high-frequency potentials at the end of the QRS complex (also known as ventricular late potentials) can be used to predict malignant ventricular arrhythmias in patients with coronary artery disease and cardiomyopathy (Fig. 3).

```
Analysis Filter : 40-250Hz
Std. QRS Duration (unfiltered):    90 ms
Total QRS Duration (filtered)  :  116 ms
Duration Of HFLA signals(40uV):    38 ms
RMS Voltage    (terminal 40ms) :   19 uV
Mean Voltage   (terminal 40ms) :   14 uV
```

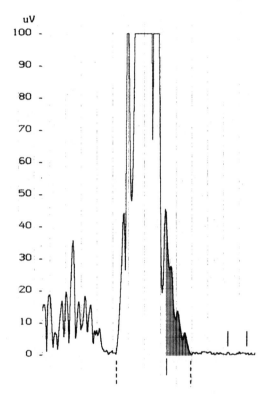

Figure 3. Signal-averaged ECG exhibiting late potentials in a patient with reentrant ventricular tachycardia. The RMS or mean terminal voltage less than 25 μV indicates a positive finding in a patient with a filtered QRS duration of 116 ms.

Uses

Although studies have been done regarding the usefulness of SAECGs in children,[58–60] the indication and utility of this particular diagnostic tool in children remains unclear at this time. It may be useful in the evaluation of ventricular arrhythmias after repair of CHD as well as in survivors of sudden cardiac death. SAECGs may or may not predict the inducibility of these arrhythmias with more invasive and provocative testing.

Advantages/Disadvantages

The major advantage of the SAECG in children at this time is that it provides noninvasive, high-resolution analysis of the characteristics of myocardial depolarization. The disadvantages include the longer time frame needed to acquire the data (compared with the conventional 12-lead ECG) and its decreased usefulness in specific ECG abnormalities including presence of bundle branch block, severe intraventricular conduction abnormalities, ventricular paced rhythms, and ventricular preexcitation (e.g., WPW).

Implications for Clinicians

When compared with the traditional 12-lead ECG, the challenge for the cardiovascular clinician of obtaining an SAECG in a child may seem monumental in several ways. The clinician must be more cognizant of proper skin preparation prior to electrode placement in order to reduce noise on the SAECG. Three additional electrodes must be placed and the child must remain quiet and still for a longer period (approximately 10 minutes). Additional precautions taken when performing a 12-lead ECG also apply when obtaining an SAECG.

Patient and Family Considerations

The patient and family considerations are the same as those for the 12-lead ECG, with the exception that the SAECG requires a longer acquisition period and may or may not provide any relevant clinical information. Again, patient and family education prior to performing the test is of utmost importance as is allowing the child to participate as much as possible.

Ambulatory Monitoring

Twenty-four-hour ambulatory (Holter) monitoring has come a long way since its initial inception in 1949.[61] Large transmitters carried around in backpacks providing real time ECG recordings from a distance were eventually downsized to approximately 4 pounds, allowing 10 to 24 hours of recording that could later be screened for analysis. Presently, ambulatory monitors weigh less than 2 pounds, allow multichannel recording with five ECG electrodes and leads, and permit computerized scanning with beat-to-beat labeling as well as compact storage for later retrieval.

Uses

Twenty-four-hour ambulatory monitors can be used for a variety of purposes in a variety of patients,[62] and can be used for 12 to 48 hours at a time. This particular diagnostic tool can be used to assess a multitude of both symptomatic and asymptomatic arrhythmias (Figs. 4 and 5). Am-

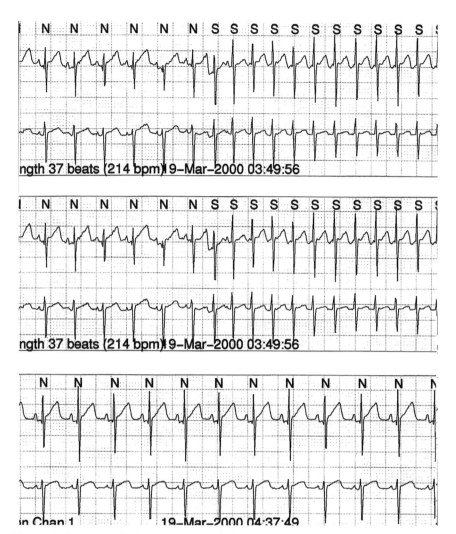

Figure 4. Supraventricular tachycardia (SVT) documented on ECG recordings of two channels each from a 24-hour ambulatory monitor. Sinus rhythm is denoted by the "N" with SVT labeled "S"; the sinus rhythm is interrupted by a premature atrial contraction that initiates an episode of SVT at 214 bpm on the top two identical panels, with sinus rhythm noted on the third panel.

bulatory monitors are generally placed for 24 hours and delineate the lowest, highest, and average heart rates seen over that period. They are particularly helpful in assessing heart rate variability and number of ectopic beats (supraventricular and ventricular) over a specific time frame. They can be useful in assessing sinus node dysfunction (especially in postoperative patients) as well as AV node function, specifically the length of pauses in both of these scenarios.

More specific uses of ambulatory monitors include the evaluation of

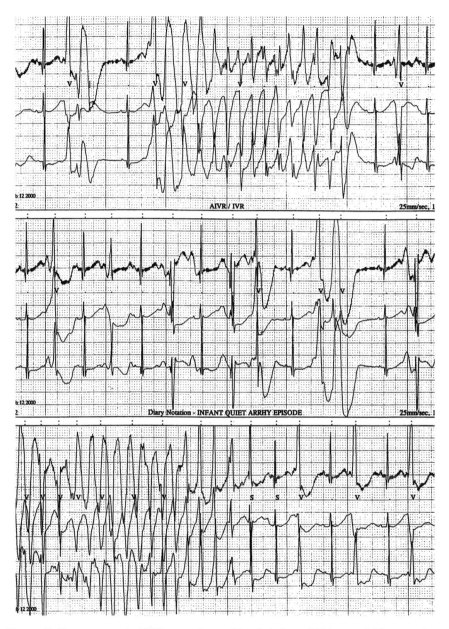

Figure 5. Three separate ECG recordings of leads I, II, and III from a 24-hour ambulatory monitor of a 3-day-old infant with familial long QT syndrome and torsades de pointes. The markedly prolonged QT interval and T wave alternans can be seen on the sinus beats. The scanner's decoder has denoted a "V" for what it interprets as a PVC and an "S" for sinus beats. Due to the rapid rate of the torsades de pointes, the beats are not automatically detected and labeled by the decoder's software.

patients with AET, PVCs, and of both preoperative and postoperative arrhythmias in children with CHD. It is especially helpful in patients after radiofrequency ablation to assess for proarrhythmia[63] or in those who confuse sinus tachycardia with an arrhythmia after the procedure. In patients with congenital complete AV block (CCAVB), 24-hour ambulatory monitoring can document junctional and ventricular escape intervals as well as the number of PVCs, which is helpful in determining the timing of permanent pacemaker implantation. Ambulatory monitors are helpful in assessing pacemaker/implantable cardioverter defibrillator (ICD) function (or dysfunction) as well as the appropriateness of rate-adaptive settings in patients with rate-adaptive devices. They can also be used to assess the efficacy of pharmacologic therapy.

Advantages/Disadvantages

The major advantage of 24-hour ambulatory monitoring is that it is noninvasive and relatively easy to use. It is a screening tool that is most useful for arrhythmias or symptoms that occur on a daily basis. Two simultaneous leads can be obtained and, in most cases, result in high-fidelity recordings.

The disadvantages include the difficulty in documenting sporadic events as well as the different computer algorithms used to analyze the data, which are occasionally inaccurate in labeling select arrhythmias in pediatric patients. Their use is limited in patients with LQTS because of the potential sources of error in detecting prolongation of the QT interval,[64] although some researchers have found them helpful in obtaining otherwise covert data in this subset of pediatric cardiology patients.[65]

Implications for Clinicians

Similar to other types of ECG recordings, the quality of the ECGs obtained from the 24-hour ambulatory monitor is dependent on the skill and expertise of the individual placing the device, as well as on its subsequent scanning. All equipment components should be evaluated prior to use on the patient to ensure that the recorder is in proper working order and that none of the lead wires are frayed. The skin should be properly cleansed prior to electrode placement, with the leads attached in such a way that the child's movement and activities will not cause them to become dislodged. The authors use a mesh cover (similar to a tank top) that slips over the child's head to protect electrode and lead placement. A new battery should be placed in the monitor itself and the clinician should ensure that the cassette is moving (i.e., the device is recording) prior to dismissing the child and family. Instructions for returning the device as well as troubleshooting techniques should be discussed with the patient and family as described below in "Patient and Family Considerations." Extra electrodes should be provided to the parents in case of dislodgment.

Although most of the equipment used for scanning the ambulatory monitor is equipped with adequate arrhythmia recognition software, the individual performing the data analysis should have some basic pediatric arrhythmia knowledge. In patients with AET, the device may label the beats as normal when indeed they are not. The clinician must also be aware of such things that can alter the accuracy of the recordings, such as tape drag or inadvertent increases in tape speed.

Patient and Family Considerations

Patients and families should receive information and education regarding the ambulatory monitor, including the following: why it is being placed, precautions to be taken while it is in place, frequently encountered problems during its use, and when and where to return the monitor. Taking the time to explore these issues with patients and their families can alleviate some of the problems that may occur after the child leaves the health care facility.

In most cases, the physician has already explained the rationale for the ambulatory monitor, whether for routine follow-up, suspected device malfunction, documentation of current arrhythmia management, documentation of a new-onset arrhythmia, or simply to rule out an arrhythmia. The clinician placing the monitor can reiterate this prior to placing the monitor as well. An explanation of how the device works is very helpful to most families.

Once the device has been placed, the clinician should explain to the patient and family when it is permissible to remove it, and clearly delineate instructions for its return. The clinician should stress that the device should not become wet, nor should the child be exposed to situations in which it may accidentally become so. It is also critical to show the parent(s) the tape speed, so that if they should look at it later, they will be knowledgeable as to how slowly it moves. Instructions should be given regarding replacement of electrodes and/or leads if they should become inadvertently dislodged. In many cases, patients and parents are given a diary in which to document the child's activities and/or symptoms that may occur while the device is in place. These diaries may or may not be helpful in the long run. In most cases, the child is encouraged to maintain all activities of daily living while the device is in place, with the exception of those previously mentioned.

Transtelephonic Electrocardiography

Transtelephonic electrocardiography has become a useful tool for the pediatric cardiovascular clinician.[66,67] The transtelephonic ECG monitoring system consists of a transmitter (of which there are various types) that is used to capture and send the ECG over the telephone to a receiving center located in the hospital or ambulatory care setting. The ECG is sent to a receiving center (either stand-alone or computer-linked) that uses either an answering machine or an acoustic coupler (Fig. 6). The answering machine allows patients and parents to call 24 hours a day, 7 days a week, while the acoustic coupler requires an individual to be present in order to answer the phone to receive the ECG.

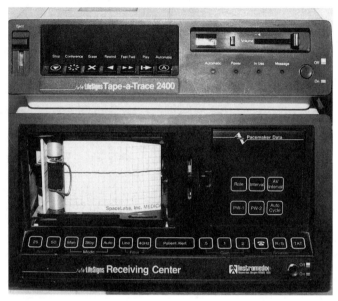

Figure 6. Older style transtelephonic receiving center and answering machine.

TTMs are available in a variety of types and sizes and should be tailored to the specific needs of each individual patient. The three basic types of TTMs that are routinely used in children include: 1) those that are used to send a *real time* ECG upon experiencing symptoms or for routine follow-up; 2) those that record and store the event and allow playback at a later time (i.e., *event recorders*); and 3) those that constantly "scan" the heart rhythm and can store data before, during, and after symptoms are experienced (i.e., *loop recorders*) (Fig. 7). Currently, there is a transmitter that can be surgically implanted and allows the clinician to obtain the data noninvasively; its disadvantage, however, is that it is not really feasible in very young patients because it must be surgically implanted. The specific type of transmitter prescribed should be chosen with the following variables in mind: the frequency of symptoms, the duration of symptoms, and the age of the child.

Uses

The usefulness and cost effectiveness of TTM has been demonstrated in children with symptomatic arrhythmias.[68] In addition to monitoring

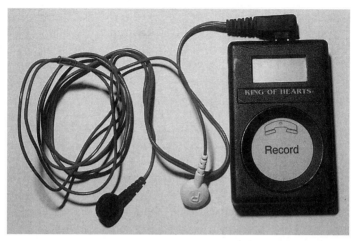

Figure 7. Transtelephonic loop recorder that uses two surface ECG leads to continuously scan the patient's rhythm. When symptoms occur, the patient simply depresses the record button located on the front of the monitor to store the ECG event.

the rhythm of patients complaining of palpitations, chest pain, dizziness, or syncope,[67,69,70] TTM can be used to routinely document asymptomatic arrhythmias such as AET, PJRT, and some IARTs.

TTM is a routine component of permanent pacemaker follow-up and is helpful in documenting asymptomatic abnormalities.[71] Parents are instructed to transmit routinely, but also if the child experiences symptoms or trauma to the pacemaker. The TTM that provides real time transmissions is most helpful in patients who are required to submit routine or scheduled transmissions, such as pacemaker patients. This type of transmitter is helpful in documenting the etiology of the child's symptoms[67,68] and is most useful in patients whose episodes last 10 to 20 minutes. The event recorder is most helpful in patients with transient episodes that are over by the time the child can reach a telephone, while the loop recorder is useful for rhythms and/or symptoms that are transient and have a prodrome.

Advantages/Disadvantages

The overall advantages of TTM include: 1) cost effectiveness, especially when compared with 24-hour ambulatory monitors; 2) rapid interpretation; and 3) portability. Each type of transmitter has specific advantages as well. The real time transmitter is less expensive than the other types of monitors; for pacemaker patients, it helps to avoid unnecessary office visits and it identifies problems needing prompt attention. It is easy to use and patients and parents can be taught to use it effectively. The event recorder has the capability of storing multiple events, allowing later playback of the event. It is excellent for documenting events or episodes that are brief or sports related and, because of its small size, it is preferred by adolescents. The loop recorder can store multiple events with hundreds of seconds of data and is helpful in determining what precedes an event.

The disadvantages of TTM include the following: 1) a telephone is required for real time transmissions or playback; 2) some monitor types are expensive; and 3) the patient must recognize the symptoms but remain conscious in order to document the event. The major disadvantage of the real time monitor is that a telephone is necessary at the time of the event. A disadvantage of the event recorder is that, because of its small size, it is sometimes difficult for the child to press the record button. The loop recorder has several disadvantages: 1) it must be worn continuously; 2) two leads that connect to the recorder must be attached to the chest; and 3) it has the propensity to alter skin integrity.

Implications for Clinicians

It is helpful for the individual receiving the transtelephonic ECG to have some knowledge of the various transmitters and how they operate. In the authors' institutions, the clinicians who provide the patient and family education regarding transmitter usage are the same individuals who receive the ECGs. On occasion, patients/parents become flustered when attempting to send the ECG and may place the telephone backward on the transmitter or in the phone cradle. Knowledge of the type of transmitter allows the receiver to solve potential problems related to technique in various cases.

The clinician receiving the transtelephonic ECG should have some basic knowledge of ECG and arrhythmia interpretation. In the event of an abnormal rhythm strip recording, the clinician should contact the patient and family to ascertain symptomatology (Figs. 8 and 9). The abnormal findings should be brought immediately to the prescribing physician's attention in order to plan treatment strategies. The use of TTM for pacemaker surveillance is discussed in depth in chapter 7 of this text.

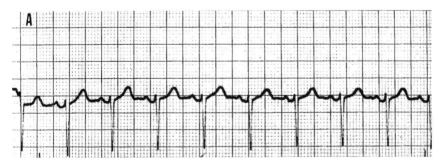

Figure 8. Transtelephonic ECG rhythm strip exhibiting normal sinus rhythm on a patient complaining of chest pain.

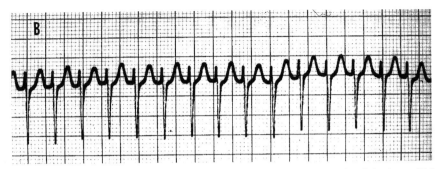

Figure 9. Same patient as that in Figure 8, but with complaints of palpitations. This modified lead II rhythm strip reveals an episode of supraventricular tachycardia at a rate of 170 bpm.

Patient and Family Considerations

In order for patients and families to obtain and send transtelephonic ECGs successfully, the cardiovascular clinician must spend an adequate amount of time performing patient and family education. This education should be transmitter specific and should include both verbal and written instructions and a return demonstration as well. Many families will momentarily panic when faced with the initial transmission at home, but some of this anxiety can be alleviated if they are allowed to handle and test the device in the presence of an expert. Not only does this teaching session provide an opportunity for patients and families to ask questions, it also allows the clinician to evaluate the effectiveness of their technique. In the authors' centers, the patient and parents are instructed verbally and then asked to send a baseline rhythm strip recording to the receiving center that is evaluated prior to the end of the teaching session. This gives the parents an idea of how the system works, with an emphasis on the importance of their technique. Instructions should be given on approximately how long they will use the monitor; this is generally dependent on the ECGs received, e.g., if SVT is documented after 1 week, the monitor can be returned. Most event monitors and loop recorders are prescribed for 30-day increments.

Exercise Stress Testing

EST is used to determine a quantitative as well as a reproducible index of the patient's cardiorespiratory performance, thus making the physiologic changes that occur during this particular diagnostic tool helpful in the noninvasive evaluation of select cardiac rhythm disturbances in children. EST is performed by attaching 10 ECG electrodes/leads, which are constantly monitored before, during, and after graded treadmill testing. The most commonly used protocol in children is the Bruce protocol,[72] in which the speed and incline increase at 3-minute intervals. Some centers will use a modified version of this protocol.

Uses

EST can be used in a variety of clinical situations and is extremely useful in patients who have experienced exercise-induced syncope or in those who experience their arrhythmia-related symptoms with exercise of any type.[73,74] EST is particularly helpful in assessing patients with known or suspected sinus node dysfunction and has actually been found to be a more sensitive indicator of sinus node dysfunction than invasive electrophysiology testing.[75] Not only is EST valuable in the initial determination of sinus node dysfunction, it can also be used in the periodic assessment of those postoperative patients who are prone to sick sinus syndrome, such as Mustard, Senning, and Fontan patients.

EST can be used to assess the antegrade accessory pathway characteristics in patients with WPW, with the sudden loss of ventricular pre-excitation during exercise a relatively good correlate to a pathway with a long antegrade refractory period. SVT is rarely precipitated by exercise in children, so EST may or may not document this particular arrhythmia. Patients with ventricular ectopy and an anatomically normal heart can benefit from EST, and if the ectopy suppresses with exercise, the arrhythmia may be considered benign. If not, further investigation may be warranted.[73]

Patients with LQTS may benefit from EST because abnormalities such as T wave alternans and ventricular arrhythmias may be exacerbated (or seen) with exercise. In patients with borderline or normal QT intervals on 12-lead ECG, the EST may result in QT prolongation with faster heart rates, assisting the clinician in making the diagnosis of a prolonged QT. Additionally, EST can be used to assess the adequacy of β-blockade in patients with LQTS or in other patients for whom these agents are used for arrhythmia suppression.

EST can be very helpful in patients with permanent cardiac devices. In patients with permanent pacemakers, EST can be used to determine the adequacy of rate-adaptive parameters, upper tracking rates, and upper rate limit behavior. It can also be helpful in assessing sensitivity settings, especially since the atrial electrogram voltage decreases with exercise in children.[76] In patients with antitachycardia devices, particularly ICDs, EST can be helpful in identifying upper sinus rates in order to allow adequate programming of tachycardia recognition rates.

Advantages/Disadvantages

The advantages of using EST as a diagnostic tool in patients with cardiac rhythm disturbances include the fact that it is generally readily available to the clinician and it partially simulates the patient's activities of daily living. The disadvantages include a low yield for SVT induction and limited use in younger patients, i.e., those younger than 5 years of age.

Implications for Clinicians

The clinician involved in EST has multiple responsibilities. He or she should ensure that all equipment is properly grounded and in proper working order prior to test initiation. Many centers require that parents sign a consent form prior to EST in case of an adverse event. The area in which the EST is to be performed should be properly equipped for any and all clinical and emergency situations and should contain the following: oxygen, suction equipment, resuscitation equipment, and a defibrillator. Personnel performing EST should, at a minimum, be trained in basic life support. The patient will require skin preparation prior to electrode placement, to aid in obtaining quality ECGs during exercise. Noninvasive blood pressure as well as pulse oximetry monitoring should be performed at predetermined intervals during the EST and compared with baseline for any changes.

Patient and Family Considerations

Patients and families should receive an explanation of what to expect during the EST prior to its implementation. It should be stressed that in order for a complete and accurate test result, the child will be encouraged to continue until exhaustion unless an arrhythmic event requires premature termination of the test. It is important to explain to the child that the speed and incline will increase periodically, and a warning just prior to this occurrence is most helpful. Also, the child should be informed of the periodic blood pressure measurements.

Telemetry Electrocardiographic Monitoring

Telemetry ECG monitoring is a type of ambulatory monitoring that is primarily used in the hospital setting. It consists of continuous radiofrequency transmission of multiple ECG leads from a battery operated radiotransmitter to a central station. The central station receiving unit captures the oncoming signal through an antenna and continuously displays the ECG on an oscilloscope.

Uses

Telemetry ECG monitoring is primarily used in postoperative cardiovascular patients, specifically patients who have undergone repair of CHD, permanent cardiac arrhythmia device placement (i.e., pacemakers and ICDs), and patients who require temporary pacing. Additional uses for telemetry monitoring include: 1) screening postoperative Mustard,

Senning, or Fontan patients who may be hospitalized for other reasons; 2) assessment of antiarrhythmic drug efficacy and/or proarrhythmia; 3) assessment of postoperative neonates or infants with feeding problems who may be at risk for bradycardia or aspiration; 4) assessment of patients with electrolyte imbalances; and 5) assessment of patients who have had drug overdoses.

Advantages/Disadvantages

The biggest advantage of telemetry monitoring is that it allows the clinician to make an immediate assessment of the child's arrhythmia, activity, and/or symptoms (Fig. 10). Since bradycardia follows apnea in only a very few seconds, telemetry monitoring has the additional advantage of being an effective apnea monitor in select patients. The disadvantages of using an attended telemetry system include the challenge of educating clinicians in basic ECG and arrhythmia interpretation and the tendency for the individual attending the monitor to over- or underreact in specific clinical situations.

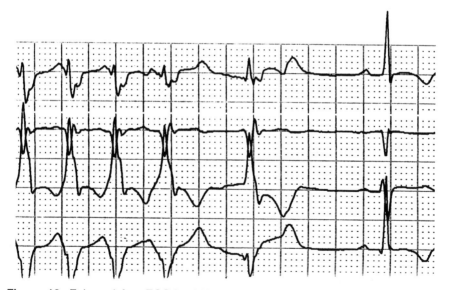

Figure 10. Enlarged four-ECG-lead rhythm strip from a patient being monitored on telemetry, exhibiting an episode of ventricular tachycardia that spontaneously terminates.

Implications for Clinicians

The cardiovascular clinician has a multitude of responsibilities when patients are placed on telemetry. Prior to attaching the telemetry unit, the clinician should make sure it is clean and in good working order. The leads should be inspected for frays and replaced as necessary. A new battery should be placed in the unit prior to its use. In order to portray the intended (and correct) monitoring lead, the clinician must place the electrodes in the correct position. In most cases, a five-lead wire system is used with a choice of a preferred monitoring lead or leads. The limb leads are the most commonly used monitoring leads in the hospital telemetry setting, requiring electrodes to be placed on the left arm (LA), right arm (RA), left leg (LL), right leg (RL), and a V lead placed at the fourth intercostal space at the right sternal border. The skin should be free of lotions and oils prior to electrode placement; alcohol pads can be used for skin preparation if necessary. The lead wire should be attached to the electrode prior to its placement on the child's skin, to enhance patient comfort as well as to prevent the conducting gel from being displaced.[77] Hebra[77] recommends "rolling" the electrode onto the chest wall also as a method for preserving the conducting gel and allowing the electrode to remain functional longer. The electrodes should be replaced every 48 hours. In patients with implanted devices, electrodes should never be placed directly over the device, since removal of the electrode can result in altered skin integrity, which increases the patient's risk for pocket infection. Once the device is in place and functioning properly, the unit itself can be placed in a pouch to allow the child increased mobility.

The physician's orders for telemetry monitoring should include alarm limits and findings that require physician notification. In most cases, the clinician will want to obtain a brief history of any previous rhythm disturbances in order to know what to look for. In patients with implanted pacemakers, the orders should include various pacemaker parameters, e.g., mode, rate, etc., which are covered in depth in chapter 7. The prescribed alarm limits should be set and not altered without a physician's order. The alarms should not be turned off for any reason. If the patient should leave the unit unmonitored, the clinician should disconnect the telemetry unit (versus turning off the alarms) and reconnect it when the patient returns. This practice will prevent the clinician from inadvertently leaving the alarms off once the patient returns to the monitoring unit.

The clinician should print a rhythm strip periodically to document the child's rhythm, as well as any time the alarms are triggered or a rhythm abnormality is detected. The child's heart rate should always be measured using a printed rhythm strip, not by using the heart rate displayed on the monitor, which can be distorted by artifact or electrode movement. In children with large P waves or T waves, the monitor may "double count" and display an incorrect heart rate; this is an additional reason for obtaining a printed rhythm strip. Clinicians should also be aware that in patients with pacemakers, the monitor may count the pacemaker stimulus as the heart rate when in fact the pacemaker may not be capturing, which results in cardiac arrest in some patients.[78] The authors do not use the pacemaker enhancement software because of the associated artifact. Astute electrode placement will result in the ability to see a pacemaker spike in most patients.

The fundamentals of ECG and arrhythmia interpretation are beyond the scope of this chapter, but it should be noted that Smith and colleagues[79] recommend the following simple steps for cardiac rhythm assessment in children: 1) evaluate the heart rate; 2) evaluate whether the rhythm is regular or irregular; 3) assess the P wave; 4) assess the PR interval; 5) assess the relationship of the P wave to the QRS complex; 6) assess the QRS duration; 7) assess the ST segment; 8) assess the T wave; 9) evaluate the QT interval; and 10) assess for the presence of U waves.

The first step in evaluating the telemetry rhythm strip, especially if it contains abnormal findings, is that the clinician should remember to assess the patient and not just the monitor. If a rhythm abnormality occurs, the clinician must assess the child's hemodynamic status. The child's vital signs should be obtained followed by an overall clinical assessment, including the child's level of consciousness (LOC), color, respiratory rate and effort (including tachypnea, nasal flaring, or use of accessory muscles), and the presence and strength of peripheral pulses. The child's physician should then be promptly notified.

Patient and Family Considerations

The patient and family should be informed of the reason for telemetry monitoring and given a brief explanation of how the system works. The clinician should emphasize that the child must remain in the monitoring area and that when electrodes become displaced, they must be replaced, even in the middle of the night or when the child is sleeping. By providing this initial information up front, the clinician can avoid upsetting the patient and family at later times.

Electrophysiology Testing

Electrophysiology testing can be accomplished in one of two ways: transesophageal studies, which are limited for atrial application only, or intracardiac testing (IEPS), in which multiple catheters can be placed inside the heart for recording and stimulation in a variety of locations. The following discussion is limited to IEPS since transesophageal testing is discussed in depth in chapter 4.

Uses

The IEPS is performed in children and young adults to assess the characteristics of the cardiac conduction system and to analyze arrhythmia mechanisms. The specific indications for electrophysiology testing in children are similar to those in adults.[80] The specific recommendations that are different from those of adults are as follows: 1) Class I indications include patients with undiagnosed narrow QRS tachycardia that cannot be distinguished from sinus tachycardia; 2) Class II indications include asymptomatic patients possibly at high risk for sudden death, especially patients who have undergone surgery for CHD as well as patients with CCAVB and a wide QRS escape rhythm; and 3) Class III indications include patients with CCAVB and a narrow QRS escape rhythm, patients with acquired complete AV block, and asymptomatic patients with surgically induced bifascicular block.[80] As a reminder, Class I indications are those in which experts agree that an IEPS is indicated, Class II are those in which experts are divided as to whether the IEPS will be beneficial or not, and Class III indications are those in which experts agree an IEPS is not indicated.

The IEPS can be used to: 1) document the function of the SA and AV nodes in anticipation of permanent pacemaker implantation; 2) assess the efficacy or proarrhythmia of antiarrhythmic drugs; 3) assess the efficacy of antiarrhythmia devices; or 4) map the substrate of an arrhythmia for ablation. In the pediatric world, it is routine practice to combine the IEPS and ablation, as this exposes the child to one rather than two stressful admissions for an invasive procedure with sedation or anesthesia.

Advantages/Disadvantages

The major advantage of intracardiac IEPS is that, if the arrhythmia is reproducible, the vast amount of data that can be obtained from the recording and stimulation is virtually unrivaled when compared with the other arrhythmia diagnostic tools. Additionally, the arrhythmia mechanisms can be further delineated and specific arrhythmia substrates identified.

The disadvantages are the complications associated with the invasiveness of the procedure (which are listed in Table 3) as well as the anxiety provoked in the patient and family. In young children, sedation and/or anesthesia must be administered; this is also considered a disadvantage when compared with other diagnostic techniques.

Table 3
Potential Complications of Intracardiac Electrophysiology Testing

Infection
Hemorrhage
Hypotension
Hematoma
Vascular/arterial injury
Thrombophlebitis
Emboli
Perforation/tamponade
Pneumothorax
Intractable arrhythmia
Death

Implications for Clinicians

The roles and responsibilities of the clinician involved in the care of children undergoing IEPS vary with the particular phase of the study. The implications for clinicians are divided into the phases of prior to, during, and immediately after the IEPS procedure. Patient and family education are discussed in the section on patient and family considerations.

Prior to the Procedure

The team of clinicians caring for the child undergoing IEPS is multifaceted and involves patient-specific and laboratory-specific responsibilities. While each individual clinician has specific duties to perform, the goal of the team should be to ensure the patient's safety at all times.

Patient Considerations

Since most IEPS procedures are performed on an outpatient or 23-hour observational stay basis, many centers require a preprocedural work-up visit on the day prior to the procedure. The clinician should ensure that all preprocedural tests specified by the physician performing the IEPS be completed at this time. The authors routinely perform pregnancy testing in all females 12 years and older who will undergo IEPS. Other preprocedural tests that may be ordered include blood work, 12-lead ECG, 24-hour ambulatory monitor, EST, and chest radiograph. It is important that the responsible clinician ensure that all ordered tests are completed and readily available on the day of the procedure.

In the authors' institutions, a specific nurse is responsible for coordinating these activities. If the child is receiving general anesthesia for the procedure, the clinician should ensure that the patient and family meet with anesthesia personnel to discuss anesthesia and sedation issues as well as when to withhold food and fluids. If sedation is to be administered by catheterization/electrophysiology laboratory personnel, these issues should be discussed with the patient and family by the physician performing the procedure. Once all tests have been completed and all consent forms signed, the clinician should reiterate when and why food and fluids are to be withheld. The patient and family should be informed at this time exactly when and where they are to report to on the day of the procedure.

Laboratory Considerations

Cardiovascular clinicians directly involved in the IEPS have the responsibility of ensuring that all equipment needed to perform the procedure is available and in proper working order. Each clinician working in the catheterization/electrophysiology laboratory must possess specific knowledge of the procedure itself as well as the equipment used throughout the procedure. All electrical equipment should be properly grounded and in excellent working order as evidenced by frequent evaluations by the institution's biomedical department.

The clinician working in the catheterization/electrophysiology laboratory should have an adequately stocked diagnostic and electrophysiologic catheter supply for any and all patient sizes and clinical situations. Smaller catheters (e.g., 2 Fr to 4 Fr) as well as catheters with closer electrode spacing are a must when caring for pediatric patients. Two external defibrillators must be available at all times, with at least one of them having the ability to temporarily pace, preferably with hands-free, self-adhesive electrodes. The procedure room should be fully equipped with airway management equipment, suction, and all necessary drugs and equipment needed for cardiopulmonary resuscitation.

Once the child is brought into the laboratory, the adequacy of the surface ECG electrodes should be verified before the patient is prepped and draped. Adequate body temperature maintenance is critical, especially in neonates and infants, and it can be maintained by manipulation of the room temperature or by using an external temperature-regulating apparatus. Adequate radiation safety precautions, such as the use of thyroid drapes and/or gonad shields, should be taken to reduce radiation exposure to the patient as well as the staff.

During the Procedure

Patient Considerations

The most important task of the clinician during IEPS is the performance of an ongoing assessment of the child's overall hemodynamic status. If conscious or deep sedation is used, the nurse managing the care of the patient should have no other responsibilities during the procedure, in order to ensure that the patient is always attended to and constantly monitored.[81,82] The clinician should always remain cognizant of the patient's tachyarrhythmia response, and should be prepared to assist with any emergency interventions. Knowledge of pediatric drug dosages is critical for nurses and other clinicians involved in the care of children undergoing invasive cardiovascular procedures.

The clinician should constantly monitor the patient for any potential complications associated with IEPS (see Table 3). Clinicians working in the cardiac catheterization/electrophysiology laboratories should be trained in basic and advanced pediatric life support and should have some basic knowledge of ECG and arrhythmia interpretation. Due to high anxiety and fear of the unknown, the authors have a designated clinician who updates the child's family on their child's progress periodically during the IEPS.

Protocol Implications

Following the course of an IEPS may seem difficult to the novice, but preparation and repetition will provide the basis for a sound understanding of most routine cases. In today's fast-paced, high-tech environment, there is little time for the clinician to learn basic electrophysiology. In order for any staff member to follow a case and anticipate the next step with confidence, the clinician must master the basic protocols used in each study, the results expected from each protocol, and the expected characteristics of the arrhythmia mechanism.

The basic IEPS involves two simple acts: pacing and recording. The stimulator functions as an external pacemaker that can be set to perform pacing protocols from the atrium or ventricle. The recording system displays surface electrograms from a standard 12-lead ECG along with intracardiac electrograms (EGMs) from each electrode catheter in real time, and captures designated parts for measurement and analysis.

Catheter Placement

A variety of catheters, from two to five, may be placed in the heart to record electrical activity as well as for stimulation. These catheters are generally made of woven Dacron, and come in various shapes and sizes. The number of electrodes on the catheter's tip varies from 3 to 14, with variable electrode spacing. Some catheters are steerable and are usually used in a bipolar configuration. The catheters are placed through venous sheaths, most commonly in the femoral veins but also in the alternative sites of the subclavian, internal jugular, and median antecubital veins.

Access to the left side of the heart can be accomplished using a transseptal or retrograde (arterial) approach. In some patients, access can be gained through a patent foreman ovale, a clinically insignificant opening from fetal circulation that generally closes at birth. The transseptal approach requires that a puncture be made in the atrial septum using a transseptal needle and a sheath (over a wire). The sheath is introduced from the femoral vein and is advanced into the left atrium.[83] This is accomplished using biplane fluoroscopy, with left atrial pressure recordings to verify placement. Once the electrophysiologic catheter has been placed, left atrial recording or stimulation can be performed or the catheter can be moved into the left ventricle through the mitral valve. The retrograde or arterial approach involves placing the catheter into the left side of the heart through the arterial system. Specifically, the catheter is positioned through the femoral artery through the aortic valve into the left ventricle. The left atrium is accessed by passing the catheter retrogradely across the mitral valve into the left atrium. Both methods require that the patient be heparinized with close observation of activated clotting times until sheath removal.

The catheters are generally placed in four sites. The atrial catheter is placed in the high right atrium (HRA) and records electrical activity in and around the SA node. The His bundle electrogram (HBE) catheter is placed across the tricuspid valve, allowing recording of low atrial and ventricular activity for evaluation of AV node function. The ventricular catheter is generally placed in the right ventricular apex (RVA) and allows electrical activity to be recorded from the right ventricle. The CS catheter records both atrial and ventricular activity from the base of the left atrium close to the AV groove, allowing determination of retrograde atrial activation sequences in patients with SVT. Occasionally catheters will be placed in the RVOT, left ventricle, and/or left atrium.

The catheters are placed in their anatomic locations using single or biplane fluoroscopy (Fig. 11) and a typical electrophysiologic tracing depicts surface ECG leads I, AVF, V_1, and V_6 along with the specific EGMs (Fig. 12). Once the catheters have been positioned, baseline intervals are measured to document the resting cardiac rhythm. Measurements of rates and intervals during IEPS are measured in milliseconds (ms) rather than the traditional beats per minute (bpm) and intervals of timing are termed "cycle lengths." These and other common electrophysiology terms and abbreviations can be found in Table 4.

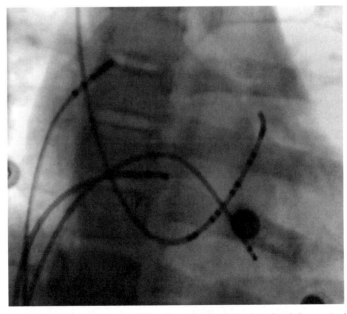

Figure 11. Intracardiac catheter position for a typical electrophysiology study shown in a posteroanterior radiograph. A catheter from the arm with 10 electrodes is positioned in the coronary sinus for left atrial and left ventricular recording. Catheters positioned from the femoral vein are for recording the high right atrium, His bundle, and right ventricular apex.

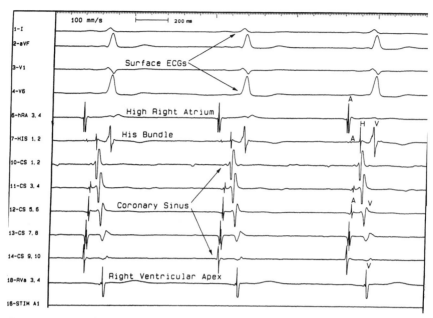

Figure 12. Typical intracardiac electrogram tracings recorded from the catheter positions noted in Figure 11. The bipolar electrograms are preceded by surface ECG leads I, aVF, V_1, and V_6 and include a high right atrial recording from electrodes 3 and 4, His bundle electrograms from electrodes 1 and 2, coronary sinus electrograms from pairs 1&2, 3&4, 5&6, 7&8, and 9&10, and the right ventricular apex electrogram from electrodes 3 and 4.

Table 4
Abbreviations and Terminology Used in Electrophysiology

A	Atrial; refers to the atrial deflection on the intracardiac electrogram
AH	AH interval; refers to the interval between the atrium (A) and the His bundle (H) deflection
Automaticity	The ability of a cell to depolarize spontaneously
CI	Coupling interval; refers to the time between paired beats
CL	Cycle length; refers to the length of a cycle or the time between one event and the next repetitive signal; represented in milliseconds
CS	Coronary sinus
CSNRT	Corrected sinus node recovery time
Drive train	The length of time between consecutive paced beats in a specific stimulation sequence; expressed in milliseconds and as S_1
EGM	Electrogram; refers to the waveforms obtained from electrodes touching the heart
Entrainment	Pacing technique used to terminate specific tachyarrhythmias; the pacing cycle length is progressively shortened until it controls each cycle of the cardiac impulse

Table 4
Abbreviations and Terminology Used in Electrophysiology (*cont.*)

Extrastimulus	An electrical impulse (extrinsic) delivered at a preset rate or programmed coupling interval; expressed as S_1, S_2, S_3, S_4, etc.
H	His; refers to His bundle deflection on intracardiac electrogram
HBE	His bundle electrogram
HRA	High right atrium
HV	His-to-ventricle interval
LSRA	Low septal right atrium
RVA	Right ventricular apex
S	Stimulus artifact
S_1	Stimulus artifact 1; refers to constant cycle length known as the drive train
S_2	Stimulus artifact 2; refers to first premature stimulus
S_3	Stimulus artifact 3; refers to second premature stimulus
S_4	Stimulus artifact 4; refers to third premature stimulus
V	Ventricle; refers to ventricular deflection on intracardiac electrogram
VA	Ventricle to atrium

Baseline Intervals

Baseline or resting intervals are recorded and measured prior to the start of programmed electrical stimulation. The three common intervals used during electrophysiology testing are the PA, AH, and HV intervals. The PA interval is an indirect measurement of atrial conduction and is performed by measuring the beginning of the earliest P wave activation on the surface ECG to the rapid deflection of the atrial EGM on the HBE catheter. Normal PA intervals range from 20 to 30 ms. The AH interval is indicative of conduction from the AV node to the His bundle and is calculated by measuring from the earliest rapid deflection of the atrial EGM to the beginning of the His bundle deflection on the HBE. Normal AH ranges have been published as age specific (from 43 to 127 ms),[84] with an average of 60 to 120 ms, which can vary with autonomic tone. The HV interval is used to assess conduction from the bundle of His to the ventricular myocardium (or distal conduction system) and is determined by measuring the beginning of the His bundle deflection to the earliest onset of ventricular activation on the surface ECG or the ventricular EGM. Again, normal ranges for the HV interval are age specific (from 17 to 56 ms),[84] with an average of 30 to 55 ms.

The AV node can be assessed using certain intervals on the intracardiac EGMs. This assessment is made by measuring the LSRA-H interval during intrinsic electrical activity, and varies according to age in children.[85] These intervals also vary with different cycle lengths as well as with autonomic tone. The function of the AV node can also be assessed by determining various refractory periods.

Programmed Electrical Stimulation

Programmed electrical stimulation protocols are performed to gather information, specifically to determine SA conduction times (SACTs), sinus and AV nodal conduction, and refractory periods of specific cardiac tissue. The primary goal of the electrophysiology study is to evaluate the patient's cardiac electrophysiology (whether normal or abnormal) while attempting to induce arrhythmias. If one knows which part(s) of the conduction system are being tested with each protocol, anticipation of the results and prompt recognition will make the study smoother and perhaps more expeditious. The following measurements and protocols are used in IEPS testing: sinus node recovery time (SNRT), SACT, refractory period determination, decremental and burst pacing, and arrhythmia induction techniques.

Sinus Node Recovery Time

SNRT is the most commonly used method for assessing sinus node automaticity, and is performed by overdrive pacing the atrium at progressively faster rates for periods of 30 seconds. The paced cycle length is decreased (which results in a faster rate) in 50-ms increments until one of the following occurs: Wenckebach and/or 2:1 block occurs, hypotension occurs, or a cycle length of 300 ms is reached. Because the SNRT is partially determined by the patient's sinus cycle length, the value is corrected to a standardized value known as a corrected SNRT or CSNRT. The CSNRT is obtained by subtracting the patient's basic sinus cycle length from the number obtained from the interval of the last paced beat to the first intrinsic sinus beat once overdrive pacing has been terminated (Fig. 13).

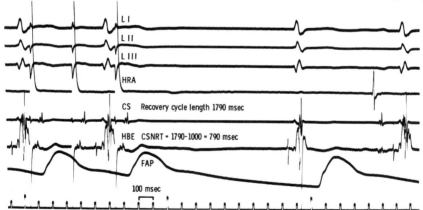

Figure 13. Programmed electrical stimulation to obtain a sinus node recovery time. After the final three drive train beats are delivered and pacing stopped, the bundle of His, rather than the sinus node, recovers first. Since there is not retrograde conduction, the recovery time of the sinus node can also be seen. The P wave seen on the coronary sinus catheter is normal with a high to low activation sequence. The corrected sinus node recovery time of 790 ms is prolonged. CS = coronary sinus; CSNRT = corrected sinus node recovery time; FAP = femoral artery pressure; HBE = His bundle electrogram; HRA = high right atrium.

The normal range for CSNRT is 100 to 250 ms, with the absolute upper limit being no more than 160% of the basic cycle length.[86] A value of 600 ms indicates moderate dysfunction, while a value of 3 seconds or greater is indicative of severe sinus node dysfunction.

Sinoatrial Conduction Time

The SACT is another method used to evaluate sinus node function. This indirect measurement is the length of time that it takes an electrical impulse (or signal) to conduct through the perinodal tissue of the sinus node. It is assessed using either of two indirect methods[87,88] or a direct method of measuring from the onset of the sinus node electrogram to the onset of the HRA electrogram.[86] A normal SACT in children using the indirect method of Strauss is 124±38 ms.[89]

Refractory Period Determination

Refractory periods of the cardiac conduction system are determined using extrastimuli or, simply, premature beats. These extrastimuli are delivered at various paced cycle lengths and can be introduced during the patient's intrinsic rhythm or into a paced rhythm known as a drive train. Both the pacing cycle length and the pacing amplitude can affect refractoriness. The first extrastimulus is delivered at a cycle length 20 ms shorter than the intrinsic or paced cycle length. Subsequent extrastimuli are decremented by 10 to 20 ms until refractoriness is reached, which occurs when a premature stimulus finds a component of the conduction system unable to conduct secondary to prematurity of that stimulus.

There are several types of refractory periods: *absolute, functional,* and *effective.* These refractory periods are used to evaluate atrial tissue, ventricular tissue, the AV node, and the His-Purkinje system as well as accessory pathways. The absolute refractory period is the length of time from the onset of an action potential until the cell can respond to a strong stimulus. The tissue being stimulated will be unresponsive during this time. The functional refractory period measures how rapidly a structure can conduct from itself to another and is the shortest coupling interval that is conducted and is measured distal to the tissue. The effective refractory period, the most commonly calculated refractory period, is indicative of how fast select tissue can conduct; it is the longest coupling interval of a premature stimulus that fails to conduct and is measured proximal to the refractory tissue. The effective refractory period is especially important in evaluating properties of accessory pathways and reveals the general health of the tissue being evaluated. The longer the effective refractory period, the more dilated and fibrotic the tissue is likely to be.

The *atrial effective refractory period* is determined by introducing an atrial extrastimulus into either an intrinsic or paced rhythm. Once the atrial stimulation fails to produce a response (i.e., fails to capture), the atrial tissue is considered refractory. Simply, it is the longest S_1S_2 that fails to depolarize the atrium. The effective atrial refractory period ranges from 159 to 360 ms. The *AV node effective refractory period* is used to assess AV node function and is accomplished as above. It is the longest A_1A_2 that fails to depolarize the His bundle. The atrium may still be captured by the extrastimulus, but there is no AV nodal conduction. The normal range for AV nodal refractoriness is 230 to 425 ms. In most cases, the AV node becomes refractory before the atrial muscle does.

The *ventricular effective refractory period* is determined by introducing a ventricular extrastimulus into either an intrinsic or paced ventricular rhythm (Fig. 14). Once this stimulus fails to capture the ventricle, the cycle length at which the extrastimulus was delivered becomes the ventricular refractory period and is the longest S_1S_2 in which the S_2 fails to depolarize the ventricle. The normal range for a ventricular muscle refractory period is from 170 to 290 ms.

Refractory periods of accessory pathways can also be obtained in both the antegrade and retrograde directions. When the antegrade refractory period of the accessory pathway is reached, the QRS complex will become

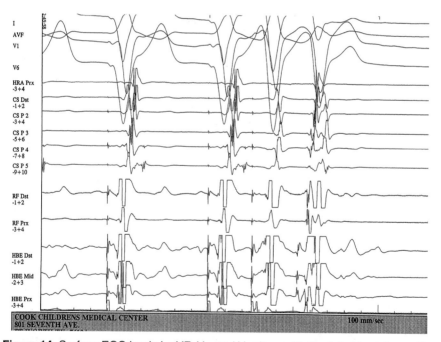

Figure 14. Surface ECG leads I, aVF, V$_1$, and V$_6$ along with the following intracardiac electrograms: high right atrium (HRA), coronary sinus (CS) ×5, RF ×2, and His bundle (HBE) x2 during programmed electrical stimulation. The last two beats of the drive train can be seen on the left followed by the introduction of an S$_2$. There is decremental conduction from the ventricle to the bundle of His that reactivates the ventricle (also known as a V$_3$).

narrow, indicating conduction through the AV node and not the accessory pathway. Retrograde refractory periods of the AV node and ventricle can be obtained as well.

Decremental and Burst Pacing

Antegrade and retrograde conduction are also assessed using decremental pacing. Antegrade conduction is evaluated by pacing the atria from the HRA catheter at a rate slightly faster than the patient's intrinsic heart rate. The pacing cycle length is gradually decreased until Wenckebach and/or 2:1 block occurs. The AH interval prolongs with faster and faster paced cycle lengths until the atrial electrogram is no longer followed by a His bundle deflection or ventricular electrogram. The normal cycle length at which this occurs ranges from 350 to 500 ms.

Retrograde conduction is assessed by pacing the ventricle at increasingly faster rates, also known as incremental pacing. Retrograde conduction can occur through the AV node or an accessory pathway. If the interval from the ventricular EGM to the atrial EGM (i.e., the VA interval) lengthens with each decrease in cycle length, it is termed "decremental conduction," which is a normal characteristic of the AV node. If decremental conduction does not occur or if there is sudden dissociation, this may indicate the presence of an accessory pathway. If there is no retrograde conduction with the initial cycle length, protocol progression is not necessary.

Burst pacing can be performed in either chamber and generally 8 to 10 beats are used. Atrial burst pacing can be used to induce supraventricular arrhythmias, whereas ventricular burst pacing is used to induce ventricular arrhythmias. The initial burst cycle length is slightly higher than the patient's intrinsic ventricular rate and each subsequent burst is decremented by 20 ms until Wenckebach or 2:1 block occurs or an arrhythmia is induced.

Arrhythmia Induction

Any of the previously described stimulation protocols may result in arrhythmia induction. Typically, attempts at arrhythmia induction begin with the least aggressive protocol and progress to more aggressive ones. In the event that the arrhythmia was not induced with a single extrastimulus, the protocol may be repeated using two or three extrastimuli, termed "doubles" and "triples," respectively. If the aforementioned protocols fail to produce an arrhythmia, isoproterenol can be administered in an attempt to simulate exercise. Isoproterenol is infused at 0.05 to 0.1 μg/kg/min to yield a 20% to 30% increase in the patient's baseline heart rate. Once this increase has been achieved, the stimulation protocols are then repeated. If this is not successful, the catheter can be moved to an alternate site, e.g., the RVA catheter is repositioned to the RVOT.

After the Procedure

The IEPS procedure, when not performed in conjunction with a catheter ablation, takes from 1 to 3 hours. The clinician assuming care for the patient after IEPS should obtain specific information from cardiac catheterization/electrophysiology laboratory personnel regarding the procedure. This "report" should include why the procedure was performed, any significant findings, the type and amount of sedation/anesthesia used, any problems or complications encountered during the procedure, and the number and condition of the puncture site(s) and dressings placed at the completion of the procedure. Upon assumption of care, these sites should be inspected for presence of hemorrhage, swelling, or hematoma, and the affected extremity evaluated for warmth, color, capillary refill, and palpable pulses. The child's LOC should be documented, as should his or her heart rate and rhythm, blood pressure, respiratory rate and effort, and body temperature.

The child's leg is generally kept straight for several hours following the procedure. If bleeding occurs at the puncture site, the clinician should hold firm pressure and have someone notify the child's physician. In most cases, this will stop the bleeding and a new dressing can be applied. The child's LOC will vary depending on the type of sedation/anesthesia used, and diet progression should proceed when the child is fully awake and alert. In most cases, following the procedure continuous ECG monitoring is performed until discharge. The clinician should evaluate the ECG for heart rate, rhythm, and intervals as well as the presence of any arrhythmia. Any changes from baseline should be should be reported to the child's physician, along with a report of the child's hemodynamic response to the arrhythmia.

Discharge Planning

Many patients are discharged the same day as the IEPS, while some may require an inpatient stay for cardiac arrhythmia management. Regardless of when the patient is discharged, the clinician must ensure that appropriate discharge planning takes place. A major component of discharge planning is patient and family education, which is discussed separately below.

An adequate return to the patient's baseline state should be the primary responsibility of the clinician prior to discharge. The child's vital signs should be stable with adequate hemostasis and the respiratory status having returned to the preprocedural state. An adequate amount of fluids should be consumed and the child should urinate prior to discharge. If specific tests have been ordered following the procedure, the clinician should ensure that they have been completed and reviewed by the discharging physician. The clinician should provide oral and written instructions regarding care of the puncture site, any prescribed medications, subacute bacterial endocarditis (SBE) prophylaxis (if applicable), signs and symptoms to report to the physician, any activity restrictions, telephone numbers for postdischarge problems or questions, and follow-up care. Patients discharged the day of the procedure should be instructed to remain quiet over night and informed about food and fluid intake and when to remove the dressing (usually the next morning).

Patient and Family Considerations

Patient and family education regarding IEPS should begin as soon as the decision is made to proceed with this particular diagnostic method. Patients and parents should be informed of the reasons for the IEPS, the potential complications associated with IEPS, the potential benefits of performing IEPS, as well as what to expect before, during, and after the IEPS.

The child should receive education at an age-appropriate level. Both verbal and written information regarding the procedure should be used in the educational process. Directions regarding when and why to withhold food and fluids should be reinforced and time frames for admission, procedure duration, recovery, and discharge clarified. Older children and adolescents may appreciate a tour of the catheterization/electrophysiology laboratory on the day before the procedure, to decrease fear and anxiety on the day of the procedure.

Postprocedure routines should be discussed with the patient and family. The child should be informed that there will be puncture sites or "poke marks" with tight bandages over them when he or she wakes up. The child should be told that he or she will need to lay flat in bed for several hours after the procedure and may slowly resume food and fluids. Information regarding any restrictions after the procedure, such as tub baths or swimming, should be provided to the patient and family before the procedure to allow necessary planning.

Home care instructions should be given to the responsible person in a quiet, relaxed, and unrushed atmosphere. Patients and families should be instructed to keep the puncture sites clean and dry and a bandaid may be used if clothing or underwear irritate the site(s). Parents should be instructed to inspect the site(s) daily for 2 to 3 days for drainage, swelling, redness, or hematoma. Activity restrictions and allowances should be discussed, with a general recommendation of light activity for 2 to 3 days following IEPS to allow puncture site healing. Other issues to be reviewed with the patient and family include medications that the child will be taking when discharged, SBE prophylaxis (if applicable), signs and symptoms requiring physician notification, and follow-up.

Principles of Educating Children and their Families

The care of children with cardiac rhythm disturbances can be quite challenging. In addition to the clinical and physical aspects of their care, clinicians must be able to provide expert patient and family education. Although much of this education is directed toward the child's parents, the child must be informed of and prepared for specific procedures.[90] This section includes an overview of the concept of family-centered care, the child's understanding of illness based on developmental level, and methods for preparing and educating the child with cardiac arrhythmias and his or her family.

Family-Centered Care

Family-centered care is a model of care delivery in which the family is recognized as a constant in the child's life. Health care professionals as well as associated service systems should strive to support, respect, encourage, and enhance the family unit by empowering them as well as providing effective helpgiving.[91] Cardiovascular caregivers should support the family by identifying and building on their strengths as opposed to their weaknesses, as individuals and as a family. This can be accomplished by allowing parents to display their abilities and to acquire new ones as necessary to meet the child's needs (known as enabling) and by allowing the family to maintain or acquire a sense of control over their lives by fostering their own strengths, abilities, and actions (known as empowerment).[91]

By developing a parent-professional partnership, the cardiovascular clinician identifies the family as having a rightful role in deciding what is important for the individual family members and for the family as a whole, while supporting and strengthening the ability of the family to nurture and promote its development. The benefits of family-centered care have been identified[92,93] and include the following: 1) the family experiences less stress in caring for their child by experiencing a greater feeling of confidence as well as competence; 2) the dependency of the family on professional caregivers decreases; 3) the cost of care decreases; 4) health care professionals experience greater job satisfaction; and 5) families and health care providers are empowered to develop new skills and expertise.[92,93]

Children's Understanding of Illness

Unlike adults, children who experience illness have different understandings of their internal body parts and disease processes based on their specific cognitive and developmental levels. These levels or stages account for common misconceptions (often not verbalized) that the child may have regarding specific illness-related issues. Crider[94] has identified seven developmental stages of the child's awareness and understanding of his or her internal body parts and how they function. These, although not always age and stage matched, are summarized in Table 5.[94]

Crider[94] has stated that children are unlikely to learn about a specific body part until it is important for an explanation of body function. Research has shown that preschoolers can identify many external body parts,

Table 5
Crider's Stages of Children's Understanding
of Body Parts and Function[94]

Stage 1 (preschool age)	• Thinks on global level • What's inside is what is seen going into and out of the body
Stage 2 (school age)	• Body parts are described according to shape, substance, and motion • Reasoning is based mostly on proximity of parts or functions
Stage 3 (approximately 9 years of age)	• Body is seen as a storage container • Body parts facilitate movement into and out of these containers
Stage 4	• Internal organs are active agents responsible for the movement of body substances
Stage 5	• Recognizes coordination among body parts and reversibility of actions
Stage 6	• Described as transformation of body substances, such as food to waste
Stage 7 (approximately 16 years of age)	• Can provide cellular/chemical explanation about specific functions of body parts

but have significantly less understanding of internal body parts.[95] Two studies, on 7 and 8 year olds[96] and 6 and 7 year olds,[97] identified the blood, bones, and heart as perceived internal organs in these age groups. The identification of their anatomic placement was noted to improve with age.

Gellert[96] found a developmental sequence associated with the understanding of the heart's function. Preschoolers (42%) and school-aged children (40% to 50%) identified the heart as essential to life, but could not elaborate. The preschoolers described the heart as thumping or beating (21%) and as making, supplying, or purifying the blood. Interestingly, 11% thought that the heart had something to do with love. The school-aged children were divided: 20% to 40% thought that the heart was responsible for circulating the blood or oxygen, and 30% to 40% described the heart's function as being related to breathing. By adolescence, 80% to 100% described the heart as the organ that circulates the blood.

In addition to being aware of the child's perception of his/her body parts, another factor to consider when educating and preparing children for cardiac arrhythmia management is the child's perception of the disease etiology.[98] This perception is based on Piaget's theory of child development. Early perceptions of disease etiology occur when children are preoperational, ranging in age from 3 to 6 or 7 years. The two illness etiologies include phenomenism and contagion. Phenomenism occurs when children identify an external influence as the cause of the illness. This external influence generally occurs around the same time as the illness, but not necessarily in close proximity to the child. With contagion, the concept is similar with more emphasis placed on the physical proximity of the child and the cause.

In the concrete operational stage of cognitive development, illness causation is described as contamination and/or internalization. In the former, the cause is *contact* with the external person, object, or event. Internalization as a disease etiology is when the child views the illness as occurring secondary to *"taking in"* the causative agent, e.g., swallowing or inhaling it.[98]

Formal operational thought involves more abstract thinking and concept manipulation. The causes are now described as physiologic or psychophysiologic. The physiologic cause is described as the malfunction or absence of function of a specific organ with an external trigger. With the psychophysiologic etiology, in addition to thinking of an external trigger, the child also recognizes that the trigger can be psychological.[98]

Patient and Family Education

With the aforementioned concepts in mind, the clinician can begin to formulate a plan for assessing, implementing, and evaluating a specific educational plan for the patient with a cardiac arrhythmia (and his or her family). The overall goals of patient and family education are to decrease anxiety, promote cooperation, and support or teach new coping skills. In synchrony with the concept of family-centered care, the parents can often guide clinicians in deciding how much information is enough for their particular child, since they know if their child is of the inquisitive type or is satisfied with short answers and/or descriptions. Taking into consideration the child's developmental age and cognitive abilities, the clinician can develop strategies to meet the needs of patients and their families. The following discussion includes basic principles for the clinician to use when assessing and planning education for patients and families. It is followed by a discussion of specific techniques to be used, based on the child's age, which is subdivided into the following groups: infant/toddler, preschool age, school age, and adolescent.

Basic Educational Principles

The initial part of the patient and family education process is the assessment phase, which should include what the patient and family may (or may not) already know about the diagnosis, procedure, or intervention. By allowing the patient and family to discuss what they already know, the clinician can tailor their education in an understandable manner in order to decrease anxiety and fear while establishing or reinforcing a trusting relationship. After the assessment phase has been initiated, the clinician can identify problems and establish goals with the patient and family.

Patient and family education should be carried out in a quiet and relaxed atmosphere with few interruptions. A basic explanation of the diagnosis, procedure, or intervention should be provided with ample opportunity given for the child and family to ask questions. Since there are many sources of patient education materials, cardiovascular clinicians should be aware of the implications associated with each. Nurses who prepare their own patient education materials must remain cognizant of the material's readability, which should be at no greater than a seventh-grade reading level.[99] Available children's literature used for patient and family education is not always accurate[100]; thus, clinicians should carefully evaluate these sources of information prior to promoting their use. Similarly, clinicians must be aware of information that patients and families obtain from the Internet. Since the information is not regulated, misinformation exists[101] and cardiovascular clinicians should warn patients and families as well as devise ways to screen this information. In addition to verbal and written information, patient education can involve the use of videotapes, dolls, heart models, puppets, and play therapy.[102] General guidelines for preparing children for procedures have been published by Wong and colleagues[103] and are summarized in Table 6.

Infant/Toddler

The patient and family education of the infant and toddler is more directed toward the child's parents. Since stress exists for the entire family when the child is diagnosed with a cardiac arrhythmia and must undergo treatment, the role of the clinician in providing information is to be able to decrease that stress in part by alleviating fear of the unknown. For example, in a neonate with newly diagnosed SVT, it is important to encourage the mother to grieve for a normal child and to be informed that the resultant arrhythmia was not her fault. Even though mothers do not verbalize these thoughts, 9 times out of 10, they are thinking them. The clinician should be as honest as possible with parents regarding their child's diagnosis, prognosis, and available treatment options. If the clinician is unsure of any specifics regarding the diagnosis, interventions, or

Table 6
Guidelines for Planning Patient and Family Education[103]

1. Review the child's/parent's present level of understanding.
2. Develop a plan based on the child's developmental age.
3. Incorporate the parents into the educational plan.
4. Allow ample time for discussion.
5. Use concrete terms to describe the procedure and use visual aids when possible.
6. Use words appropriate to the child's level of understanding.
7. Clarify all unfamiliar words.
8. Emphasize the sensory aspects of the procedure, i.e., what the child will hear, see, feel, smell, and touch.
9. Allow the child to practice procedures that require cooperation.
10. Introduce anxiety-provoking information last.
11. Be honest with the child, especially regarding painful and/or unpleasant procedures or interventions.

treatment plans, he or she should be comfortable in saying so. When new information arises, the clinician should share this information with patients and families as soon as possible. Often, parents just want someone to listen to their fears and concerns, and the clinician should make every attempt to make time to do this, with the end result a less anxious and more informed parent.

Preschool Age

The preschool-aged child is egocentric, has increased language skills (when compared to the toddler age), a limited concept of time, a low tolerance for frustration, fears of bodily harm, intrusion, and castration, and a potential viewpoint that illness and hospitalization is a form of punishment. The education directed at the school-aged child should include the use of play, demonstration of equipment whenever possible, and explanations in simple terms and in relation to how it will affect the child. The child should be encouraged to verbalize ideas and concerns. The clinician should use 10- to 15-minute teaching sessions that may be divided into multiple sessions, and should avoid overestimating the child's ability to comprehend certain words and concepts. The clinician should clarify why the procedure is being performed and state that the procedure is NOT a form of punishment. Because of the child's fear of bodily harm, the clinician should use dolls and drawings when possible for explanations, and should emphasize what body parts are involved in the procedure realizing that procedures involving the child's genitalia provoke increased anxiety in this age group.

School Age

The school-aged child now has increased language skills and an interest in acquiring knowledge. The child now has an improved concept of time, increased self-control, and is developing relationships with peers. The clinician should explain procedures to the school-aged child using correct medical terminology, and should explain reasoning for him or her using simple drawings of anatomy and physiology. The function and operation of equipment should be expressed in concrete terms and the child should be allowed to manipulate equipment when necessary. A longer teaching session can be used (20 minutes) and the child should be told exactly what to expect, with allowance of time for questions. If possible, the child should be included in decision making and active participation encouraged. All clinicians involved in the care of the school-aged should strive to maintain privacy.

Adolescent

The adolescent is more capable of abstract thought and reasoning, is extremely appearance conscious, is more concerned with the present versus the future, is independence minded, and is continuing to develop relationships with peers and group identity. The clinician should expand on the adolescent's education by providing rationale for why a specific test or intervention is necessary or beneficial as well as explaining the long-term consequences of the intervention or procedure. The clinician should remain cognizant of the fact that the adolescent may fear death and/or disability and should encourage questions regarding the teenager's fears as well as treatment options and/or alternatives. Privacy is a major issue and should be protected at all times. A discussion of how the intervention or procedure may affect the adolescent's appearance as well as an emphasis on potential benefits of the procedure or intervention should be included in the educational plan. One important issue to remember when caring for adolescents is the realization that the immediate effects of the procedure or intervention are more significant than any future benefits. In striving for independence, the adolescent should be allowed to participate in the decision-making process whenever possible, but the clinician should be aware of the fact that regression to more childish coping methods is likely in some cases. Last, the clinician should allow the adolescent to talk with other adolescents who have a similar diagnosis and who may have undergone the same or similar procedures.

By using the concepts of family-centered care and incorporating the child's developmental age and cognitive abilities, the clinician can formulate an educational plan designed to meet the needs of patients and families. The clinician should also keep in mind that patient and family education is not primarily to disseminate information, but to support the family by decreasing anxiety and allowing them to position themselves as comfortable and cooperative caregivers.

In summary, cardiovascular clinicians can improve the care provided to children with cardiac arrhythmias by becoming knowledgeable about the specific arrhythmia mechanisms and substrates, the associated diagnostic tools, and the provision of expert patient and family education. Incorporating these concepts into the child's overall plan of care can make caring for these children and their families a positive and rewarding experience.

References

1. Mines GR: On circulating excitations in heart muscles and their possible relation to tachycardia and fibrillation. Trans Roy Soc Canada 1914; 4:43–53.
2. Janse MJ: Mechanisms of arrhythmias. In Camm AJ (ed.): Clinical Approaches to Tachyarrhythmias. Vol. 1. Mount Kisco, NY: Futura Publishing Company, Inc.; 1993:1–56.
3. Cranefield PR, Wit AL, Hoffman RB: Genesis of cardiac arrhythmias. Circulation 1973; 47:190–196.
4. Wit AL, Cranefield PF: Triggered activity in cardiac muscle fibers of the simian mitral valve. Circ Res 1976; 38:85–91.
5. Rosen M: Is the response to programmed electrical stimulation diagnostic of mechanisms for arrhythmias? Circulation 1986; 73:II18.
6. Rosen M, Wit A: Triggered activity. In Zipes D, Rowlands D (eds.): Progress in Cardiology: Arrhythmias, Part III. Philadelphia: Lea & Febiger; 1998:39–46.

7. Gillette PC: The mechanisms of supraventricular tachycardia in children. Circulation 1976; 54:133–139.

8. Ko JK, Deal BJ, Strasburger JF, et al: Supraventricular tachycardia mechanisms and their age distribution in pediatric patients. Am J Cardiol 1992; 69:1028–1032.

9. Deal BJ: Supraventricular tachycardia mechanisms and natural history. In Deal BJ, Wolff GS, Gelband H (eds.): Current Concepts in Diagnosis and Management of Arrhythmias in Infants and Children. Armonk, NY: Futura Publishing Company, Inc.; 1998:117–143.

10. Akhtar M, Jazayeri MR, Sra J, et al: Atrioventricular nodal reentry. Clinical, electrophysiological, and therapeutic considerations. Circulation 1993; 88: 282–295.

11. Sung RJ, Lauer MR, Chun H: Atrioventricular node reentry: Current concepts and new perspectives. Pacing Clin Electrophysiol 1994; 17:1413–1430.

12. McGuire MA, Bourke JP, Robotin MC, et al: High resolution mapping of Koch's triangle using sixty electrodes in humans with atrioventricular junctional (AV nodal) reentrant tachycardia. Circulation 1993; 88:2315–2328.

13. Naheed ZJ, Strasburger JF, Deal BJ, et al: Fetal tachycardia: Mechanisms and predictors of hydrops fetalis. J Am Coll Cardiol 1996; 27:1736–1740.

14. Beerman LB, Neches WH, Fricker FJ, et al: Arrhythmias in transposition of the great arteries after the Mustard operation. Am J Cardiol 1983; 51:1530–1534.

15. Vetter VL, Tanner CS, Horowitz LN: Inducible atrial flutter after the Mustard repair of complete transposition of the great arteries. Am J Cardiol 1988; 61:428–435.

16. Muller GI, Deal BJ, Strasburger JF, et al: Electrocardiographic features of atrial tachycardias after operation for congenital heart disease. Am J Cardiol 1993; 71:122–124.

17. Chinitz LA, Bernstein NE, O'Connor B, et al: Mapping reentry around atriotomy scars using double potentials. Pacing Clin Electrophysiol 1996; 19:1978–1983.

18. Waldo AL: Mechanisms of atrial fibrillation, atrial flutter, and ectopic atrial tachycardia—A brief review. Circulation 1987; 75:37–40.

19. Wells JL Jr., Karp RB, Kouchoukos NT, et al: Characterization of atrial fibrillation in man: Studies following open heart surgery. Pacing Clin Electrophysiol 1978; 1:426–438.

20. von Bernuth G, Engelhardt W, Kramer HH, et al: Atrial automatic tachycardia in infancy and childhood. Eur Heart J 1992; 13:1410–1415.

21. Mehta AV, Ewing LL: Atrial tachycardia in infants and children: Electrocardiographic classification and its significance. Pediatr Cardiol 1993; 14: 199–203.

22. Levine JH, Michael JR, Guarnieri T: Treatment of multifocal atrial tachycardia with verapamil. N Engl J Med 1985; 312:21–25.

23. Wit AL, Rosen MR: Cellular electrophysiology of cardiac arrhythmias. I. Arrhythmias caused by abnormal impulse generation. Mod Concepts Cardiovasc Dis 1981; 50:1–6.

24. Wit AL, Rosen MR: Cellular electrophysiology of cardiac arrhythmias. II. Arrhythmias caused by abnormal impulse generation. Mod Concepts Cardiovasc Dis 1981; 50:7–12.

25. Wellens HJJ, Schuilenburg RM, Durrer D: Electrical stimulation of the heart in patients with ventricular tachycardia. Circulation 1972; 46:216–226.

26. Wellens HJJ, Durer DR, Lie KI: Observations on mechanisms of ventricular tachycardia in man. Circulation 1976; 54:237–244.

27. Yabek SM: Ventricular arrhythmias in children with an apparently normal heart. J Pediatr 1991; 119:1–11.

28. Noh CI, Gillette PC, Case CL, et al: Clinical and electrophysiologic characteristics of ventricular tachycardia in children with normal hearts. Am Heart J 1990; 120:1326–1333.
29. Vetter VL, Josephson ME, Horowitz LN: Idiopathic recurrent sustained ventricular tachycardia in children and adolescents. Am J Cardiol 1981; 47: 315–322.
30. Vetter VL: Ventricular arrhythmias in pediatric patients with and without congenital heart disease. In Horowitz LN (ed.): Current Management of Arrhythmias. Philadelphia: BC Decker; 1990:208.
31. Garson A Jr.: Ventricular arrhythmias after repair of congenital heart disease: Who needs treatment? Cardiol Young 1991; 1:177–181.
32. Dunnigan A, Pritzker MR, Benditt DG, et al: Life threatening ventricular tachycardias in late survivors of surgically corrected tetralogy of Fallot. Br Heart J 1984; 52:198–206.
33. Deanfield J, McKenna W, Rowland E: Local abnormalities of right ventricular depolarization after repair of tetralogy of Fallot: A basis for ventricular arrhythmia. Am J Cardiol 1985; 55:522–525.
34. Dick M II, Russell MW: Ventricular tachycardia. In Deal B, Wolff G, Gelband H (eds.): Current Concepts in Diagnosis and Management of Arrhythmias in Infants and Children. Armonk, NY: Futura Publishing Company, Inc.; 1998: 181–222.
35. Shimizu W, Ohe T, Kurita T, et al: Early afterdepolarizations induced by isoproterenol in patients with congenital long QT syndrome. Circulation 1991; 84:1915–1923.
36. Zhou JT, Zheng LR, Liu WY: Role of early afterdepolarizations in familial long QTU syndrome and torsade de pointes syndrome. Pacing Clin Electrophysiol 1992; 15:2164–2168.
37. Bouman LN, Jongsma HJ: Structure and function of the sino-atrial node: A review. Eur Heart J 1986; 7:94–104.
38. Vetter VL, Tanner CS, Horowitz LN: Electrophysiologic consequences of Mustard repair of d-transposition of the great arteries. J Am Coll Cardiol 1987; 10:1265–1273.
39. Kurer CC, Tanner CS, Vetter VL: Electrophysiologic findings after Fontan repair of functional single ventricle. J Am Coll Cardiol 1991; 17:174–181.
40. Feltes TF, Friedman RA: Transesophageal echocardiographic detection of atrial thrombi in patients with non-fibrillation atrial tachyarrhythmias and congenital heart disease. J Am Coll Cardiol 1994; 24:1365–1370.
41. Freedberg RS, Kronzon I, Rumancik WM, et al: The contribution of magnetic resonance imaging to the evaluation of intracardiac tumors diagnosed by echocardiography. Circulation 1988; 77:96–103.
42. Denfield SW, Gajarski RJ, Towbin JA: Cardiomyopathies. In Garson A Jr., Bricker JT, Fisher DJ, Neish SR (eds.): The Science and Practice of Pediatric Cardiology. 2nd ed. Baltimore: Williams & Wilkins; 1998:1851–1883.
43. Strain JE, Grose RM, Factor SM, et al: Results of endomyocardial biopsy in patients with spontaneous ventricular tachycardia but without apparent structural heart disease. Circulation 1983; 68:1171–1181.
44. Wiles HB, Gillette PC, Harley RA, et al: Cardiomyopathy and myocarditis in children with ventricular ectopic rhythm. J Am Coll Cardiol 1992; 20:359–362.
45. Mendelsohn JS, Quinn MT, McNabb WL: Interview strategies commonly used by pediatricians. Arch Ped Adolesc Med 1999; 153:154–157.
46. Dunnigan A: Clinical evaluation of the child with an arrhythmia. In Deal BJ, Wolff GS, Gelband H (eds.): Current Concepts in Diagnosis and Management of Arrhythmias in Infants and Children. Armonk, New York, Futura Publishing Company, Inc., 1998:1–16.
47. Bates B, Hoekelman RA: Interviewing and the health history. In Bates B (ed.):

A Guide to Physical Examination and History Taking. 4th ed. Philadelphia: JB Lippincott Company; 1997:1–27.
48. Barness LA: The pediatric history and physical examination. In Oski FA, DeAngelis CD, Feigin RD, Warshaw JB (eds.): Principles and Practice of Pediatrics. Philadelphia: JB Lippincott Company; 1990:28–43.
49. Pacia SV, Devinsky O, Luciano DJ, et al: The prolonged QT syndrome presenting as epilepsy: A report of two cases and literature review. Neurology 1994; 44:1408–1410.
50. Einthoven W, Fahr G, Dewaart A: Über die richtung und die manifest grosse der potentialschwankungen im menschlichen herzen und über den einfluss der herzlage auf der form des electrocardiograms. Arch Gestame Physiol 1913; 150:275. Hoff H, Sekelju P (transl.) Am Heart J 1950; 40:163–180.
51. Goldberger E: Unipolar Lead Electrocardiography. 2nd ed. Philadelphia: Lea & Febiger; 1950:23–35.
52. Wilson FN, Johnston FD, Macleod AG, et al: Electrocardiograms that represent the potential variations of a single electrode. Am Heart J 1934; 9: 447–458.
53. Garson A Jr.: The Electrocardiogram in Infants and Children. A Systematic Approach. Philadelphia: Lea & Febiger; 1983:19–35.
54. Xie B, Heald SC, Bashir Y, et al: Localization of accessory pathways from the 12-lead electrocardiogram using a new algorithm. Am J Cardiol 1994; 74: 161–165.
55. Liebman J, Plonsey R, Gillette PC: Pediatric Electrocardiography. Baltimore: Williams & Wilkins; 1982:60–133.
56. Lander P, Berbari EJ, Lazarra R: Optimal filtering and quality control of the signal-averaged ECG: High fidelity 1 minute recordings. Circulation 1995; 91:1495–1505.
57. Breithardt G, Cain ME, El-Sherif N, et al: Standards for analysis of ventricular potentials using high resolution or signal averaged electrocardiography: A statement by a Task Force of the European Society of Cardiology, the American Heart Association, and the American College of Cardiology. J Am Coll Cardiol 1991; 17:999–1006.
58. Zimmerman M, Freidli B, Adamec R, et al: Ventricular late potentials and induced ventricular arrhythmias after surgical repair of tetralogy of Fallot. Am J Cardiol 1991; 67:873–878.
59. Vaksmann G, Kohen ME, Lacroix D, et al: Influence of clinical and hemodynamic characteristics on signal-averaged electrograms in postoperative tetralogy of Fallot. Am J Cardiol 1993; 71:317–321.
60. Fallah-Najmabadi H, Dahdah NS, Palcko M, et al: Normal values and methodologies: Recommendations for signal-averaged electrocardiography in children and adolescents. Am J Cardiol 1996; 77:408–412.
61. Holter NJ, Gengerelli JA: Remote recording of physiological data by radio. Rocky Mountain Med J 1949; 46:747–751.
62. Crawford MH, Bernstein SJ, Deedwania PC, et al: ACC/AHA guidelines for ambulatory electrocardiography. A report of the American College of Cardiology/American Heart Association Task Force on Practice Guidelines. J Am Coll Cardiol 1999; 34:912–948.
63. Johnson TB, Varney FL Jr., Gillette PC, et al: Lack of proarrhythmia as assessed by Holter monitor after atrial radiofrequency ablation of SVT in children. Am Heart J 1996; 132:120–124.
64. Christiansen JL, Guccione P, Garson A Jr.: Difference in QT interval measurement on ambulatory ECG compared with standard ECG. Pacing Clin Electrophysiol 1996; 19:1296–1303.
65. Neyroud N, Maison-Blanche P, Denjoy I, et al: Diagnostic performance of QT interval variables from 24-hour electrocardiography in the long QT syndrome. Eur Heart J 1998; 19:158–165.

66. Fyfe DA, Holmes DR, Neubauer SA, et al: Transtelephonic monitoring in pediatric patients with clinically suspected arrhythmias. Clin Pediatr 1984; 23:139–143.

67. Houyel L, Fournier A, Centazzo S, et al: Use of transtelephonic electrocardiographic monitoring in children with suspected arrhythmias. Can J Cardiol 1992; 8:714–744.

68. Karpawich PP, Cavitt DL, Sugalski JS: Ambulatory arrhythmia screening in symptomatic children and young adults: Comparative effectiveness of Holter and telephone event recordings. Pediatr Cardiol 1993; 14:147–150.

69. Cumbee SR, Pryor RE, Linzer M: Cardiac loop ECG recording: A new noninvasive diagnostic test in recurrent syncope. South Med J 1990; 83:39–43.

70. Linzer M, Comegno A: Long-term ambulatory ECG monitoring in syncope: The state of the art. Cardiovasc Rev Reports 1993; 14:11–29.

71. Wiles HB, Buckles DS, Zeigler VL: Noninvasive diagnostic techniques. In Gillette PC, Garson A Jr. (eds.): Pediatric Arrhythmias: Electrophysiolgy and Pacing. Philadelphia: WB Saunders Company; 1990:205–215.

72. Cumming GR, Everatt D, Hastman L: Bruce treadmill test in children: Normal values in a clinic population. Am J Cardiol 1978; 41:69–75.

73. Rozanski JJ, Dimich I, Steinfeld L, et al: Maximal exercise stress testing in evaluation of arrhythmias in children: Results and reproducibility. Am J Cardiol 1979; 43:951–956.

74. Weigal TJ, Porter CJ, Mottram CD, et al: Detecting arrhythmias by exercise electrocardiography in pediatric patients: Assessment of sensitivity and influence on clinical management. Mayo Clin Proc 1991; 66:379–386.

75. Garson A Jr., Gillette PC, Gutgesell HP, et al: Stress-induced ventricular arrhythmias after repair of tetralogy of Fallot. Am J Cardiol 1980; 46:1006–1012.

76. Ross BA, Zeigler V, Zinner A, et al: The effect of exercise on the atrial electrogram voltage in young patients. Pacing Clin Electrophysiol 1991; 14: 2092–2097.

77. Hebra JD: Continuous monitoring and lead selection. In Paul S, Hebra JD (eds.): The Nurse's Guide to Cardiac Rhythm Interpretation: Implications for Patient Care. Philadelphia: WB Saunders Company; 1998:40–56.

78. Brownlee JR, Serwer GA, Dick M II, et al: Failure of electrocardiographic monitoring to detect cardiac arrest in patients with pacemakers. Am J Dis Child 1989; 143:105–107.

79. Smith JB, Ley SJ, Curley MAQ, et al: Tissue perfusion. In Curley MAQ, Smith JB, Moloney-Harmon PA (eds.): Critical Care Nursing of Infants and Children. Philadelphia: WB Saunders Company; 1996:155–248.

80. Zipes DP, DiMarco JP, Gillette PC, et al: ACC/AHA Task Force Report. Guidelines for clinical intracardiac electrophysiological and catheter ablation procedures. Circulation 1995; 92:673–691.

81. Bubien R, Fisher J, Gentzel J, et al: NASPE Expert Consensus Document: Use of IV (conscious) sedation and analgesia by nonanesthesia personnel in patients undergoing arrhythmia specific diagnostic, therapeutic, and surgical procedures. Pacing Clin Electrophysiol 1998; 21:375–384.

82. Association of Operating Room Nurses: Proposed recommended practice: Monitoring the patient receiving IV conscious sedation. AORN J 1992; 56: 316–324.

83. Gillette PC, Blair HL: Intracardiac electrophysiology studies. In Gillette PC, Garson A Jr. (eds.): Clinical Pediatric Arrhythmias. 2nd ed. Philadelphia: WB Saunders Company; 1999:36–47.

84. Lau KC, Ross DL: Invasive electrophysiological studies in children. In Wren C, Campbell RWF (eds.): Paediatric Cardiac Arrhythmias. Oxford: Oxford University Press; 1996:68–93.

85. Gillette PC, Buckles D, Harold M, et al: Intracardiac electrophysiology studies. In Gillette PC, Garson A Jr. (eds.): Pediatric Arrhythmias: Electrophysiology and Pacing. Philadelphia: WB Saunders Company; 1990:216–248.

86. Kugler JD: Sinus node dysfunction. In Gillette PC, Garson A Jr. (eds.): Pediatric Arrhythmias: Electrophysiology and Pacing. Philadelphia: WB Saunders Company; 1990:250–300.

87. Strauss HC, Saroff AL, Bigger JT Jr., et al: Premature atrial stimulation as a key to the understanding of sinoatrial conduction in man. Circulation 1973; 47:86–93.

88. Narula OS, Shantha N, Vasquez M, et al: A new method for measurement of sinoatrial conduction time. Circulation 1978; 58:706–714.

89. Kugler JD, Gillette PC, Mullins CE, et al: Sinoatrial conduction in children: An index of sinoatrial node function. Circulation 1979; 59:1266–1276.

90. Rollins JH, Brantly DK: Preparing the child for procedures. In Smith DP (ed.): Comprehensive Child and Family Nursing Skills. St. Louis: Mosby-Year Book, Inc.; 1991:1–8.

91. Dunst CJ, Trivette C: Empowerment, effective helpgiving practices, and family centered care. Pediatr Nurs 1996; 22:334–337.

92. Curley M, Wallace J: Effects of the nursing mutual participation model of care on parental stress in the pediatric intensive care unit: A replication. Pediatr Nurs 1992; 7:377–385.

93. Johnson BH, Jeppson ES, Redburn L: Caring for Children and Families: Guidelines for Hospitals. Bethesda, MD: Association for Care of Children's Health; 1992.

94. Crider C: Children's conceptions of the body interior. In Bibace R, Walsh ME (eds.): New Directions for Child Development: Children's Conceptions of Health, Illness, and Bodily Functions. San Francisco: Jossey-Bass; 1981:49–66.

95. Youngblut JM: Children's understanding of illness: Developmental aspects. AACN Clin Issues 1994; 5:42–48.

96. Gellert E: Children's conceptions of the content and functions of the human body. Genet Psychol Monogr 1962; 65:293–411.

97. Glaun D, Rosenthal D: Development of children's concepts about the interior of the body. Psychother Psychosom 1987; 48:63–67.

98. Bibace R, Walsh ME: Children's conceptions of illness. In Bibace R, Walsh ME (eds.): New Directions for Child Development: Children's Conceptions of Health, Illness, and Bodily Functions. San Francisco: Jossey-Bass; 1981:31–48.

99. Owen PM, Johnson EM, Frost CD, et al: Reading, readability, and patient education materials. Cardiovasc Nurs 1993; 29:9–13.

100. Manworren RCB, Woodring B: Evaluating children's literature as a source for patient education. Pediatr Nurs 1998; 24:548–553.

101. McClung HJ, Murray RD, Heitlinger LA: The Internet as a source for patient education. Pediatrics 1998; 101:E2.

102. Manion J: Preparing children for hospitalization, procedures, or surgery. In Craft MJ, Denehy JA (eds.): Nursing Interventions for Infants & Children. Philadelphia: WB Saunders Company; 1990:74–92.

103. Wong DL, Hockenberry-Eaton M, Wilson D, Winkelstein ML, Ahmann E, DiVito-Thomas PA (eds.): Whaley & Wong's Nursing Care of Infants and Children. 6th ed. St. Louis: Mosby-Year Book, Inc., 1999:1210–1282.

Chapter 2

Supraventricular Arrhythmias

Sarah S. LeRoy RN, MSN, CPNP and Macdonald Dick II, MD

Supraventricular arrhythmias comprise the majority of arrhythmias seen in the pediatric population. In the last decade, progress in the diagnosis and management of arrhythmias as well as complex congenital heart disease (CHD) dramatically changed the field of pediatric electrophysiology. The ability to definitively treat supraventricular tachycardia (SVT) using radiofrequency ablation and concurrent innovations in biotechnology have resulted in remarkable advances in understanding arrhythmia mechanisms and substrates. Prior to the era of radiofrequency ablation, treatment for most patients was limited to the use of antiarrhythmic medications, surgery, or permanent pacemakers, and relatively few patients underwent invasive electrophysiologic testing. Definitive therapy with radiofrequency ablation is now a first-line therapy for patients with SVT without associated heart disease, and is increasingly used to treat complex atrial arrhythmias such as intraatrial reentry tachycardia (IART) and atrial fibrillation.

Complex atrial arrhythmias remain a common cause of morbidity in patients who have undergone surgical repair of complex CHD, a population that is growing due to significant advances in cardiovascular surgery. As a result, an increasing number of patients seen in the pediatric electrophysiology laboratory are young adults with CHD, blurring the distinction between pediatric and adult electrophysiology and increasingly impacting the delivery of services.

The following discussion is subdivided into the headings of "Tachyarrhythmias" and "Bradyarrhythmias." The section on tachyarrhythmias includes those that incorporate the atrioventricular (AV) node and those that are confined to the atria. The section on bradyarrhythmias includes both congenital and acquired AV block as well as sinus node dys-

From Zeigler VL, Gillette PC: *Practical Management of Pediatric Cardiac Arrhythmias.* Armonk, NY: Futura Publishing Co., Inc.; ©2001.

function. The clinical presentation and electrocardiographic (ECG) findings associated with each substrate are discussed, followed by a discussion on diagnostic tools, management strategies, and implications for clinicians. A separate section at the end of the chapter presents the patient and family considerations for children with supraventricular arrhythmias.

Tachyarrhythmias

Tachyarrhythmias that originate in the atria or incorporate atrial tissues as an integral part of the arrhythmia substrate are the most frequently diagnosed sustained arrhythmias during childhood. Comprising approximately 95% of arrhythmias diagnosed in children with structurally normal hearts,[1] these arrhythmias also predominate in children with congenital and acquired heart disease.[2,3] While usually not life threatening, they are a significant source of medical expense,[4] of morbidity following repair of complex CHD,[2,3] and of distress for children and families.[5]

Increased precision in diagnostic terminology has evolved with advances in knowledge of arrhythmia mechanisms and substrates. Earlier nomenclature employed the terms "paroxysmal atrial tachycardia" and "paroxysmal SVT" as general and inclusive labels describing intermittent narrow complex tachycardias. More recently, the term "supraventricular tachycardia (SVT)" has been advocated for narrow complex tachyarrhythmias, and in the clinical arena it is used in reference to patients with intermittent, narrow complex tachycardias with an undetermined mechanism. More precise diagnostic terminology is used for tachyarrhythmias that are electrophysiologically proven or distinguished by ECG characteristics (e.g., IART, automatic atrial tachycardia, or the permanent form of junctional reciprocating tachycardia [PJRT]).

SVT can be defined as a sustained, accelerated, nonsinus cardiac rhythm originating above the level of the AV junction or above the bifurcation of the bundle of His.[6] Proven cellular electrophysiologic mechanisms of supraventricular arrhythmias include reentry and abnormal or enhanced automaticity (see chapter 1). Automatic (or ectopic) supraventricular arrhythmias are less common in children, are often persistent or incessant, and are frequently resistant to medical therapy.[7] Due to the inherent chronic nature of these arrhythmias, patients with untreated automatic tachyarrhythmias are at risk for development of arrhythmia-related cardiomyopathies that often resolve with definitive treatment.[8] A classification of supraventricular tachyarrhythmias by arrhythmia mechanism can be found in Table 1.

Approximately 90% of pediatric supraventricular tachyarrhythmias are supported by a reentrant mechanism that incorporates the AV node.[9] The majority of these arrhythmias can be further delineated as AV reentry tachycardia (AVRT) or AV nodal reentry tachycardia (AVNRT). In

Table 1.
Classification of Supraventricular Tachyarrhythmias

Automatic
Atrial ectopic tachycardia (AET)
Junctional ectopic tachycardia (JET)
Chaotic or multifocal atrial tachycardia (CAT or MAT)

Reentrant
Atrioventricular reentry tachycardia (AVRT)
  Wolff-Parkinson-White (WPW)
  Concealed WPW
Atrioventricular nodal reentry tachycardia (AVNRT)
Atrial flutter
  Intraatrial reentry tachycardia (IART)
Atrial fibrillation
Permanent junctional reciprocating tachycardia (PJRT)
Sinoatrial nodal reentry tachycardia (SNRT)
Lown-Ganong-Levine tachycardia (LGL)
Mahaim tachycardia

AVRT, an accessory pathway extrinsic to the AV node completes the reentrant circuit, while in AVNRT the circuit is composed of fibers adjacent to and in continuity with the AV node. In contrast, the arrhythmia mechanism of the remaining 10% of SVT does not incorporate the AV node as part of the arrhythmia circuit. This group includes the reentrant rhythms atrial flutter, IART, and atrial fibrillation as well as the ectopic rhythms atrial ectopic tachycardia (AET), also known as atrial automatic tachycardia, and chaotic or multifocal atrial tachycardia (CAT or MAT, respectively).

Estimates of the incidence of SVT in children with structurally normal hearts range from 1 in 250 to 1 in 1000 children.[10] Natural history studies suggest that there are three age categories in which the incidence of symptomatic SVT episodes increase: 1) the neonatal period; 2) middle childhood; and 3) adolescence.[11–13] Approximately 50% of children with SVT are diagnosed during the neonatal period, and of these, 30% to 50% will have no recurrence of their arrhythmia after 18 months of age.[14,15] In contrast, spontaneous resolution for children who experience their first symptomatic episode later in childhood is quite low.[12]

Pediatric patients with supraventricular arrhythmias in the presence of congenital or acquired heart disease present unique management challenges. For many of these patients, the arrhythmias are either persistent or recurrent, are refractory to medical management, and are associated with significant symptoms particularly if cardiac function is compromised. The use of many antiarrhythmic medications is limited in these patients due to negative inotropic effects. Perioperative supraventricular arrhythmias in this patient population represent an aspect of arrhythmia management that can be extremely problematic.

Tachyarrhythmias that Incorporate the Atrioventricular Node

As previously noted, there are specific supraventricular tachyarrhythmias that incorporate the AV node within the circuit. These arrhythmia mechanisms include AVRT associated with manifest or concealed Wolff-Parkinson-White (WPW), PJRT, Lown-Ganong-Levine (LGL) tachycardia, Mahaim tachycardia, and AVNRT. Their clinical presentation and ECG characteristics are discussed below.

Wolff-Parkinson-White Syndrome

As originally described in 1930,[16] WPW syndrome consisted of ventricular preexcitation on the surface ECG, SVT, and young age at initial presentation. The clinical diagnosis of WPW is predicated on a short PR interval, slurred upstroke of the QRS complex (known as delta wave or preexcitation), and a prolonged QRS duration for age during normal sinus rhythm. Twenty percent to 50% of patients with the characteristic ECG findings during normal sinus rhythm never experience AVRT,[17,18] hence the use of the nomenclature "WPW syndrome" in those patients who do have associated SVT.

The substrate supporting SVT in patients with WPW is an embryologic remnant[19] histologically described as a muscle bundle that traverses the fibrous AV valve.[20] This muscle bundle provides an alternative electrical connection between the atria and ventricles, hence the use of the terms "accessory connection" or "accessory pathway." Conduction through the accessory pathway may be either *manifest* or *concealed. Manifest* conduction refers to the specific findings on the surface ECG during normal sinus rhythm, including a short PR interval and delta wave resulting in a prolonged QRS duration for age. These findings reflect early activation or preexcitation of the ventricles through the accessory pathway, and constitute the clinical diagnosis of WPW. Patients with an electrophysiologic proven accessory pathway without preexcitation have a *concealed* accessory connection. In these patients the accessory pathway is only capable of retrograde conduction; therefore, during sinus rhythm, there is a normal PR interval, a narrow QRS complex, and no delta wave, thus, concealed WPW.

Estimates of the prevalence of WPW syndrome range from 1.6 per 1000 individuals to 4 per 100,000 individuals per year.[18] Approximately 10% to 30% of infants with WPW have associated cardiac disease,[21] most commonly Ebstein's anomaly, l-transposition, and cardiomyopathy.[11,12,21] While most cases are sporadic, a rare familial inheritance pattern has been reported.[22]

Approximately 50% of infants with documented SVT have ventricular preexcitation on surface ECG during normal sinus rhythm. In 20% to 35% of these infants, preexcitation resolves within the first year of life,[11,13] although a significant number of these children have future episodes of

SVT.[11] In children with persistence of preexcitation, there is a significantly higher incidence of recurrent episodes, particularly during adolescence.[13]

A small number of patients with WPW are at risk for catastrophic events. The reported incidence of a catastrophic event as the presenting symptom ranges from 0.3% to 4.8%.[17,23] Prior clinical symptoms are not helpful in predicting which patients with WPW are at high risk for catastrophic events[24]; however, a history of syncope in patients with WPW is correlated with rapid antegrade conduction in the presence of atrial flutter-fibrillation[25] but is not independently predicative of sudden cardiac death (SCD).[26] Intermittent preexcitation is linked with slow antegrade conduction, suggesting a low risk for catastrophic events in the presence of atrial flutter or atrial fibrillation.[27]

The mechanism of cardiac arrest in patients with WPW is very rapid antegrade conduction across the accessory pathway (>300 beats per minute [bpm]) during an episode of atrial flutter or fibrillation which degenerates into ventricular fibrillation (VF).[28] Variables associated with catastrophic events include a shortest preexcited R-R interval of ≤220 ms during atrial flutter or fibrillation (suggesting rapid antegrade conduction across the accessory connection), a history of atrial fibrillation, presence of underlying heart disease, male adolescence, and multiple accessory pathways.[17,23,25,29]

Atrioventricular Reentry Tachycardia Associated with Concealed and Manifest Wolff-Parkinson-White Syndrome

The term "AVRT" is used as an inclusive term for SVT in patients with an accessory pathway. Concealed and manifest WPW are the two most common forms of AVRT seen in the pediatric population. Other forms of AVRT include PJRT, Mahaim tachycardia, and LGL.

During episodes of AVRT, the electrical impulse is usually conducted from the atria to the ventricles antegrade via the normal conduction system (i.e., the AV node and His-Purkinje system) and retrograde to the atria via the accessory pathway. In some patients, the tachycardia is supported by antegrade conduction through the accessory pathway to the ventricles with return to the atria via the AV node.

The prevalence of an accessory pathway supporting AVRT varies with age at diagnosis, comprising approximately 93% of fetal-onset tachyarrhythmias,[30] 75% of childhood-onset SVT,[9,31] and 70% of adolescent-onset SVT.[9] The most frequent initiating even for paroxysmal SVT of this type in a child is a premature beat.[32]

Clinical Presentation

Children with AVRT generally present with paroxysmal episodes of tachycardia ranging from 220 to 320 bpm in neonates[14,15] and from 160 to 280 bpm in older children.[13] Infants are more likely to present with congestive heart failure (CHF) than are older children,[33] although the arrhythmia in this age group can be well tolerated for hours without overt symptoms that might alert parents to a problem. Retrospectively, parents often give a 24- to 48-hour history of vague but progressive symptoms including poor feeding, lethargy, irritability, vomiting, and/or pallor. Interestingly, approximately 20% of infants with SVT are diagnosed during routine office visits during asymptomatic episodes.[11,14,34]

In older children, the presenting symptom is usually palpitations that may be related to physical exertion or emotional excitement. The frequency and duration of episodes vary greatly. Some children experience one or two episodes a year, lasting seconds or minutes, that resolve spontaneously or with simple vagal maneuvers, while others experience frequent and/or severe episodes, lasting hours, that require medical or electrical cardioversion. Children as young as 3 or 4 years of age may alert their parents by complaining that "my heart is beeping" or "my heart is beating out of my chest." Older children may be able to describe whether the onset and termination of the episodes are abrupt or gradual, which is helpful in distinguishing SVT from sinus tachycardia. In addition to palpitations, symptoms in older children may include dizziness, difficulty breathing, chest pain, and/or syncope. A small percentage of patients with manifest WPW present with cardiac arrest or SCD. The clinical manifestations for patients with concealed WPW are similar to those described for patients with manifest WPW, except that these patients are not at an increased risk for sudden catastrophic events because of the absence of antegrade conduction across the accessory pathway.

Electrocardiographic Characteristics

As previously described, characteristic ECG criteria for WPW include a short PR interval, slurred upstroke of the QRS complex (or delta wave), and prolonged QRS duration for age (Fig. 1). In some patients, preexcitation may be subtle or even intermittent. Additional clues for patients with subtle preexcitation include: 1) no Q wave in the left chest leads; 2) a PR interval less than 100 ms; and 3) left axis deviation.[35]

Patients with manifest WPW and SVT may exhibit two distinct forms of tachycardia, *orthodromic* and/or *antidromic*. *Orthodromic* SVT, the most common form, occurs when conduction proceeds antegrade through the AV node and retrograde through the accessory pathway (Fig. 2). *Antidromic* SVT, present in less than 10% of patients,[9] occurs when the impulse is conducted antegrade through the accessory pathway and retrograde through the AV node, resulting in an altered ventricular activation sequence and a wide QRS complex pattern (Fig. 3). Unless AV dissociation is present, indicating ventricular tachycardia (VT), it is difficult to distinguish antidromic SVT from VT.

In patients with concealed WPW, the findings on surface ECG during normal sinus rhythm are normal. During tachycardia, the ECG charac-

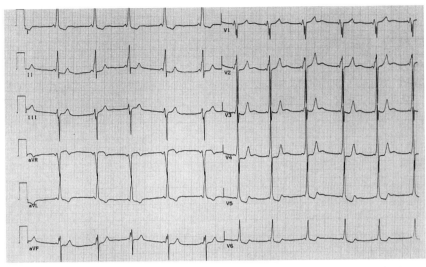

Figure 1. Twelve-lead ECG in a patient with Wolff-Parkinson-White exhibiting the typical features of a short PR interval, a wide QRS complex, and a slurred upstroke of the QRS complex known as a delta wave, all of which can be seen in multiple leads.

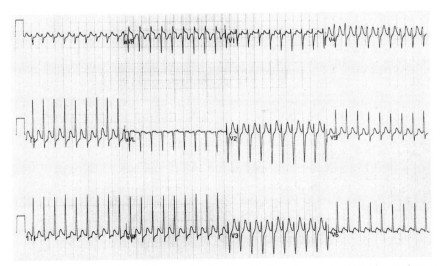

Figure 2. Twelve-lead ECG in a patient with orthodromic supraventricular tachycardia (SVT). The SVT exhibits a narrow QRS indicating retrograde conduction through the accessory pathway.

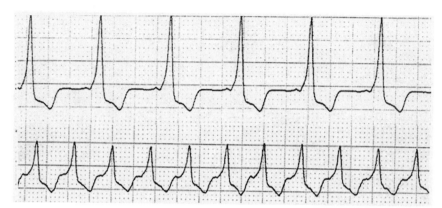

Figure 3. Two ECG rhythm strips from the same patient with Wolff-Parkinson-White. The top panel shows normal sinus rhythm with ventricular preexcitation. The bottom panel shows antidromic supraventricular tachycardia in which the tachycardia is conducted antegrade over the accessory pathway.

teristics are the same as those for the orthodromic SVT associated with WPW. The ECG characteristics of WPW during normal sinus rhythm and the associated tachycardias, both orthodromic and antidromic, include the following:

	During Normal Sinus Rhythm	Orthodromic SVT	Antidromic SVT
Rate	Within normal limits for age	220–320 bpm in neonates; 160–280 bpm in older children	Same as for orthodromic SVT
Rhythm	Regular	Regular	Regular
P wave	Normal	Absent or negative with an RP interval of >70 ms in lead II	Absent
PR interval	Short (<90 ms); P wave may merge into QRS complex	Not applicable	Not applicable
QRS complex	Wider than normal for age due to the slurred upstroke of the QRS complex known as a delta wave	Narrow, except in cases of rate-related bundle branch block or in patients with pre-existing bundle branch block	Wide (>120 ms)

Several methods to identify the location of accessory pathways based on ECG waveform polarities during normal sinus rhythm have been reported.[36-38] Early efforts identified two categories determined from the polarity recorded from the right precordial leads, primarily V_1 and V_2. Patients with a Type A pattern demonstrate a dominant R wave in these leads, suggesting a left-sided accessory pathway; patients with a Type B pattern have a dominant S or QS deflection, suggesting a right-sided pathway.[36] Recently, more elaborate algorithms have been developed aimed at predicting pathway location from the polarity of the delta wave in various leads as recorded by the ECG during normal sinus rhythm.[37,38]

Permanent Junctional Reciprocating Tachycardia

PJRT, originally described by Coumel and colleagues in 1967,[39] is an uncommon type of AVRT affecting approximately 1% of pediatric arrhythmia patients.[40] This arrhythmia is virtually incessant at rates ranging from 120 to 250 bpm and is the most common form of incessant SVT in children. Supported by a reentrant circuit involving an accessory pathway, the cardiac impulse is conducted antegrade through the AV node and His-Purkinje system, with retrograde conduction through a slowly conducting accessory pathway that is usually located near the ostium of the coronary sinus[41] (Fig. 4).

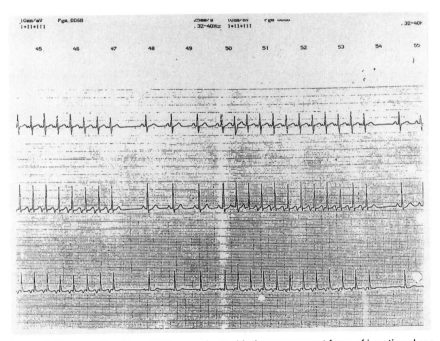

Figure 4. ECG leads I, II, and III in a patient with the permanent form of reciprocating tachycardia. The classic negative P waves are visible in leads II and III, with temporary cessation of the tachycardia followed by tachycardia resumption, which is typical of the incessant nature of this arrhythmia.

Clinical Presentation

Dorostkar and colleagues[40] reviewed the clinical course of 21 patients with PJRT seen at two institutions between 1989 and 1995. There was an equal distribution between males and females, and more than 50% of the patients presented at birth, with a mean age at presentation of 3 to 4 years. Decreased ventricular function was common, particularly in infants, but improved with age (attributed to decreasing tachycardia rates) and following definitive therapy via surgical or radiofrequency ablation.[40] There is no reported association with congenital or acquired heart disease. The presenting symptoms associated with PJRT can vary from child to child and are usually mild. Due to its incessant nature, it can result in cardiomegaly on chest radiograph, decreased ventricular function on echocardiogram, and CHF if undetected for a long period.

Electrocardiographic Characteristics

The ECG characteristics of PJRT include the following:

Rate	120–250 bpm; the tachycardia cycle length increases with age, resulting in lower tachycardia rates[40]
Rhythm	Incessant, regular rhythm with periods of interruption secondary to block in the retrograde accessory pathway followed by a sinus beat with resumption of tachycardia
P wave	Negative P waves in leads II, III, aVF, and the left lateral leads
PR interval	Normal PR but long RP interval consistent with slow retrograde conduction
QRS complex	Narrow QRS duration (<120 ms)

Lown-Ganong-Levine Syndrome

Lown, Ganong, and Levine[42] first described a group of patients with intermittent SVT with a short PR interval in the absence of a delta wave on the surface ECG (Fig. 5). This diagnosis, also called "enhanced AV nodal conduction," is included, along with WPW and Mahaim tachycardia, as one of the preexcitation syndromes.

Possible explanations for the ECG findings in patients with LGL include partial bypass of the AV node[43] or antegrade conduction via the fast pathway in patients with dual AV nodal physiology.[44] It may also be explained by an AV node malformation or a functional abnormality unaccompanied by an abnormal anatomic substrate.[45] The clinical presentation of patients with LGL is similar to those described for patients with AVRT. In addition to the narrow complex SVT associated with LGL, associated arrhythmias include atrial fibrillation with a rapid ventricular re-

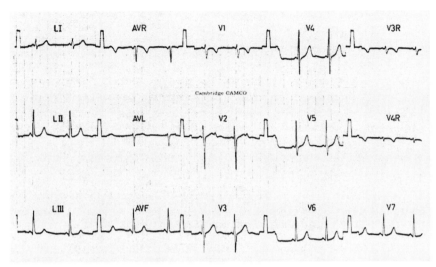

Figure 5. Fifteen-lead ECG demonstrating Lown-Ganong-Levine. This arrhythmia is characterized by a short PR interval with a narrow QRS complex.

sponse.[44,46] This diagnosis is uncommon in pediatric patients, but in patients with these ECG findings and symptomatic SVT, electrophysiology study and treatment with either antiarrhythmic medications or radiofrequency ablation may be indicated.

Electrocardiographic Characteristics

Aside from the short PR interval, the surface ECG during normal sinus rhythm is normal. During tachycardia, the ECG characteristics are the same as those identified for orthodromic SVT. The basic ECG characteristics for patients with LGL include the following:

	During Normal Sinus Rhythm	During SVT
Rate	Normal for age	220–320 bpm in neonates 160–280 bpm in older children
Rhythm	Regular	Regular
P wave	Normal	Absent or negative with RP >70 ms (lead II)
PR interval	Short (<90 ms)	Not applicable
QRS complex	Normal	Narrow

Mahaim Tachycardia

Mahaim conduction describes a rare reentrant mechanism that produces a wide QRS complex SVT. This tachycardia is supported by an accessory pathway that either partially or completely bypasses the normal AV node-His-Purkinje system. A *nodoventricular* Mahaim fiber originates in the AV node and inserts in the ventricular myocardium; a *fasciculoventricular* Mahaim fiber originates from the bundle of His with insertion into the ventricular myocardium. An *atriofascicular* bypass tract originates in the right atrial free wall near the tricuspid valve beginning with an AV-node-like structure that inserts into or near the right bundle branch. A Mahaim fiber may provide the antegrade limb of a reentrant circuit during SVT or may be entirely a bystander. The first two types of fibers, nodoventricular and fasciculoventricular, are usually bystanders. In patients with an atriofascicular Mahaim fiber, the reentrant circuit comprises the atriofascicular fiber as the antegrade limb and the His-Purkinje system as the retrograde limb[47] (Fig. 6). Importantly, all three forms of Mahaim fibers do not conduct in a retrograde manner.

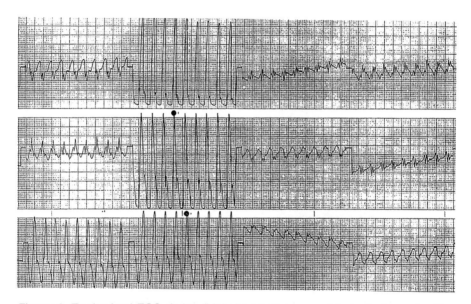

Figure 6. Twelve-lead ECG during "Mahaim type" supraventricular tachycardia. The QRS complex has a left bundle branch block morphology due to insertion of the atrio-fascicular fiber into the mid right ventricular septum. In this type of tachycardia, there is no visible atrioventricular dissociation. Reproduced from Perry JC: Supraventricular tachycardia. In Garson A Jr., Bricker JT, Fisher DJ, Neish SR (eds.): The Science and Practice of Pediatric Cardiology. 2nd ed. Baltimore: Williams & Wilkins; 1998: 2094, with permission.

Electrocardiographic Characteristics

The ECG during normal sinus rhythm in patients with Mahaim conduction depends on the site of origin of the Mahaim fiber. The ECG may exhibit a normal or somewhat shortened PR interval with a slightly wide QRS duration usually with a left bundle branch block configuration. The QRS pattern during the tachycardia of all three forms is also that of left bundle branch block configuration.

Patients with fasciculoventricular Mahaim conduction and SVT may exhibit AV dissociation, making the differentiation between it and VT difficult to discern. The ECG characteristics of patients with Mahaim fibers include the following:

	During Normal Sinus Rhythm	During SVT
Rate	Normal for age unless other cardiac pathology	220–320 bpm in neonates 160–280 bpm in older children
Rhythm	Regular	Regular
P wave	Normal	Absent or negative with RP >70 ms (lead II)
PR interval	Normal or short	Not applicable
QRS complex	Wider than normal for age due to ventricular preexcitation, with left bundle branch block pattern and left axis deviation	Wide, same as during normal sinus rhythm, with left bundle branch block pattern and left axis deviation

Atrioventricular Nodal Reentry Tachycardia

AVNRT is less common than AVRT during childhood but increases in frequency with older age at time of first presentation. It is the second most common type of SVT in children and accounts for 8% to 13% of paroxysmal SVT in neonates,[33,48] 30% in adolescents,[9] and greater than 50% in adults.[49] There is no reported association with congenital or acquired heart disease.

The reentrant circuit in AVNRT is composed of two functionally but not anatomically distinct pathways immediately adjacent to the AV node. Most authors subscribe to the concept that the circuit consists of a fast pathway positioned just anterior to the bundle of His and a slow pathway lying more inferiorly and posteriorly between the os of the coronary sinus and the posterior rim of the tricuspid valve in the triangle of Koch.[50] Thus, the ventricle is not a critical part of the circuit. There are two types of AVNRT, *typical* and *atypical* (Fig. 7). In the majority of patients, *typical* AVNRT (also known as the "slow-fast" form) is supported by antegrade conduction through the slow pathway and retrograde conduction through the fast pathway. *Atypical* AVNRT (also known as the "fast-slow" form) is supported by antegrade conduction across the fast pathway and retro-

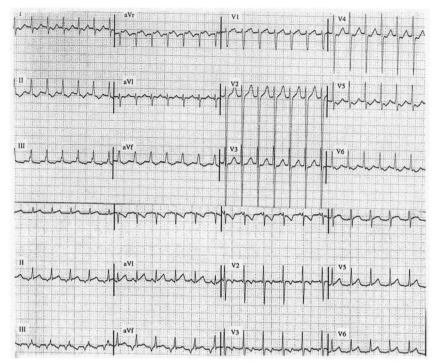

Figure 7. Two 12-lead ECGs exhibiting typical and atypical atrioventricular node reentry tachycardia. The top 12-lead ECG shows a rapid, narrow QRS tachycardia with no visible P waves (typical), while the bottom 12-lead ECG shows a rapid, narrow QRS tachycardia with negative P waves in leads II, III, and aVF with a "normal" PR interval (atypical).

grade conduction across the slow pathway. Since retrograde conduction occurs via the slow pathway, retrograde atrial activation is delayed compared to that seen during typical AVNRT, resulting in the characteristic ECG findings during SVT of a short PR interval and longer RP interval. Atypical AVNRT occurs infrequently but can be the underlying mechanism for an incessant tachycardia in children.[51]

Clinical Presentation

The clinical presentation of patients with AVNRT is similar to that of patients with AVRT. Symptoms include those previously described for children with AVRT, with the addition of visible neck pulsations during SVT, which supports AVNRT as the arrhythmia substrate.[52]

Electrocardiographic Characteristics

The ECG characteristics of patients with typical and atypical AVNRT include the following:

	During Normal Sinus Rhythm	During Atypical AVNRT	During Typical AVNRT
Rate	Within normal limits for age	150–280 bpm	150–280 bpm
Rhythm	Regular	Regular	Regular
P wave	Normal	Absent; retrograde P waves may be within or at the terminal portion of the QRS complex	Negative P waves in leads II, III, aVF, and V_4 through V_6
PR interval	Normal	P wave in QRS complex or very short RP interval (<70 ms)	Normal (or slightly long) and with a long RP interval
QRS complex	Normal duration	Narrow (<120 ms)	Narrow (<120 ms)

Diagnostic Tools for Patients with Tachyarrhythmias that Incorporate the Atrioventricular Node

Obviously, the most critical diagnostic tool for the diagnosis of any arrhythmia is an ECG, preferably a 12-lead ECG, taken during the arrhythmia episode. Other tools can document the arrhythmia and aid in determining its mechanism. Twenty-four-hour ambulatory monitoring can be helpful in identifying SVT, but only if an episode occurs while the monitor is in place. Incessant SVT, such as PJRT, may be elucidated with use of this diagnostic tool, which shows the arrhythmia to be present more than three quarters of the day in most patients.[53] Transtelephonic monitors can be helpful for patients who have brief episodes, while exercise stress testing can be helpful for patients with WPW, to assess antegrade accessory pathway properties. Transthoracic echocardiography can be used to determine if associated structural defects are present or to determine if the arrhythmia has resulted in decreased ventricular function. When administered as an intravenous (IV) bolus, adenosine transiently blocks AV nodal conduction and unmasks those arrhythmias not dependent on the AV node for perpetuation. In patients with a wide QRS tachycardia that is thought to be SVT, an esophageal atrial recording may help to identify the substrate. These and other diagnostic tools are discussed in more detail in chapter 1.

Management Strategies for Tachyarrhythmias that Incorporate the Atrioventricular Node

The management strategy for SVT of this type comprises a broad range of long- and short-term treatments. The choice of initial treatment strategy is based on the child's hemodynamic response to the SVT. If the child is hemodynamically compromised, as evidenced by poor perfusion, lethargy, pallor, hypotension, CHF, or shock, the treatment method of choice is synchronized, direct current cardioversion.

Immediate management strategies that can be used with patients exhibiting SVT include a variety of techniques that are discussed in chapter 4. The first of these strategies is the use of vagal maneuvers, such as the diving reflex, the Valsalva maneuver, and carotid massage.[54–57] These maneuvers induce a vagally mediated negative dromotropic effect on the AV node. IV adenosine, when used in patients with SVT that incorporates the AV node, interrupts the reentry circuit by slowing AV nodal conduction to the point of block.[58] Other pharmacologic agents used in the immediate management of SVT include IV amiodarone,[59] esmolol,[60] and procainamide. Other immediate management strategies include recording and/or overdrive pacing either via a transesophageal electrode catheter[61] or during the immediate postoperative period via epicardial pacing wires. Finally, synchronized direct current cardioversion is indicated for hemodynamically unstable patients.

Long-term treatment for children with SVT that incorporates the AV node includes pharmacologic therapy and radiofrequency catheter ablation, which are described in detail in chapters 5 and 6, respectively. Pharmacologic therapy is the preferred treatment method of choice in neonates and infants, since 30% to 50% of children diagnosed with SVT in the neonatal period will have no arrhythmia recurrence after 18 months of age.[14,15] In children with medically refractory SVT, SVT associated with significant symptomatology, or decreased cardiac function secondary to SVT, radiofrequency catheter ablation is the treatment method of choice.

Implications for Clinicians for Tachyarrhythmias that Incorporate the Atrioventricular Node

Nurses and other clinicians caring for children with SVT must have a basic knowledge of supraventricular arrhythmia mechanisms. Identification of the specific substrate is not as important as the assessment of the arrhythmia's hemodynamic effect on the patient. Although the majority of patients with SVT are hemodynamically stable, the clinician should constantly assess the patient for any changes in baseline status. If the patient begins to experience signs of decompensation, the clinician must identify and report these changes. Significant changes in the patient's level of consciousness (LOC), vital signs, color, respiratory status, and/or changes in perfusion should be documented and communicated to the child's physician.

Clinicians caring for patients with SVT must be knowledgeable regarding available treatments and must be ready to assist with any emergency maneuvers. If pharmacologic agents are to be used, the clinician should be aware of the drug's mechanism of action, dosage, duration of action, potential adverse effects, any known drug reactions, and reversal agents (if available).

Patient and family education is pivotal in caring for children with SVT. This education should include information about the arrhythmia itself, any nursing or medical procedures that the child must undergo, use of vagal maneuvers, other treatment options, and indications for seeking medical attention. For most patients, the arrhythmia is not life threatening; this is an important reassurance to be communicated to the parents. All explanations should be brief, simple, repeated often, and accompanied by clear, relevant written materials on a level that each individual patient and family can understand.

Tachyarrhythmias that are Confined to the Atria

Tachyarrhythmias that are confined to the atria include those arrhythmias that do not require the AV node for perpetuation. These arrhythmias include AET, CAT or MAT, atrial flutter, atrial fibrillation, and junctional ectopic tachycardia (JET). The following discussion includes the clinical presentation, the ECG characteristics, diagnostic tools, and management strategies for each. The implications for clinicians are discussed as they pertain to tachyarrhythmias that are confined to the atria.

Atrial Ectopic Tachycardia

AET is one of the most common causes of incessant tachycardia during childhood and accounts for 11% to 16% of pediatric SVT.[9] As the name implies, the underlying mechanism is presumed to be enhanced automaticity or triggered activity. This arrhythmia is characterized by prolonged or incessant episodes of rapid atrial tachycardia. Unlike reentrant SVT, in which episodes start and stop abruptly, AET is characterized by warming up (slowly accelerating) and warming down (slowly decelerating), without an initiating event such as a premature beat. In a series reported by Mehta and colleagues,[62] no association with underlying cardiac disease was found; however, Dhala and colleagues[63] identified cardiac disease in 38% (6/16) of their pediatric population.

Clinical Presentation

Atrial ectopic/automatic tachycardia presents as an incessant or persistent arrhythmia that may result in tachycardia-induced cardiomyopathy. In the pediatric population, this arrhythmia usually presents during early childhood[62,63] and approximately 50% of children with incessant AET exhibit overt symptoms of CHF at the time of initial presentation.[63] Similar to other SVT, children with AET may present with palpitations, exercise intolerance, dizziness, and, occasionally, syncope. Often, children with AET are referred secondary to cardiomegaly on chest radiograph and are later found to have decreased ventricular function. AET rates vary widely from 100 to 300 bpm.[63] AV block may be present even at lower heart rates, perhaps due to rate-related cardiomyopathy. Lack of normal heart rate variability is common in these patients and can be a clue in patients who do not exhibit particularly fast tachycardia rates. On the other hand, the AET mechanism is sensitive to autonomic tone and may exhibit variation in rate throughout the day. Although uncommon, spontaneous resolution has been reported.[64] The arrhythmia is often refractory to medical management, and in older children radiofrequency ablation is usually recommended.

Electrocardiographic Characteristics

AET is characterized by an abnormally fast heart rate and, usually, an abnormal P wave vector on the surface ECG. Although the ectopic focus can originate in either the left or right atrium, more than half of them are localized to the right side (Figs. 8 and 9). The P wave vector of high

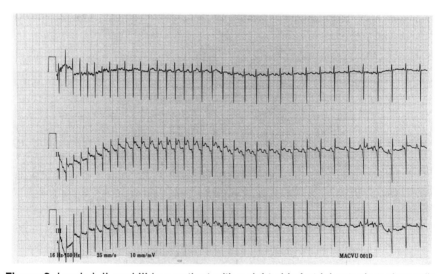

Figure 8. Leads I, II, and III in a patient with a right-sided atrial ectopic tachycardia. The first half of the recording shows the rapid rate followed by the classic deceleration of the tachycardia, making the upright, sinus-looking P waves easier to identify.

right-sided AET is the same as that seen in sinus rhythm (or sinus tachycardia), making it difficult to discriminate between the two. The ECG characteristics of AET include the following:

	Right AET	Left AET
Rate	100–250 bpm	100–250 bpm
Rhythm	Regular, unless AV block, then irregular; AET "warms up" with gradual acceleration and "warms down" with gradual deceleration	Regular, unless AV block, then irregular; AET "warms up" with gradual acceleration and "warms down" with gradual deceleration
P wave	Positive in leads I and aVL; similar to sinus P wave if near sinus node, negative P wave if low right atrial origin	Negative in leads I and aVL, positive in V_1
PR interval	Relatively short to normal; shortens with faster rates unless AV block is present	Relatively short to normal; shortens with faster rates unless AV block is present
QRS complex	Narrow or normal for age, unless bundle branch block is present	Narrow or normal for age, unless bundle branch block is present

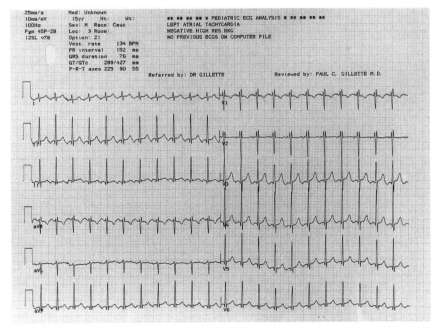

Figure 9. Twelve-lead ECG in a patient with a left-sided atrial ectopic tachycardia. The negative P waves can be seen in leads I, aVL, and V_6. Because this focus is located in the lower left atrium, negative P waves can also be seen in leads II, III, and aVF.

Diagnostic Tools

Two of the most helpful tools used to identify patients with AET include 24-hour ambulatory monitoring and echocardiography. Because children's heart rates are often relatively fast, the initial heart rate determination by the clinician may not suggest an abnormal heart rhythm. The 24-hour ambulatory monitor will reveal that the heart rate does not slow down appropriately (especially at night) as well as minimal heart rate variability. The echocardiogram will identify those patients with tachycardia-induced ventricular dysfunction.

Management Strategies

Because of its automatic nature, unlike reentrant SVT, AET will not respond to direct current cardioversion or atrial overdrive pacing, specifically because of its automatic nature. AET is often difficult to manage medically, so initial efforts are usually directed at ventricular rate control and improvement/support of cardiac function. Pharmacologic therapy may include digoxin and afterload reducers to manage ventricular dysfunction and antiarrhythmic medications such as Class Ic agents, sotalol, and amiodarone to manage the tachycardia. In acute situations, IV amiodarone has proven beneficial for some patients.[59,65] Definitive therapy can be achieved with radiofrequency catheter ablation.

Chaotic Atrial Tachycardia

Chaotic atrial tachycardia (CAT), also referred to as multifocal atrial tachycardia (MAT), is an uncommon tachyarrhythmia in children, accounting for only 0.2% of pediatric arrhythmias.[66] It is most commonly diagnosed during early infancy, presents as incessant or persistent, and usually follows a benign course,[67–69] although unexpected sudden death has been reported.[68,70] In the adult population, this arrhythmia is associated with chronic hypoxic pulmonary disease[71]; however, this has not been a dominant finding in the pediatric population. In some series, there is a high incidence of underlying cardiac disease[70] with cardiomyopathy as the most prevalent diagnosis,[69,72] although this has not been a universal finding.[73] In the absence of underlying cardiac disease, most children have normal ventricular function. The arrhythmia is often refractory to medical therapy, but spontaneous resolution is common.[68] The mechanism has not been conclusively determined and may involve abnormal atrial automaticity, triggered activity, or reentry.[74]

Clinical Presentation

Most children with CAT are diagnosed during early childhood, usually before the age of 3 years.[68] The most common presenting symptom is respiratory distress[66,67] or CHF, although many children are asymptomatic at the time of presentation[73] with an irregularly rapid heart rate as the only clinical finding.

In a series of seven infants with CAT reported by Fish and colleagues,[73] atrial rates were between 250 and 700 bpm and ventricular rates between 240 and 375 bpm. One patient was identified prenatally and the oldest age at initial diagnosis was 11 months. Symptoms included varying degrees of lethargy, tachypnea, and poor perfusion. Three patients had a viral upper respiratory infection at the time of initial presentation. A rapid ventricular response was associated with serious hemodynamic compromise in one patient. No patient had significant underlying heart disease or cardiac enlargement on chest radiograph. Long-term outcome was excellent, with spontaneous resolution of the arrhythmia seen in the majority of patients.

Electrocardiographic Characteristics

CAT is characterized by five distinct criteria: 1) a minimum of three P wave morphologies; 2) a lack of a dominant atrial rhythm; 3) isoelectric intervals between P waves; 4) varying P-P, R-R, and RP intervals; and 5) average atrial tachycardia rates of greater than 100 bpm (Fig. 10). Additional ECG characteristics include the following:

Rate	Atrial rate 250–700 bpm[62]
Rhythm	Irregular with varying P-P, PR, and R-R intervals
P wave	Well formed and discrete with three or more P wave morphologies
PR interval	Variable
QRS complex	Variable, often with aberrant QRS morphology

Atrial Flutter

Atrial flutter is an IART with considerably more heterogeneity than was initially appreciated.[75] Current categories of atrial flutter based on distinct ECG and electrophysiologic properties as well as anatomic substrates include *typical* atrial flutter, *atypical* atrial flutter, and *incisional* IART.[76,77] The substrate for atrial flutter consists of a macroreentrant circuit around fixed or functional barriers with areas of relatively slow conduction and unidirectional block. An abnormal atrial tissue substrate (e.g., atrial distention and/or intraatrial conduction delay) is often present.[78]

In *typical* atrial flutter, the electrical impulse (usually confined to the right atrium) follows a counterclockwise circuit around the tricuspid valve. Atrial anatomic structures that function as barriers forming the corridor in which the circuit travels include the crista terminalis, the eustachian valve, the inferior vena cava, the coronary sinus os, and the tricuspid valve

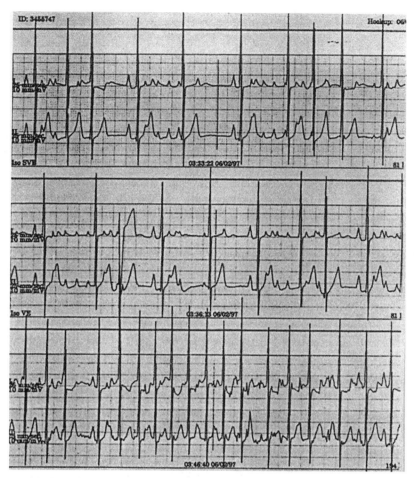

Figure 10. Ambulatory monitor ECG tracings from a 10-month-old child with chaotic atrial tachycardia. Reproduced from Sokoloski M: Tachyarrhythmias confined to the atrium. In Gillette PC, Garson A Jr. (eds.): Clinical Pediatric Arrhythmias. 2nd ed. Philadelphia: WB Saunders Company; 1999:92, with permission.

annulus.[77,79] The characteristics of typical atrial flutter include sudden onset/termination, the ability to initiate/terminate the arrhythmia with pacing, and the possibility of termination with direct current cardioversion. The pattern of atrial activation during typical atrial flutter results in the classic "sawtooth" pattern most prominent in the inferior leads.

Atypical atrial flutter travels in a clockwise manner around the tricuspid valve in a pattern of electrical activation that transcribes broad flutter waves that are positive in the inferior leads. The term "IART" can cause confusion, as it is used to describe other tachyarrhythmias that fulfill the previously described criteria for atrial flutter. When used diagnostically, "IART" generally refers to atrial reentrant rhythms in the presence of postoperative CHD. It is usually slower with lower amplitude P waves and lacks the classic "sawtooth" flutter waves.[80] If an atrial incision provides a barrier bordering the reentrant circuit in which the impulse travels, the term *"incisional* IART" is correctly used.

Atrial flutter is uncommon in children with structurally normal hearts. Limited primarily to infancy, atrial flutter accounts for 30% of fetal tachyarrhythmias,[81] 11% to 18% of neonatal tachyarrhythmias,[9,13] and 8% of supraventricular tachyarrhythmias in children greater than 1 year of age[82] (Fig. 11). The incidence of associated CHD at the time of the initial episode

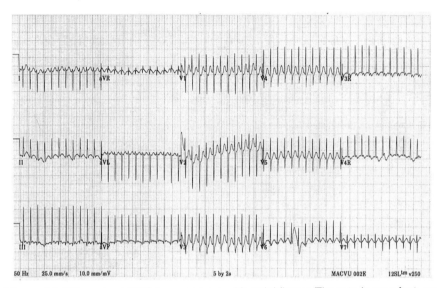

Figure 11. Fifteen-lead ECG in a newborn with atrial flutter. The rate is very fast, approximately 300 bpm, making this substrate initially difficult to discern.

of atrial flutter is 6% in fetal-onset tachyarrhythmias,[81] 50% with onset during infancy,[83] and 92% with onset in children greater than 1 year of age.[83] The clinical outcome for infants with isolated flutter is excellent and recurrence is rare after initial conversion.[84,85]

Intraatrial reentrant arrhythmias are a significant source of morbidity following surgery for complex CHD. Affecting 10% to 35% of children after the Fontan operation[86,87] for single ventricle anatomy, it is also a known sequelae following the Mustard and Senning procedures for d-transposition of the great arteries.[2,88] Factors associated with the development of atrial flutter after the Fontan procedure include older age at operation, AV valve abnormality, and the type of Fontan connection.[86,87]

Usually, the rate of IART in children with underlying heart disease is slower than that of typical atrial flutter, with P-P cycle lengths ranging from 260 to 460 ms[76] (Fig. 12). In postoperative patients, advances in mapping have identified atrial incisions as the anatomic substrates supporting this reentrant tachyarrhythmia.[89,90] For example, in Fontan patients, there are data to suggest that the suture line of the lateral cavopulmonary

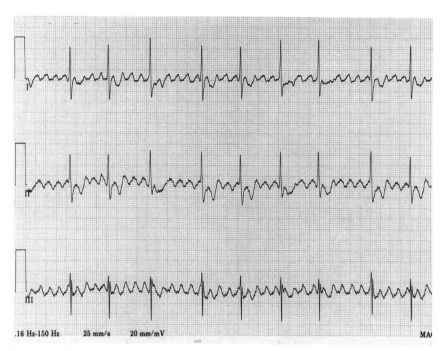

Figure 12. Simultaneous leads I, II, and III in a postoperative congenital heart disease patient with atrial flutter. The typical flutter waves can be seen in all leads.

connection and the natural anatomic right atrial boundaries (vena cava orifices, coronary sinus orifice, and the AV groove) serve as barriers creating a corridor with areas of slow conduction.[91] Current efforts at prevention include alterations in surgical technique,[92] e.g., strategic placement of surgical incisions traversing potential anatomic pathways.

Clinical Presentation

During infancy, atrial flutter cycle lengths can range from 125 to 200 ms with 2:1 or 3:1 conduction resulting in heart rates between 150 and 300 bpm.[84] Infants are often asymptomatic but may present with tachypnea, poor feeding, and diaphoresis.[83] In older children, atrial flutter cycle lengths range from 125 to 300 ms with corresponding atrial rates of 200 to 450 bpm, although the atrial rates may be slower in patients treated with antiarrhythmic medications. The classic findings in a patient with atrial flutter include a heart rate of 150 bpm, an atrial (flutter) rate of 300 bpm, and 2:1 AV conduction. Older children and adolescents may be asymptomatic particularly if AV conduction ratios preclude an elevated ventricular rate. Possible symptoms include palpitations, shortness of breath, and decreased stamina.[93] Garson and colleagues[82] report the following presenting symptoms in a collaborative study: 30% of patients were asymptomatic, 28% had dyspnea or other signs of CHF, 24% had palpitations, 9% had syncope, 8% had presyncope or dizziness, and 1% had been resuscitated from sudden death.

Atrial flutter is often sustained, requiring direct current cardioversion or overdrive atrial pacing for conversion. In adult patients with chronic atrial flutter, irrespective of the presence or absence of structural heart disease, there is a significant risk for thromboembolism (14%, with an approximate annual risk of 3%), suggesting the need for anticoagulation in these patients.[94]

Electrocardiographic Characteristics

The ECG characteristics of the various forms of atrial flutter include the following:

	Typical Atrial Flutter	Atypical Atrial Flutter	IART
Rate	Atrial rate 230–450 bpm, slower if structural heart disease or taking anti-arrhythmic drugs	Atrial rate 200–300 bpm	Atrial rate 150–300 bpm
Rhythm	Regular if fixed degree of AV block, otherwise irregular	Regular or irregular depending on degree of AV block	Regular or irregular depending on degree of AV block
P wave	Negative "saw-tooth" flutter waves in leads II, III, and aVF	Positive flutter waves in leads II, III, and aVF	Small, more discreet, and difficult to see P waves; may be hidden in QRS complex or T wave
PR interval	Not applicable	Not applicable	Not applicable
QRS complex	Narrow, unless bundle branch block or ventricular preexcitation	Narrow, unless bundle branch block or ventricular preexcitation	Narrow, unless bundle branch block

Diagnostic Tools

In addition to the 12-lead ECG, other tools may enable the clinician to delineate atrial flutter. If the arrhythmia is not of the classic atrial flutter pattern, P waves may be difficult to discern. Adenosine administration can help by inducing temporary AV block in order to unmask "flutter" P waves. Additionally, transesophageal atrial recordings can also aid in delineating the P-QRS relationship. In patients with implanted pacemakers or defibrillators, intracardiac electrograms are useful.

Management Strategies

Patients with hemodynamically unstable atrial flutter, especially infants, should undergo immediate direct current cardioversion. When considering this option in postoperative CHD patients, clinicians should remain cognizant of the risk of transient bradycardia or asystole after cardioversion as well as the risk of atrial thrombus dislodgment with cardioversion. Regarding the latter, there is currently no consensus among experts regarding the use of prophylactic anticoagulation in this situation.

Transesophageal overdrive pacing can be used to terminate atrial flutter, especially in newborns. In the newborn with an anatomically normal heart, digoxin is often administered for 6 months and then discontinued. Other antiarrhythmic medications used to manage atrial flutter include sodium channel blockers, β-blockers (in the absence of depressed ventricular function), calcium channel blockers, and Class III agents. For chronic atrial flutter, permanent atrial antitachycardia pacing is an option. Radiofrequency ablation and surgical options can also be considered.[95,96]

Atrial Fibrillation

Atrial fibrillation is uncommon in children and is extremely unusual as an isolated finding. A genetic locus for familial atrial fibrillation has been identified[97] and there are rare case reports of isolated atrial fibrillation in the fetus[98] and the child.[99] In one series, findings on atrial tissue biopsies from young adult patients with isolated atrial fibrillation were uniformly abnormal, with evidence for myocarditis, noninflammatory localized cardiomyopathy, and patchy fibrosis.[100] Known risk factors for atrial fibrillation include sick sinus syndrome, cardiomyopathy (dilated and hypertrophic), mitral valve abnormalities, late repair of atrial septal defect, WPW syndrome, and hyperthyroidism.[28,101,102]

The mechanism of atrial fibrillation is thought to be multiple circus movements or "wavelets" propagating in a substrate of abnormal atrial tissue. Factors contributing to sustained atrial fibrillation include an enlarged atrium (or atria), a short atrial refractory period, and slow conduction velocity. Recently, in older patients, initiation of atrial fibrillation has been related to triggering ectopic beats arising in the pulmonary veins,[103] and these ectopic foci have been treated with intracardiac catheter ablation.

Clinical Presentation

As noted previously, atrial fibrillation is rare in infants and children, and is generally associated with underlying cardiac pathology. Factors affecting the clinical presentation of children with atrial fibrillation include age at presentation, ventricular rate, and underlying cardiac function. Fetal atrial fibrillation is associated with a rapid ventricular response and fetal hydrops and is often treated with maternal digoxin administration. In older children and adults, intermittent episodes of atrial fibrillation are associated with palpitations and syncope. Most patients seem to be able to adapt to chronic atrial fibrillation with a slow ventricular response but may report problems with easy fatigability, low stamina, palpitations, and lightheadedness.

Electrocardiographic Characteristics

Atrial fibrillation is characterized by fine, irregular undulations of the baseline on the surface ECG (Fig. 13). The specific ECG characteristics of atrial fibrillation include:

Rate	Atrial rate between 450 and 600 bpm; ventricular rate is variable
Rhythm	Irregularly irregular (due to variable AV conduction)
P wave	Usually low-voltage chaotic pattern, difficult to discern and discrete P waves
PR interval	Not applicable
QRS complex	Narrow QRS complex, unless patient has existing bundle branch block or ventricular preexcitation

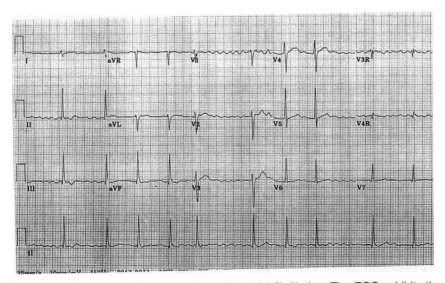

Figure 13. Fifteen-lead ECG in a patient with atrial fibrillation. The ECG exhibits the undulating baseline classic of atrial fibrillation with an irregular ventricular response. The ventricular response is slow because the patient is taking digoxin, which has slowed the ventricular rate.

Diagnostic Tools

The 12-lead ECG is usually the only diagnostic tool necessary for identifying atrial fibrillation. Asymptomatic patients, such as postoperative CHD patients, may require 24-hour (or longer) ambulatory monitoring to document episodes.

Management Strategies

The immediate management of atrial fibrillation is dependent on the child's hemodynamic response to the arrhythmia. In cases of significant hemodynamic compromise, the treatment method of choice is direct current cardioversion. Because patients with atrial fibrillation are at risk for thromboembolic events, the clinician should make an effort to determine the duration of the atrial fibrillation episode. If atrial fibrillation has been present for greater than 48 hours, the risk of a thromboembolic event is increased and transesophageal echocardiography is recommended to attempt to identify any existing clots, since the risk of their incidence is higher than once appreciated.[104] Transesophageal echocardiography should not be solely relied on and if the need for cardioversion is urgent, anticoagulation should be instituted with IV heparin, followed by oral anticoagulation afterward. If clots are visualized, efforts aimed at slowing the ventricular response (with AV nodal blocking agents such as digoxin, calcium channel blockers, or β-blockers) should be undertaken until adequate anticoagulation can be achieved. In patients with hemodynamically stable atrial fibrillation, pharmacologic conversion may be tried using Class Ic agents or amiodarone.[105]

Patients undergoing elective cardioversion for atrial flutter or atrial fibrillation after surgery for CHD should undergo 3 weeks of warfarin administration, unless the onset was clearly within the preceding 48 hours. Oral anticoagulation in these patients should be continued for 1 to 2 months afterward with warfarin (aspirin alone is inadequate) to achieve an international normalized ratio (INR) of greater than 2. Black and colleagues[106] raised the issue of whether clots form after direct cardioversion in patients with atrial fibrillation due to poor atrial function, despite a previously negative transesophageal echocardiogram.

The long-term management of atrial fibrillation is varied among pediatric electrophysiologists. Of utmost importance is the consideration of long-term oral anticoagulation therapy in patients with chronic or paroxysmal atrial fibrillation in an effort to lessen the incidence of thromboembolic events. The goal of long-term therapy in children is to restore normal sinus rhythm versus ventricular rate control. Pharmacologic agents such as digoxin and select Class Ic agents have been used to treat atrial fibrillation in the past. Newer treatments include radiofrequency catheter ablation,[103] multisite atrial pacing,[107] and creation of surgical lines of conduction block via the Maze procedure,[108] and its variations.

Junctional Ectopic Tachycardia

JET is a rare pediatric arrhythmia that is associated with significant mortality. It occurs in two distinct settings: 1) as a *congenital* and often familial arrhythmia, and 2) during the early *postoperative* period after CHD surgery involving the right atrium, and/or right ventricle. The underlying mechanism in both settings is automaticity,[109] with postoperative JET occurring due to irritation/damage of the AV junction and/or His bundle (e.g., from edema, suturing, or incision lines) during the surgical repair (Fig. 14). As is characteristic of automatic rhythms, there may be a "warming up" or gradual increase in tachycardia rates at the time of initiation, and "warming" down or gradual slowing prior to termination.

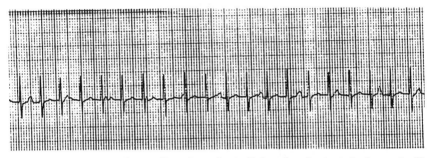

Figure 14. Single channel recording of a patient with junctional ectopic tachycardia. The QRS complex is narrow with an abnormally fast rate and atrioventricular dissociation.

Clinical Presentation

Villain and colleagues[110] reported a series of 26 patients with congenital JET. The age at the time of initial presentation ranged from birth to 6 months, and 18 of 26 patients presented at or before 4 weeks of age. Heart rates ranged from 140 to 370 with a mean of 230 bpm. Sixteen patients presented with CHF and shock. All symptomatic children had decreased ventricular function, which was also present in 5 of 8 asymptomatic children. The symptomatic children had significantly higher tachycardia rates than did the asymptomatic children. No associated cardiac malformations were identified in this series. Fifty percent of the children had a family history of JET.

The overall mortality rate in this group of patients was 35% with 19% of deaths directly attributed to the arrhythmia.[110] The remaining deaths occurred in association with surgery or other invasive procedures. There were two sudden deaths in patients in whom the arrhythmia was thought to be well controlled, an occurrence that has also been reported in other series.[111,112]

Postoperative JET is most frequently seen in neonates and infants with CHD following complex surgical repair.[7] This arrhythmia has been reported as a complication following repair of tetralogy of Fallot, Fontan procedure, closure of ventricular septal defect, and other complex repairs.[111,113,114] The median heart rate is 210 bpm.[112] This arrhythmia is often refractory to medical management and there is significant associated mortality.[114,115] JET usually presents during the immediate postoperative period but can occur 24 to 72 hours following surgery.[7,115] If the hemodynamic state can be managed and the ventricular rate slowed, the arrhythmia is usually self-limiting.[7]

Electrocardiographic Characteristics

The ECG characteristics of JET include the following:

	Postoperative	Congenital
Rate	Incessant tachycardia between 110 and 250 bpm	Incessant tachycardia between 110 and 250 bpm
Rhythm	Regular	Regular
P wave	Normal amplitude P wave; atrial rate somewhat slower than ventricular rate	Large amplitude distinct P waves; very slow atrial rate
PR interval	Not applicable due to AV dissociation	Not applicable due to AV dissociation
QRS complex	Narrow unless bundle block is present	Narrow unless bundle block is present

Diagnostic Tools

A multichannel ECG recording is generally sufficient to identify congenital or postoperative JET. In cases in which the AV relationship is unclear, a transesophageal electrode can be used to determine if there is AV dissociation or retrograde conduction. In postoperative patients, the temporary epicardial pacing wires can be used for this same purpose. The echocardiogram is a useful adjunct in the evaluation of the arrhythmia's overall effect on hemodynamics.

Management Strategies

The management strategies vary depending on whether the JET is *congenital* or *postoperative*. The *congenital* form is often refractory to antiarrhythmic drugs and can result in tachycardia-induced ventricular dysfunction.[110] Management strategies for congenital JET include antiarrhythmic drug therapy (often requiring a combination of agents), permanent pacing, and, rarely, radiofrequency ablation.[116]

Postoperative JET is potentially fatal if not promptly recognized and treated. The overall treatment goals for patients with postoperative JET include 1) increase vagal tone; 2) decrease adrenergic/sympathetic tone; and 3) increase cardiac output.

With the aforementioned treatment goals in mind and the fact that the arrhythmia is self-limiting, management strategies should be aimed at keeping the child sedated, chemically paralyzed, and with minimal stimulation. Serum electrolytes, such as potassium, magnesium, and calcium, should be maintained at their upper limits of normal. Induced hypothermia (i.e., between 33°C and 35°C) in conjunction with procainamide decreases automaticity and has been helpful in some cases.[117] Postoperative JET is difficult to treat because it is unaffected by overdrive pacing and direct current cardioversion and responds poorly to most antiarrhythmic medications, with the recent exception of IV amiodarone.[59] Atrial pacing at high enough rates to produce 2:1 AV block can assist in improving cardiac output in some cases by decreasing the ventricular rate. Paired ventricular pacing may also be beneficial.[118] In general, these methods are usually successful, but as a last resort, His bundle ablation and subsequent placement of a permanent cardiac pacemaker can be undertaken.

Implications for Clinicians for Tachyarrhythmias that are Confined to the Atria

Clinicians caring for children with SVT must have a fundamental understanding of SVT mechanisms. The chief concern for the clinician caring for the child with SVT confined to the atria should be the child's hemodynamic response to the arrhythmia. An overall clinical assessment should include the child's heart rate and rhythm; blood pressure (although hypotension is often a late sign of hemodynamic compromise in children); oxygen saturation; respiratory status including rate, nasal flaring, and retractions; peripheral pulses; color; and LOC. Once a baseline has been established, the clinician should compare any new findings to this baseline and report any significant changes to the child's physician.

Since patients with AET and CAT may not always exhibit overt symptoms of hemodynamic compromise, the clinician must constantly assess for significant changes in baseline status as well as for signs of CHF, e.g., diminished peripheral pulses, diaphoresis, tachypnea, and decreased urine output. Atrial flutter and atrial fibrillation can be a challenge to the entire health care team, especially in patients who have undergone surgery for CHD. Although the ventricular rate in these patients is generally not as fast as in those with structurally normal hearts, this SVT may have a more detrimental effect on overall hemodynamics, making ongoing assessment critical.

The clinician caring for the child with JET has responsibilities similar to those previously mentioned. Since congenital JET occurs infrequently, the treatment plan may vary from institution to institution. The clinician should explain the treatment plan to parents as soon as one has been established.

The child with postoperative JET presents unique challenges necessitating proactive management following surgery for CHD.[119] Many of these children are in critical condition following cardiac surgery, so a constant assessment of hemodynamics is pivotal. A vigilant assessment of serum electrolytes should be maintained with care to keep serum potassium, calcium, and magnesium at their upper limits of normal. The use of catecholamines should be minimized, and if the child is in the process of being extubated when JET is diagnosed, this plan should be delayed. If hypothermia is to be used as a treatment modality, the clinician should monitor the core temperature closely. An explanation to the parents in terminology that they can understand is certainly important. All findings in patients with postoperative JET should be shared with all clinicians involved in the patient's care.

Clinicians caring for any patient with tachycardia that is confined to the atria should be knowledgeable regarding specific treatment options. The clinician should be able to assist with any emergency interventions and if pharmacologic agents are used; he or she should be knowledgeable regarding the dosage, mechanism of action, potential adverse effects, and any known drug interactions. Patient and family education should include information regarding the specific arrhythmia, any nursing or medical interventions/procedures that are necessary, and any treatment that is under consideration.

Bradyarrhythmias

Bradyarrhythmias comprise a minority of the arrhythmias diagnosed in the pediatric population but are a significant problem for children with complex CHD. The most prevalent cause of bradyarrhythmias in this population is damage to the conduction system incurred during cardiac surgery, including surgically acquired second- or third-degree AV block and most cases of sinus node dysfunction. The second largest category of bradyarrhythmias is congenital complete AV block (CCAVB). Rare causes of chronic bradyarrhythmias in children include hypothyroidism, severe malnutrition (seen in association with anorexia nervosa), and isolated sinus node dysfunction (i.e., in the absence of underlying structural heart disease).

The following discussion includes sinus node dysfunction and a brief overview of all types of AV block, with an emphasis on acquired second- and third-degree AV block as well as CCAVB. Included in this discussion are the clinical presentation, ECG characteristics, and management strategies for each followed by the implications for clinicians who care for children with bradyarrhythmias.

Sinus Node Dysfunction

Sinus node dysfunction (also referred to as sick sinus syndrome) is a broad term that describes arrhythmias resulting from abnormal sinus node function. It includes a wide array of specific bradyarrhythmias including sinus bradycardia, sinus pause/arrest, sinoatrial (SA) exit block, slow escape rhythm (including junctional bradycardia), and the bradycardia-tachycardia (simply known as brady-tachy) syndrome seen in patients after atrial repair of CHD. Although there are nonsurgical causes of sinus node dysfunction, the primary underlying cause in the pediatric population is surgery for CHD. Nonsurgical causes include idiopathic or congenital etiologies, cardiomyopathies, inflammatory diseases, ischemic diseases, medications (especially antiarrhythmic agents), endocrine/metabolic diseases/states, and hypervagotonia.[120]

The brady-tachy syndrome results from anatomic pathology of the SA node and is characterized by sinus or junctional bradycardia, sinus arrest, and an increased risk for atrial tachyarrhythmias. It is rarely seen in the absence of underlying cardiac pathology[121] in the pediatric population, but it is a common long-term sequelae of procedures that require extensive atrial surgery, including atrial septal defect repair, the atrial switch operations (i.e., the Mustard and Senning), and the Fontan procedure.[122–124] Surgically acquired sinus node dysfunction is usually a chronic, progressive disorder with sinus bradycardia as the initial finding.[125–127] Development of sinus exit block, sinus arrest, intermittent atrial fibrillation/flutter, and junctional escape rhythms suggests progressive sinus node dysfunction. Associated AV conduction disease as evidenced by prolonged AV conduction times and the development varying degrees of AV block is not uncommon.[125,128] High-grade ventricular ectopy is relatively infrequently observed in association with sinus node dysfunction.[128]

An inadvertent consequence of atrial surgery is the creation of a substrate conducive to sinus node dysfunction, junctional escape rhythms, and reentrant tachyarrhythmias. Pathologic studies following the atrial switch operation describe hemorrhage and compression of the SA node, thrombosis of the SA node artery, and damage to perinodal tissues.[129–131] Surgical alteration of atrial anatomy and damage to atrial muscle tissue prolong intraatrial conduction, alter atrial anatomy, and result in heterogeneity in tissue refractoriness. Electrophysiologic studies after extensive atrial surgery demonstrate prolongation of sinus node recovery times[132,133] that is progressive,[132] prolonged SA conduction times,[132–134] prolonged atrial functional and effective refractory periods,[134] and exceptionally late activation in the portions of the systemic venous atrium nearest the inferior vena cava.[134]

A progressive decrease in the prevalence of sinus rhythm is reported for patients after atrial switch operations.[124] In a large series reported by Gelatt and colleagues,[2] the predominant rhythm as assessed by serial ECGs was sinus in 77% at 5 years and 40% at 20 years postoperatively. Freedom from atrial flutter was 92% at 5 years and 73% at 20 years. Loss of sinus rhythm was associated with previous septectomy, postoperative bradycardia, and late atrial flutter. A normal sinus rate and rhythm during the early postoperative period does not ensure normal sinus node function in the later years,[134] and the incidence of late sudden death is small but not insignificant.[124]

Sinus node dysfunction and associated tachyarrhythmias are a significant source of morbidity after the Fontan procedure. Predisposing factors are similar to those described for the atrial switch operations and include exposure of the sinus node to relatively high pressures within the Fontan baffle and preoperative conduction abnormalities associated with complex single ventricle anatomy. In an early follow-up study of patients 1 to 3 years after the Fontan procedure,[122] normal sinus rhythm was predominant in 70% of patients although sinus node dysfunction was documented via electrophysiology study in 50% of patients. In longer term follow-up studies of patients 5 to 15 years post Fontan procedure, noninvasive ECG studies report sinus node dysfunction in 13% to 26% of patients studied.[87,135] The proportion of patients remaining in normal sinus rhythm continues to decline over time.[135] Bradycardia and/or loss of AV synchrony is not well tolerated in the Fontan patient, and 10% to 47% of these patients require pacemaker implantation by 5 to 15 years.[87,135,136] Due to the direct anastomosis of the systemic venous return to the pulmonary circulation, Fontan patients with symptomatic sinus node dysfunction requiring a ventricular lead must undergo epicardial pacemaker implantation. These patients would theoretically benefit from the AV synchrony afforded by dual chamber pacing.

Clinical Presentation

Most children with sinus node dysfunction are asymptomatic,[121,137] making detection of this bradyarrhythmia incidental or identified on routine follow-up. The most common (and perhaps the most difficult to correlate) symptoms of sinus node dysfunction in children are fatigue, exercise intolerance, and dizziness. Fatigue may be exhibited in infants by poor feeding, lethargy, or symptoms of CHF, while older children may exhibit the inability to keep up with peers in everyday activities, and may require frequent naps.[138] Other symptoms of sinus node dysfunction include syncope, lightheadedness, chest pain, and, rarely, sudden death.

Electrocardiographic Characteristics

According to Kugler,[120] the surface ECG criteria for sinus node dysfunction can include one or more of the following: 1) sinus bradycardia; 2) severe sinus arrhythmia; 3) sinus pause or arrest; 4) slow escape rhythms; 5) SA exit block; 6) bradyarrhythmias/tachyarrhythmias; 7) sinus node reentry tachycardia; and 8) atrial reentry tachycardia (e.g., atrial flutter/fibrillation), the latter of which may be found in some patients in the absence of sinus node dysfunction. The ECG characteristics associated with the most common presentation of sinus node dysfunction in children include the following (Figs. 15 and 16):

	Sinus Bradycardia	Junctional Bradycardia
Rate	0–3 years, <100 bpm 3–9 years, <60 bpm 9–16 years, <50 bpm >16 years, <40 bpm	0–3 years, <100 bpm 3–9 years, <60 bpm 9–16 years, <50 bpm >16 years, <40 bpm
Rhythm	Regular, but slow	Regular, but slow
P wave	Small, but present	Absent or retrograde (i.e., behind each QRS complex)
PR interval	Normal	Not applicable
QRS complex	Narrow, unless bundle branch block is present	Narrow, unless bundle branch block is present

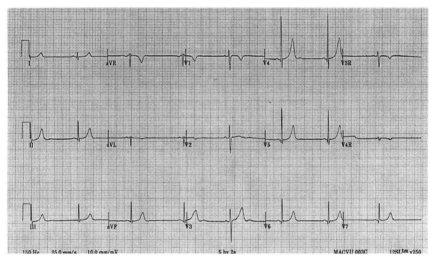

Figure 15. Fifteen-lead ECG in a school-aged child with sinus bradycardia. The P wave morphology is normal in each lead and the rate is 46 bpm.

Diagnostic Tools

The diagnosis of sinus node dysfunction in children depends on many factors and can be quite variable. Patients generally exhibit a lower mean resting heart rate and a blunted heart rate response during exercise stress testing,[139,140] making the surface ECG, 24-hour ambulatory ECG, and exercise stress testing important diagnostic tools. A careful history is often a useful adjunct. Transesophageal atrial electrophysiology testing can be used to determine sinus node recovery times, but rarely is intracardiac testing used today as a primary or standard technique for diagnosing sinus node dysfunction, since noninvasive methods have proven to be equally effective.[140]

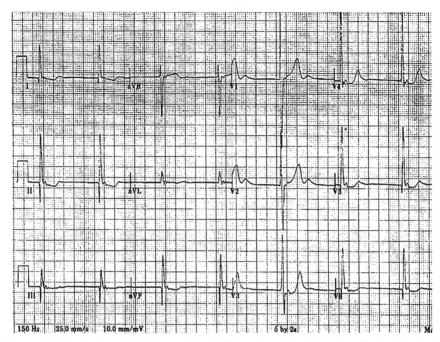

Figure 16. Twelve-lead ECG in a patient with junctional bradycardia after the Mustard procedure. The sinus rate is nearly the same as the junctional rate, as demonstrated by the apparent sinus P waves following each QRS complex.

Management Strategies

Martin and Kugler[138] recommend prevention as a management strategy for sinus node dysfunction and urge cardiovascular surgeons to adhere to three basic principles during CHD surgery: 1) know the anatomy of the sinus node and sinus node artery; 2) pay close attention to the cannulation of the superior vena cava for cardiopulmonary bypass; and 3) increase myocardial preservation by decreasing cardioplegia and ischemic times during the surgical repair.[138]

Immediate management strategies for patients with profound sinus or junctional bradycardia include atropine, isoproterenol, and temporary pacing, each of which is discussed in depth in chapter 4. In most cases, long-term treatment of sinus node dysfunction depends on each patient's specific symptomatology. Permanent pacemaker implantation is indicated for those patients with CHF, symptomatic bradycardia, exercise intolerance, syncope, asymptomatic bradycardia (resting heart rate <35 bpm), and ventricular pauses of ≥3 seconds' duration.[141]

Atrioventricular Block

AV block is a general diagnostic category used to describe abnormalities of AV conduction ranging from prolongation to complete block of impulse propagation across the AV node. *First-degree* AV block refers to slowed AV conduction as measured by an age-dependent prolonged PR interval (generally, >180 ms in children and >200 ms in adults) and, in the absence of underlying heart disease, is considered a benign finding (Fig. 17). *Second-degree* AV block refers to intermittent failure of impulse propagation and is

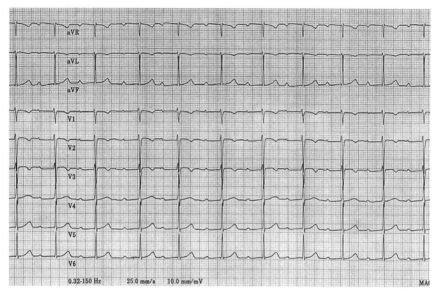

Figure 17. Nine simultaneous leads in a patient with first-degree atrioventricular block. The PR interval is greater than 200 ms and the QRS complex is normal.

categorized as Mobitz Type I (Wenckebach) or Mobitz Type II second-degree AV block. In Mobitz Type I second-degree AV block, there is progressive prolongation of the PR interval with eventual failure of AV conduction as evidenced on the surface ECG by a P wave that is not followed by a QRS complex (Fig. 18). This finding is not uncommon in healthy individuals, particularly during sleep, and, in the absence of underlying heart disease or symptoms, is usually a benign finding. In Mobitz Type II second-degree AV block, there is intermittent failure of impulse propagation that is NOT preceded by progressive prolongation of the PR interval and simply consists of a P wave that is NOT followed by a QRS complex on the surface ECG (Fig. 19). It is an unusual finding in patients without underlying heart disease, requires careful evaluation and monitoring, and may progress to *third*-degree (or complete) AV block. Risk factors for second-degree AV block (Mobitz Type II) include presence of cardiac defects (particularly those involving abnormalities of the AV junction such as l-transposition), secundum atrial septal defects, cardiomyopathy, rheumatic carditis, Lyme disease, intracardiac tumors, progressive familial AV block, and long QT syndrome.[142–147] *Third*-degree AV block refers to complete failure of impulse propagation across the AV node and can be either congenital or acquired (Fig. 20).

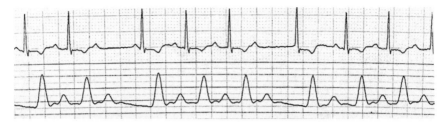

Figure 18. Single lead ECG in a patient with Mobitz Type I second-degree atrioventricular block. The PR interval progressively lengthens until a QRS is "dropped." The first sequence is 3:2 (three P waves to two QRS complexes) and the second is 4:3 followed by a junctional escape beat.

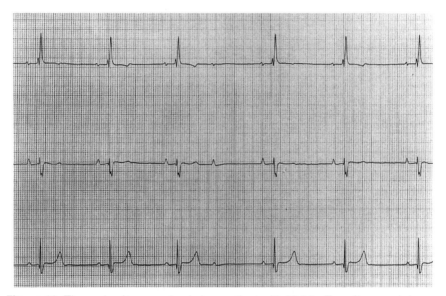

Figure 19. Three simultaneous leads in a patient with Mobitz Type II second-degree atrioventricular block. Note the sudden "dropping" of the QRS complex without progressive PR prolongation.

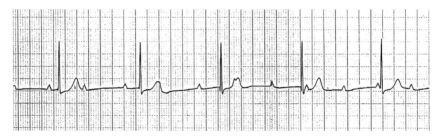

Figure 20. Telemetry rhythm strip on a patient with third-degree (complete) atrioventricular block. The QRS complex is narrow, the P waves are normal, and there is complete dissociation between the P waves and QRS complexes.

Two other types of AV block have been described, but are relatively uncommon in children. *Two-to-one* (2:1) AV block, which can be in the AV node or proximal His-Purkinje system, is the inability of alternate (i.e., every other one) atrial impulses to conduct to the ventricle. *Advanced second-degree* AV block occurs when there is loss of conduction for several consecutive P waves; this type of AV block generally progresses to third-degree or complete AV block.

Electrocardiographic Characteristics

The basic ECG characteristics of AV block include the following:

	First-Degree AV Block	Second-Degree, Mobitz Type I AV Block	Second-Degree, Mobitz Type II AV Block	Third-Degree AV Block
Rate	Regular, normal for age	**Atrial:** regular and normal for age **Ventricular:** irregular, less than atrial rate due to intermittent "dropped" QRS	**Atrial:** regular and normal for age **Ventricular:** irregular due to intermittent "dropped" QRS	**Atrial:** regular and normal for age unless CHF is present **Ventricular:** regular, but much slower than atrial rate
Rhythm	Regular	Irregular	Irregular	Regular
P wave	Normal	Normal	Normal	Normal
PR interval	Prolonged: >180 ms	Progressive prolongation with eventual "dropped" QRS	Fixed, which may or may not be prolonged; P wave occasionally not followed by QRS without progressive PR prolongation	Not applicable; complete AV dissociation
QRS complex	Narrow, unless bundle branch block is present	Narrow, unless bundle branch block is present	Narrow, unless bundle branch block is present	Narrow, unless bundle branch block is present

The following discussion focuses on the two most common types of AV block seen in the pediatric population: congenital complete (third-degree)

AV block and surgically acquired second- or third-degree AV block. The clinical presentation, diagnostic tools, and management strategies for each are included, followed by the implications for clinicians who care for children with bradyarrhythmias.

Congenital Complete Atrioventricular Block

CCAVB is relatively rare, with a prevalence estimated between 1:15,000 and 1:20,000.[146] It is associated with maternal connective tissue disorders and the presence of circulating anti-Ro/La antibodies in genetically predisposed individuals.[147] The prevalence of maternal connective tissue disease in infants with congenital complete heart block ranges from 33% to 64%. Maternal diagnoses associated with CCAVB include systemic lupus erythematosus, Sjögren syndrome, rheumatoid arthritis, and undifferentiated connective tissue disorder, with half of the mothers having only serologic evidence for connective tissue disease.[148] In a recent study of offspring of mothers with serologic evidence for maternal autoantibodies reported by Byron and colleagues,[149] 82% (71/113) exhibited CCAVB and there was a 19% (22/113) mortality rate. The majority of deaths occurred within the first 3 months of life and the cumulative probability of survival was estimated to be 79%. Sixty-seven (63%) of 107 live born children required pacemakers: 35 within 9 days of life, 15 within 1 year, and 17 after 1 year. Infants with serologically associated CCAVB usually have otherwise structurally normal hearts.

Passage of maternal antibodies to the fetal circulation is thought to occur at about 20 weeks' gestation, causing immunologic injury and fibrous replacement of the AV conduction tissue that usually spares the sinus node.[150] The diagnosis is commonly made prenatally between 20 and 30 weeks' gestation[149,151] due to fetal bradycardia and/or a history of maternal connective tissue disease. The incidence of fetal demise is not insignificant and is associated with fetal heart rates less than 55 bpm, a progressive decrease in heart rate during the pregnancy, and development of fetal hydrops.[152] Improved fetal outcomes may be achieved with improvements in monitoring and treatment.[151]

Clinical Presentation

The clinical presentation of children with CCAVB varies and is dependent on the junctional or ventricular escape rate as well as the presence or absence of structural heart disease. Children with CCAVB may be totally asymptomatic or may exhibit any of the following symptoms: fetal hydrops, fatigue, low stamina, exercise intolerance, dizziness, and syncope. Although very rare, SCD can be the presenting symptom.[146,153] Studies indicate that the average age at diagnosis for children with CCAVB is approximately 7 months of age,[146,153] although this condition is often well tolerated for many years and some individuals remain asymptomatic well into adulthood. Symptoms of CHF may present in the infant or young child[142,143] and cardiomegaly, left ventricular dilation, and increased stroke volume are not uncommon findings.[154] These latter symptoms may occur despite physiologic pacing, perhaps indicating more extensive myocardial damage.

Diagnostic Tools

There are several diagnostic tools that are helpful in identifying patients with CCAVB. In the fetus exhibiting bradycardia, a fetal echocardiogram can be used to determine heart rate and the AV relationship (by assessing the timing of mitral valve opening and ventricular contraction). Obviously, once the child is born, a 12- or 15-lead ECG can be used to document this bradyarrhythmia. Twenty-four-hour ambulatory monitors can be used to assess junctional and ventricular escape rates as well as the incidence and severity of any ventricular ectopy. Exercise stress testing is an important diagnostic tool in older children, especially those who are asymptomatic. It can be used to assess exercise tolerance and the presence of ventricular ectopy, the latter of which may be associated with sudden death in these patients.[155] Follow-up echocardiography is useful to detect myocardial dysfunction or AV valve regurgitation.

Management Strategies

Immediate management strategies for the neonate, infant, or child with CCAVB with CHF, low cardiac output, or severe symptoms involves the use of chronotropic agents and temporary pacing until arrangements can be made for a permanent pacemaker. The indications for permanent pacing vary according to symptomatology and presence of CHD. The Class I indications for a permanent pacemaker in a child with CCAVB include: 1) third-degree AV block with a wide QRS escape rhythm or ventricular dysfunction, and 2) third-degree AV block in an infant with a ventricular rate less than 50 to 55 bpm *or* with CHD and a ventricular rate of less than 70 bpm.[141] Class II indications for the child with CCAVB include: 1) third-degree AV block beyond the age of 1 year with an average heart rate less than 50 bpm or abrupt pauses in ventricular rate that are two to three times the basic cycle length, and 2) third-degree AV block in the asymptomatic neonate, child, or adolescent with CHD and a resting heart rate less than 35 bpm or pauses in ventricular rate of greater than 3 seconds.[141]

In children who do not immediately require permanent pacing due to absence of symptoms and who have an acceptable heart rate, regular outpatient follow-up is critical. Pacemaker indications in these patients include syncope, CHF, ventricular ectopy, cardiomegaly, and decreased ventricular function. Michaelsson and colleagues[156] recommend permanent pacing in children with CCAVB prior to adolescence, regardless of symptoms, in order to avoid syncope, irreversible myocardial damage, and/or death.[156]

Acquired Second- or Third-Degree Atrioventricular Block

Acquired AV block can occur as a complication of open heart surgery,[157] catheter ablation,[158] secondary to myocardial disease processes (viral cardiomyopathy, Lyme disease, intracardiac tumors, diphtheria), toxins, or as an adverse effect of some medications. Paroxysmal complete AV block has been reported during anesthesia induction,[159] head-up tilt table testing,[160] and cardiac catheterization.[161]

Acquired AV block in children is most commonly a sequela of cardiac surgery and is the most common indication for pediatric pacemaker implantation.[162] Surgically induced AV block was once a significant source of mortality and morbidity for children undergoing repair of CHD during both the early and late postoperative periods. Currently, the routine placement of temporary epicardial pacemaker wires at the time of open heart surgery and the ability to pace temporarily in the DDD mode has greatly improved the management of transient postoperative AV block in children.

In a recently published series, Weindling and colleagues[163] report a 3% incidence of complete AV block for patients with CHD undergoing cardiac surgery with cardiopulmonary bypass. Procedures associated with the greatest risk were surgery for left ventricular outflow tract obstruction (17%), l-transposition of the great arteries (11%), repair of ventricular septal defect (4%), and tetralogy of Fallot (3%). In 63% (32/51), complete AV block was transient with intact AV conduction almost always regained within 10 days postoperatively. The authors suggest that if intact AV conduction is not regained by postoperative day 10, permanent pacemaker implantation is indicated because of the increased risk for profound bradycardia and sudden death.[164–166] Late recurrence of complete AV block has been reported,[167,168] highlighting the need for long-term follow-up in order to assess for conduction abnormalities.

Clinical Presentation

The child with acquired second- or third-degree AV block may be totally asymptomatic or may exhibit any of the symptoms previously described for children with CCAVB. The child who has second- or third-degree AV block as a result of surgery for CHD may exhibit more profound symptoms in the early postoperative period, due to the overall stress of the operative repair and the lack of AV synchrony. In these patients, the lack of symptoms does not necessarily negate the need for permanent pacing, because of the potential risk of sudden death.

Diagnostic Tools

The diagnostic tools for use in patients with acquired second- or third-degree AV block are the same as those previously mentioned for patients with CCAVB. Nonsurgically acquired AV block can usually be delineated with a 12- or 15-lead ECG. In some patients after surgery for CHD, the temporary epicardial pacing wires placed at the time of surgery may help to determine the AV relationship. Routine electrophysiology studies are not performed in these patients to determine the site of block. Echocardiography can be used to assess the hemodynamic effects of the bradyarrhythmia; exercise stress testing and 24-hour ambulatory monitoring can be useful adjuncts.

Management Strategies

In patients with acquired AV block, the decision to implant a permanent pacemaker is based on the patient's symptomatology and underlying pathology. In patients with surgically acquired second- or third-degree AV block, temporary pacing should be used (if symptoms necessitate it) for 10 to 14 days after surgery in order to determine if the block is temporary or permanent. In patients who rely on temporary pacing for improved hemodynamics, the pacing thresholds of the temporary wires should be assessed daily (see chapter 4). The specific Class I permanent pacemaker indication for the patient with surgically acquired AV block is postoperative advanced second- or third-degree AV block that is not expected to resolve or that persists 7 days after cardiac surgery.[141]

Implications for Clinicians for Bradyarrhythmias

Clinicians caring for children with bradyarrhythmias must have a basic understanding of the commonly seen bradyarrhythmias in the pediatric population as well as the potential outcomes for these rhythm disturbances. The clinician should constantly assess the child's hemodynamic response to the bradyarrhythmia and document any changes in the child's baseline. Any changes in the child's LOC, vital signs, color, respiratory status, and/or perfusion should be documented and relayed to the treating physician. Any other arrhythmias, such as ventricular ectopy, should be documented as well.

Clinicians caring for children with bradyarrhythmias must be knowledgeable regarding potential management strategies for these patients, including medications, temporary pacing modalities, and permanent pacing. If pharmacologic agents are used, the clinician should be informed regarding the drug's intended mode of action, dosage, duration of action, potential adverse effects, and any known drug interactions. When using temporary pacing modalities, the clinician should be aware of the nuances of each in order to better prepare patients and their families. Patient and family education is critical for these patients and their families.

Patient and Family Considerations

Comprehensive care of the child with a supraventricular arrhythmia should address the psychosocial needs of the child and of his or her family.

Treatment goals include the facilitation of child and family adaptation and the prevention of avoidable negative psychosocial outcomes. Achievement of these goals is predicated on a positive working partnership between parents, children, and their health care providers. This section outlines some of the factors that contribute to the child's adjustment to a chronic illness, and applies them to the child with a supraventricular arrhythmia.

A comprehensive plan of care requires assessment of key variables anticipated to affect short- and long-term outcomes. For most children and families, the diagnosis of an arrhythmia and surrounding events represents a cause of stress and requires mobilization of family resources and adaptation to novel circumstances.

Considerable research has examined biomedical, child, and social-environmental factors associated with psychosocial adjustments for children with chronic illness. Many of the factors identified represent a continuum with one end representing risk and the other resiliency. Children's adjustments reflect a complex interaction of these variables over time. Examples of biomedical factors include severity of illness, prognosis, and chronicity, while child factors include gender, developmental stage, age at onset, temperament, cognitive processes, and coping methods. Social-environmental factors include family functioning, parental adjustment, social support, and socioeconomic status.[169]

Disease severity, chronicity, and prognoses for the arrhythmias discussed in this chapter vary widely, ranging from the self-limited but initially troubling CAT of infancy, to the child with AV block who requires a permanent pacemaker, to atrial flutter in the postoperative Fontan patient. Disease-related medical factors affecting children's adaptations to chronic illness include diagnosis (disease severity, prognosis, and treatment), functional impairment, cognitive abilities, and visibility (physical changes). Although important, the severity of the disease has been found to be a less critical predictor of adaptation than other factors such as family functioning and parental adjustment.[169]

There is a paucity of studies examining the psychosocial effects of a diagnosis of arrhythmia during childhood; however, heart disease, for reasons not understood, appears to place children at particular risk for psychosocial problems. In a meta-analysis of psychosocial outcomes for children with chronic illness, a diagnosis of heart disease was associated with a "large" risk for psychosocial problems while the diagnoses of cancer and asthma predicted a "moderate" risk category.[170] These findings must be interpreted with caution; however, the data suggest that the burden of heart disease poses a considerable challenge to children and their parents.

Most children with arrhythmias are not impaired in their functional abilities and in many cases the heart condition rather than the arrhythmia is the limiting factor. Most are able to participate in the usual activities that children enjoy, including regular school attendance, social activities, and recreational sports. Some of the diagnoses preclude participation in vigorous competitive sports, a category that includes the adolescent male with WPW and the Fontan patient. In the patient with WPW, this may be an appropriate rationale to pursue radiofrequency ablation for definitive treatment of the condition. For the child who has undergone the Fontan procedure, guidance by parents and health professionals toward other appropriate meaningful activities is needed. The adolescent or young adult with complex CHD and recurrent arrhythmias experiences varying degrees of functional limitations and, because of arrhythmia recurrence, often experiences many unanticipated interruptions in his or her activities of daily living.

Children with pacemakers are faced with unusual challenges, including body image changes from surgical scarring, lifelong need for an implanted device, and the need for periodic generator and/or lead replacements. In a study of psychosocial effects of pacemakers in children,[171] no significant differences were found on standardized measures of trait anxiety, self-competence, and self-esteem. Children with pacemakers were more external in their locus of control orientation than were healthy controls, but no significant differences were found between children with pacemakers and children with comparable heart disease but without a pacemaker. Peers of children with pacemakers did report negative stereotypes about children with pacemakers. This study is consistent with other data that suggest that the majority of children who have a chronic health problem make a positive adjustment; however, the risk of adjustment problems is not insignificant and is estimated to affect approximately 30% of children by the age of 15.[172]

Child factors affecting adaptation include developmental stage, age at onset, gender, temperament, and coping processes. Developmental stage is a significant determinant of children's needs and, therefore, parenting roles. During infancy, the child's inability to communicate symptoms and his or her complete dependency places a significant burden of responsibility on the parents. As described previously, infants with SVT often present with symptoms of cardiac decompensation, and a significant number are diagnosed because of the presence of an arrhythmia during a routinely scheduled office visit. Parents may experience guilt about not having detected the problem earlier and many are apprehensive that they will not accurately detect future episodes. Many parents are concerned that the child will have a prolonged undetected episode during sleep and are hesitant to let the child sleep unobserved. Education of the parents regarding the signs and symptoms of SVT in an infant, techniques for assessing heart rate, use of vagal maneuvers, and parameters for when to contact the physician or emergency room are of utmost importance. Use of a transtelephonic monitor may be helpful to confirm episodes of SVT. Linking anxious parents to other parents who have successfully navigated the issues related to having an infant with SVT can also be beneficial.

The diagnosis of an arrhythmia in a school-aged child poses different challenges and may require that school personnel be included in the plan of care. Frequently, the use of a transtelephonic monitor during school hours is needed in order to document the presence or recurrence of an arrhythmia. Use of the monitor in school is often the first indication that the child may have a "heart problem," and results in concern about what to do if the child reports symptoms such as palpitations. Use of a standardized instruction sheet, as well as written information describing guidelines for participation in gym and athletics, may be helpful for school personnel.

Developmental interruptions for the adolescent or young adult with recurrent supraventricular arrhythmias secondary to CHD can vary from the occasional episode to frequent, chronic interruptions in school and work activities. Cardioversions can be frightening and painful afterward, medications are often only marginally effective with unpleasant side effects, and the lack of timely solutions to the problem can be extremely frustrating for the young person and his or her family. An adequate support network of family and health care providers is extremely important as the patient travels this rocky and often discouraging path.

The effects of gender, temperament, and coping methods on the child's adjustment to chronic illness have not been carefully examined. Temperament describes a child's distractibility and mood as well as his or her response to novel situations, and has been shown to influence maternal behaviors.[173] Coping methods are the processes used to accomplish disease-related tasks and to maintain normal functioning. Coping is a dynamic process that may help or hinder adjustment to life circumstances. Methods of coping may be problem-focused or emotion-focused, with both methods generally used by individuals under stress. Problem-focused methods are actions taken to address the illness, such as learning to use vagal maneuvers. Emotion-focused coping methods change the emotional reaction to the experience, such as altering perceptions, blunting, or denial. For example, a child with a serious chronic heart problem could perceive an otherwise negative experience as a way to help others in similar circumstances. Children's coping strategies reflect developmental stage, and problem-focused strategies precede emotion-focused strategies.[174]

Social-environmental factors affecting the child's adjustment include socioeconomic status, family functioning, parental adjustment, and parental social support. Significant problems or deficits in any of these areas represent a risk factor for the child and suggest the need for intervention. Important tasks for parents include participating in diagnostic evaluation and treatment plans while preserving emotional well being for themselves and their children. The addition of a serious health problem to the challenges already encountered by those who lack adequate economic resources can be overwhelming. Pediatric electrophysiology is usually only available at large medical centers, and transportation, meals, parking, and accommodations represent a considerable expense. Issues such as these make the services of social work a vital component of the health care services provided.

Family functioning has proven to be an important factor in the child's ability to adjust positively to a variety of stressful life experiences. Families that are adaptable, cohesive, and communicate positively support positive adjustment in children, while families that are rigid or lack supportive boundaries for their members are less conducive to child adjustments.[175,176] Parental adjustment problems, including psychological disorders, are important predictors of child adjustment. The presence of significant maternal depression and/or anxiety poses a significant risk factor[177,178] and warrants therapeutic intervention.

Parents' perceptions of disease severity may be widely divergent from the health providers' perceptions.[177] It is the authors' experience that for many parents, "heart problems" are seen as inherently life threatening, a perception that is fostered by highly publicized reports of SCD in athletes. Parents' misperceptions regarding severity of the diagnosis may result in considerable stress, anxiety, and parenting behaviors that appear to be "overprotective" for the child, as well as excessive use of medical services and repeated contact of medical providers in the absence of significant findings. This situation indicates the need for a sensitive and in-depth assessment of the family situation. The sources of distress in such situations are probably as numerous as the families that are trying to cope with them. Contributing factors may include parental psychiatric disorder such as anxiety and/or depression, family history of SCD (particularly if the family perceives that there was medical mismanagement or a "missed diagnosis"), or gaps in parental education regarding the child's diagnosis, prognosis, or significant symptoms that need to be communicated to the child's physician. Lack of trust and communication problems frequently contribute to parent and provider frustration. In most situations, once identified, these issues can be addressed in one or two sessions focused on listening to and addressing parents' concerns and providing parental education. It is often helpful to link parents with experienced parents who have successfully navigated similar circumstances and who can act as role models and provide a support system. Cardiovascular health care providers must also remain cognizant of the fact that some patients and families will require professional help, and should not hesitate to refer them to the appropriate services, e.g., a psychologist or psychiatrist.

Identification of risk factors for a child with an arrhythmia is supported by a growing body of literature supporting the efficacy of interventions targeted at improving psychosocial outcomes for high-risk children.[179,180] Positive outcomes are predicated on the development of working partnerships between providers, children, and parents fostered by education, support, and communication. For many clinicians, the processes of assessment and intervention to promote child and family adjustments occur almost without conscious thought. Educational issues related to the diagnosis of an arrhythmia include issues related to the diagnosis itself, the etiology and prognosis associated with the specific arrhythmia, treatment modalities, and home care. Often, the teaching plan should include techniques to assess heart rate, signs and symptoms that need to be communicated to the health care professional, and the relative urgency of the signs and symptoms. It is important that health care professionals take the time to provide this education to patients and their families in order to facilitate positive outcomes.

An integral component of caring for a child with an arrhythmia (and for his or her parents) is the provision of emotional support. Health care professionals provide emotional support in a myriad of ways including attentive listening, promoting a hopeful outlook, and acknowledging the stresses and burdens encountered as well as successes in overcoming these obstacles. The authors have a collection of pictures of children with pacemakers that have been given to them by families over the years. When a child needs a pacemaker, it has been most reassuring to the child and the parents to see this collection of pictures of children pursuing various activities, including one young woman with CCAVB participating in a marathon. Hope is an important part of well being[181] and health care professionals are in a position to link families for purposes of support and/or to provide role models for positive adaptation. More formal interventions include sponsoring ongoing support groups or seminars for patients and families. Effective communication is necessary to establish a positive working partnership with children and families. Due to the episodic nature of many of the arrhythmias discussed, delivery of services must include ready phone availability.

In summary, children with supraventricular arrhythmias present with specific needs requiring specialized, highly knowledgeable care. Clinicians should strive to provide exceptional care to these patients and their families by maintaining current knowledge regarding arrhythmia mechanisms, diagnostic tools, and management strategies. Additionally, clinicians caring for children and their families must incorporate psychosocial implications and patient and family education into the child's physical plan of care.

References

1. Campbell RM, Dick M, Rosenthal A: Cardiac arrhythmias in children. Ann Rev Med 1984; 35:397–410.
2. Gelatt M, Hamilton RM, McCrindle BW, et al: Risk factors for atrial tachyarrhythmias after the Fontan operation. J Am Coll Cardiol 1994; 24:1735–1741.
3. Gelatt M, Hamilton RM, McCrindle BW, et al: Arrhythmia and mortality after the Mustard procedure: A 30 year single center experience. J Am Coll Cardiol 1997; 29:194–201.
4. Case CL, Gillette PC, Crawford FA Jr., et al: Comparison of medical care costs between successful radiofrequency catheter ablation and surgical ablation of accessory pathways in the pediatric age group. Am J Cardiol 1994; 73:600–601.
5. Wood KA, Drew BJ, Scheinman MM: Frequency of disabling symptoms in supraventricular tachycardia. Am J Cardiol 1997; 79:145–149.
6. Ludomirsky A, Garson A Jr.: Supraventricular tachycardia. In Gillette PC, Garson A Jr. (eds.): Pediatric Arrhythmias: Electrophysiology and Pacing. Philadelphia: WB Saunders Company; 1990:380–426.
7. Case CL, Gillette PC: Automatic atrial tachycardia and junctional tachycardia in the pediatric patient: Strategies for diagnosis and management. Pacing Clin Electrophysiol 1993; 16:1323–1335
8. Cruz FES, Cheriex EC, Smeets JL, et al: Reversibility of tachycardia-induced

cardiomyopathy after cure of incessant supraventricular tachycardia. J Am Coll Cardiol 1990; 16:739–744.

9. Ko JK, Deal BJ, Strasburger JF, et al: Supraventricular tachycardia mechanisms and their age distribution in pediatric patients. Am J Cardiol 1992; 69:1028–1032.

10. Garson A Jr., Ludomirsky A: Supraventricular tachycardia. In Garson A Jr., Bricker JT, McNamara DG (eds.): The Science and Practice of Pediatric Cardiology. Philadelphia: Lea & Febiger; 1990:1809–1848.

11. Deal BJ, Keane JF, Gillette PC, et al: Wolff-Parkinson-White syndrome and supraventricular tachycardia during infancy: Management and follow-up. J Am Coll Cardiol 1985; 5:130–135.

12. Perry JC, Garson A Jr.: Supraventricular tachycardia due to Wolff-Parkinson-White syndrome in children: Early disappearance and late recurrence. J Am Coll Cardiol 1990; 16:1215–1220.

13. Lundberg A: Paroxysmal tachycardia in infancy: Follow-up study of 47 subjects ranging in age from 10 to 26 years. Pediatrics 1973; 51:26–35.

14. Nadas AS, Daeschner CW, Roth A, et al: Paroxysmal tachycardia in infants and children. Study of 41 cases. Pediatrics 1952; 9:167–181.

15. Lubbers WJ, Losekoot TG, Anderson RH, et al: Paroxysmal supraventricular tachycardia in infancy and childhood. Eur J Cardiol 1974; 2:91–99.

16. Wolff L, Parkinson J, White PD: Bundle-branch block with short PR interval in healthy young people prone to paroxysmal tachycardia. Am Heart J 1930; 5:685–704.

17. Russel MW, Dorostkar PC, Dick M II: Incidence of catastrophic events associated with the Wolff-Parkinson-White syndrome in young patients: Diagnostic and therapeutic dilemma. Circulation 1993; 88I:484. Abstract.

18. Munger TM, Packer DL, Hammill SC, et al: A population study of the natural history of Wolff-Parkinson-White syndrome in Olmsted County, Minnesota 1953–1989. Circulation 1993; 87:866–873.

19. Anderson RH, Becker AE, Wenink AC: The development of the conducting tissues. In Roberts NK, Gelband H (eds.): Cardiac Arrhythmias in the Neonate, Infant, and Child. New York: Appleton-Century-Crofts; 1977:1–28.

20. Becker AE, Anderson RH, Durrer D, et al: The anatomical substrate of Wolff-Parkinson-White syndrome. A clinicopathologic correlation in seven patients. Circulation 1978; 57:870–879.

21. Mantakas ME, McCue CM, Miller WW: Natural history of Wolff-Parkinson-White syndrome discovered in infancy. Am J Cardiol 1978; 41:1097–1103.

22. Vidaillet HJ, Pressley JC, Henke E, et al: Familial occurrence of accessory atrioventricular pathways (preexcitation syndrome). N Engl J Med 1987; 317:65–69.

23. Deal BJ, Dick MD, Beerman L, et al: Cardiac arrest in young patients with Wolff-Parkinson-White syndrome. Pacing Clin Electrophysiol 1995; 18:815. Abstract.

24. Bromberg BI, Lindsay BD, Cain ME, et al: Impact of clinical history and electrophysiologic characterization of accessory pathways on management strategies to reduce sudden death among children with Wolff-Parkinson-White syndrome. J Am Coll Cardiol 1996; 27:690–695.

25. Paul T, Guccione P, Garson A Jr.: Relation of syncope in young patients with Wolff-Parkinson-White syndrome to rapid ventricular response during atrial fibrillation. Am J Cardiol 1990; 65:318–321.

26. Auricchio A, Klein H, Trappe HJ, et al: Lack of prognostic value of syncope in patients with Wolff-Parkinson-White syndrome. J Am Coll Cardiol 1991; 17:152–158.

27. Klein GK, Gulamhusein SS: Intermittent pre-excitation in the Wolff-Parkinson-White syndrome. Am J Cardiol 1983; 52:292–296.

28. Chien P, Pressley JC, Tang AS, et al: New observations on atrial fibrillation before and after surgical treatment in patients with the Wolff-Parkinson-White syndrome. J Am Coll Cardiol 1992; 19:974–981.
29. Klein GJ, Bashore TM, Sellers TD, et al: Ventricular fibrillation in the Wolff-Parkinson-White syndrome. N Engl J Med 1979; 301:1080–1085.
30. Naheed ZJ, Strasburger JF, Deal BJ, et al: Fetal tachycardia: Mechanisms and predictors of hydrops fetalis. J Am Coll Cardiol 1996; 27:1736–1740.
31. Weindling SN, Saul JP, Walsh EP: Efficacy and risks of medical therapy for supraventricular tachycardia in neonates and infants. Am Heart J 1996; 131:66–72.
32. Dunnigan A, Benditt DG, Benson DW: Modes on onset ("initiating events") for paroxysmal atrial tachycardia in infants and children. Am J Cardiol 1986; 57:1280–1287.
33. Garson A Jr., Gillette PC, McNamara DG: Supraventricular tachycardia in children: Clinical features, response to treatment, and long-term follow-up in 217 patients. J Pediatr 1981; 98:875–882.
34. Sreeram N, Wren C: Supraventricular tachycardia in infants: Response to initial treatment. Arch Dis Child 1990; 65:127–129.
35. Perry JC, Giuffre RM, Garson A Jr.: Clues to the electrocardiographic diagnosis of subtle Wolff-Parkinson-White syndrome in children. J Pediatr 1990; 117:871–875.
36. Rossenbaum FF, Hecht HH, Wilson FN, et al: The potential variations of the thorax and the esophagus in anomalous atrioventricular excitation. Am Heart J 1945; 29:281–326.
37. Fitzpatrick AP, Gonzales RP, Lesh MD, et al: New algorithm for the localization of accessory atrioventricular connections using a baseline electrocardiogram. J Am Coll Cardiol 1994; 23:107–116.
38. Arruda MS, McClelland JH, Wang X, et al: Development and validation of an ECG algorithm for identifying accessory pathway ablation site in Wolff-Parkinson-White syndrome. J Cardiovasc Electrophysiol 1998; 9:2–12.
39. Coumel P, Cabrol C, Fabiato A, et al: Tachycardie permanet par rhythm reciproqu. Arch Mal Coeur 1967; 60:1830–1864.
40. Dorostkar PC, Silka MJ, Morady F, et al: Clinical course of persistent junctional reciprocating tachycardia. Am J Cardiol 1999; 33:366–375.
41. Ticho BS, Saul JP, Hulse JE, et al: Variable location of accessory pathways associated with the permanent form of junctional reciprocating tachycardia and confirmation with radiofrequency ablation. Am J Cardiol 1992; 70:1559–1564.
42. Lown B, Ganong WF, Levine SA: The syndrome of short PR interval, narrow QRS complex and paroxysmal rapid heart action. Circulation 1952; 5:663–670.
43. Mandel WJ, Danzig R, Haykawa H: Lown-Ganong-Levine syndrome: A study using His bundle electrograms. Circulation 1971; 44:696–708.
44. Denes P, Wu D, Rosen K: Demonstration of dual A-V pathways in a patient with Lown-Ganong-Levine syndrome. Chest 1974; 65:343–346.
45. Gallagher JJ, Pritchet EL, Sealy WC, et al: The preexcitation syndromes. Prog Cardiovasc Dis 1978; 20:285–327.
46. Castellanos A, Vagueiro MC, Befeler B, et al: Syndrome of short P-R, narrow QRS and repetitive supraventricular tachyarrhythmias: The possible occurrence of the R-on-T phenomena and the limits of this syndrome. Eur J Cardiol 1975; 2:337–342.
47. Miles WM, Klein LS, Rardon DP, et al: Atrioventricular reentry and variants: Mechanisms, clinical features, and management. In Zipes DP, Jalife J (eds.): Cardiac Electrophysiology: From Cell to Bedside. Philadelphia: WB Saunders Company; 1995:638–655.

48. Crosson JE, Hesslein PS, Thilenius OG, et al: AV node reentry tachycardia in infants. Pacing Clin Electrophysiol 1995; 18:2144–2149.

49. Wu P, Denes P, Amat-y-Leon F, et al: Clinical, electrocardiographic, and electrophysiologic observations in patients with paroxysmal supraventricular tachycardia. Am J Cardiol 1978; 41:1045–1051.

50. Wu D, Yeh SJ, Wang CC, et al: Nature of dual atrioventricular node pathways and the tachycardia circuit as defined by radiofrequency ablation technique. J Am Coll Cardiol 1992; 20:884–895.

51. Wolff GS, Sung RJ, Pickoff A, et al: The fast-slow form of atrioventricular nodal reentrant tachycardia in children. Am J Cardiol 1979; 43:1181–1188.

52. Gursoy S, Steurer G, Brugada J, et al: Brief report: The hemodynamic mechanism of pounding in the neck in atrioventricular nodal tachycardia. N Engl J Med 1992; 327:772–774.

53. Perry JC: Supraventricular tachycardia. In Garson A Jr., Bricker JT, Fisher DJ, Neish SR (eds.): The Science and Practice of Pediatric Cardiology. 2nd ed. Baltimore: Williams & Wilkins; 1998:2059–2101.

54. Waxman MB, Wald RW, Sharma AD, et al: Vagal techniques for termination of paroxysmal supraventricular tachycardia. Am J Cardiol 1980; 46:655–663.

55. Lown B, Levine SA: The carotid sinus: Clinical value of its significance. Circulation 1961; 23:766–789.

56. Müller G, Deal BJ, Benson DW Jr.: "Vagal maneuvers" and adenosine for termination of atrioventricular reentrant tachycardia. Am J Cardiol 1994; 74:500–502.

57. Wildenthal K, Atkins JM, Leshin SJ, et al: The diving reflex used to treat paroxysmal atrial tachycardia. Lancet 1975; 1:12–14.

58. Opie LH, Chatterjee K, Frishman W, et al (eds.): Drugs for the Heart. 4th ed. Philadelphia: WB Saunders Company; 1995:207–246.

59. Perry JC, Fenrich AL, Hulse JE, et al: Pediatric use of intravenous amiodarone: Efficacy and safety in critically ill patients from a multicenter protocol. J Am Coll Cardiol 1996; 27:1246–1250.

60. Trippel DL, Wiest DB, Gillette PC: Cardiovascular and antiarrhythmic effects of esmolol in children. J Pediatr 1991; 119:142–147.

61. Dick M II, Scott WA, Serwer GS, et al: Acute termination of supraventricular tachyarrhythmias in children by transesophageal pacing. Am J Cardiol 1988; 61:925–927.

62. Mehta AV, Sanchez GR, Sacks EJ, et al: Ectopic automatic atrial tachycardia in children: Clinical characteristics, management and follow-up. J Am Coll Cardiol 1988; 11:379–385.

63. Dhala AA, Case CL, Gillette P: Evolving treatment strategies for managing atrial ectopic tachycardia in children. Am J Cardiol 1994; 74:283–286.

64. Koike K, Hesslein PS, Finlay DC, et al: Atrial automatic rhythms in children. Am J Cardiol 1988; 61:1127–1130.

65. Perry JC, Knilans TK, Marlow D, et al: Intravenous amiodarone for life threatening tachyarrhythmias in children and young adults. J Am Coll Cardiol 1993; 22:95–98.

66. Salim MA, Case CL, Gillette PC: Chaotic atrial tachycardia in children. Am Heart J 1995; 129:831–833.

67. Ming-Yi W, Zhi-fang W, Xiu-Yu C: Chaotic atrial rhythm in 22 infants. Chin Med J 1984; 97:500–503.

68. Bisset GS, Seigel SF, Gaum WE, et al: Chaotic atrial tachycardia in childhood. Am Heart J 1981; 101:268–272.

69. Bradley DJ, Fischbach PS, Law IH, et al: Multifocal tachycardia in children: Clinical course and long term outcome. Pacing Clin Electrophysiol 1999; 22:831. Abstract.

70. Yeager SB, Hougen TJ, Levy AM: Sudden death in infants with chaotic atrial tachycardia. Am J Dis Child 1984; 138:689–692.
71. Scher DL, Arsura EL: Multifocal atrial tachycardia: Mechanisms, clinical correlates, and treatment. Am Heart J 1989; 118:574–580.
72. Garson A, Gillette PC, Moak JP, et al: Supraventricular tachycardia due to multiple atrial ectopic foci: A relatively common problem. J Cardiovasc Electrophysiol 1990; 1:132–138.
73. Fish FA, Mehta AV, Johns JA: Characteristics and management of chaotic atrial tachycardia of infancy. Am J Cardiol 1996; 78:1052–1055.
74. Kastor JA. Multifocal atrial tachycardia. N Engl J Med 1990; 322:1713–1717.
75. Lesh MD, Van Hare GF, Epstein LM, et al: Radiofrequency catheter ablation of atrial arrhythmias: Results and mechanisms. Circulation 1994; 89:1074–1089.
76. Haines DE, DiMarco JP: Sustained intraatrial reentrant tachycardia: Clinical electrocardiographic and electrophysiologic characteristics and long-term follow-up. J Am Coll Cardiol 1990; 15:1345–1354.
77. Olshanky B, Wilber DJ, Hariman RJ: Atrial flutter–update on the mechanism and treatment. Pacing Clin Electrophysiol 1992; 15:2308–2335.
78. Waldo AL: Pathogenesis of atrial flutter. J Cardiovasc Electrophysiol 1998; 9(8 suppl):S18–S25.
79. Lesh MD, Kalman JM, Olgin JE, et al: The role of atrial anatomy in clinical atrial arrhythmias. J Electrophysiol 1996; 29:101–113.
80. Josephson ME: Clinical Cardiac Electrophysiology: Techniques and Interpretation. Philadelphia: Lea & Febiger; 1993:256–258.
81. Jaeggi E, Fouron JC, Drblik SP: Fetal atrial flutter: Diagnosis, clinical features, treatment, and outcome. J Pediatr 1998; 132:335–339.
82. Garson A, Bink-Boelkens M, Hesslein PS, et al: Atrial flutter: A collaborative study 380 cases. J Am Coll Cardiol 1985; 6:871–878.
83. Dunnigan A, Benson DW, Benditt DG: Atrial flutter in infancy: Diagnosis, clinical features, and treatment. Pediatrics 1985; 75:725–729.
84. Mendelsohn A, Dick M, Serwer G: Natural history of isolated atrial flutter infancy. J Pediatr 1991; 119:386–391.
85. Drago F, Mazz A, Garibaldi S, et al: Isolated neonatal atrial flutter: Clinical features, prognosis, and therapy. Giornale Italiano di Cardiologia 1998; 28:365–368.
86. Gewillig M, Wyse RK, de Leval RM, et al: Early and late arrhythmias after the Fontan operation: Predisposing factors and clinical consequences. Br Heart J 1992; 67:72–79.
87. Fishberger SB, Wernovsky G, Gentles TL: Factors that influence the development of atrial flutter after the Fontan operation. J Thorac Cardiovasc Surg 1997; 113:80–86.
88. Bink-Boelkens M, Velvis H, van der Heide JJ, et al: Dysrhythmias after atrial surgery in children. Am Heart J 1983; 106:125–130.
89. Lesh MD, Kalman JM, Saxon LA, et al: Electrophysiology of 'incisional' reentrant atrial tachycardia complicating surgery for congenital heart disease. Pacing Clin Electrophysiol 1997; 20:2107–2111.
90. Van Hare GF, Lesh MD, Ross BA, et al: Mapping and radiofrequency ablation of intraatrial reentrant tachycardia after the Senning or Mustard procedure for transposition of the great arteries. Am J Cardiol 1996; 77:985–991.
91. Kalman JM, VanHare GF, Olgin JE, et al: Ablation of "incisional" reentrant atrial tachycardia complicating surgery for congenital heart disease. Circulation 1996; 93:502–512.
92. Robotin MC, Serraf A, Houyel L, et al: Prevention of unbalanced lung perfusion and atrial arrhythmias after the lateral tunnel operation. Ann Thorac Surg 1997; 64:1389–1395.

93. Wood KA, Drew BJ, Scheinman MM: Frequency of disabling symptoms in-supraventricular tachycardia. Am J Cardiol 1997; 79:145–151.

94. Wood KA, Eisenberg SJ, Kalman JM: Risk of thromboembolism in chronic atrial flutter. Am J Cardiol 1997; 79:1043–1047.

95. Balaji S, Johnson TB, Sade RM, et al: Management of atrial flutter after the Fontan procedure. J Am Coll Cardiol 1994; 23:1209–1215.

96. Triedman JK, Bergau DM, Saul JP, et al: Efficacy of radiofrequency ablation for control of intraatrial reentrant tachycardia in patients with congenital heart disease. J Am Coll Cardiol 1997; 30:1032–1038.

97. Brugada R, Tapscott T, Czernuszewicz GZ, et al: Identification of a genetic locus for familial atrial fibrillation. N Engl J Med 1997; 336:905–911.

98. Tikonaja R, Kirkinen P, Nikolajev K, et al: Familial atrial fibrillation with fe-tal onset. Heart 1998; 79:195–197.

99. Bertram H, Paul T, Beyer F, et al: Familial idiopathic atrial fibrillation with bradyarrhythmia. Eur J Pediatr 1996; 155:7–10.

100. Frustaci A, Chimente C, Bellocci F, et al: Histological substrate of atrial biop-sies in patients with lone atrial fibrillation. Circulation 1997; 96:1180–1184.

101. Levy S: Factors predisposing to the development of atrial fibrillation. Pacing Clin Electrophysiol 1997; 20:2670–2674.

102. Brugada J, Mont L, Mata M, et al: Atrial fibrillation induced by atrioven-tricular reentrant tachycardia. Am J Cardiol 1997; 79:681–682.

103. Haissaguerre M, Jais P, Shah D, et al: Spontaneous initiation of atrial fib-rillation by ectopic beats originating in the pulmonary veins. N Engl J Med 1998; 339:659–666.

104. Feltes TF, Friedman RA: Transesophageal echocardiographic detection of atrial thrombi in patients with nonfibrillation atrial tachyarrhythmias and congenital heart disease. J Am Coll Cardiol 1994; 24:1365–1370.

105. Talajic M, MacDonald RG, Nattel S: Restoration of sinus rhythm in patients with atrial fibrillation. Can J Cardiol 1996; 12:29A–35A.

106. Black IW, Fatkin D, Sagar KB, et al: Exclusion of atrial thrombus by trans-esophageal echocardiography does not preclude embolism after cardioversion of atrial fibrillation: A multicenter study. Circulation 1994; 89:2509–2513.

107. Ramdat M, Beukema WP, Oude Luttikhuis HA: Multisite or alternate site pac-ing for the prevention of atrial fibrillation. Am J Cardiol 1999; 83:237D–240D.

108. Cox JL, Sundt TM: The surgical management of atrial fibrillation. Annu Rev Med 1997; 48:511–523.

109. Garson A, Gillette PC: Junctional ectopic tachycardia in children: Electro-cardiography, electrophysiology and pharmacologic response. Am J Cardiol 1979; 44:298–302.

110. Villain E, Vetter VL, Garcia JM, et al: Evolving concepts in the management of congenital junctional ectopic tachycardia: A multicenter study. Circulation 1990; 81:1544–1549.

111. Gillette PC: Evolving concepts in the management of congenital junctional ectopic tachycardia. Circulation 1990; 81:1713–1714.

112. Gillette PC, Garson A, Porter CJ, et al: Junctional automatic ectopic tachy-cardia: New proposed treatment by transcatheter ablation. Am Heart J 1983; 106:619–623.

113. Balaji S, Sullivan I, Deanfield J, et al: Moderate hypothermia in the man-agement of resistant automatic tachycardias in children. Br Heart J 1991; 66:221–224.

114. Till JA, Rowland E: Atrial pacing as an adjunct to the management of post-surgical His bundle tachycardia. Br Heart J 1991; 66:225–229.

115. Grant JW, Serwer GA, Armstrong BE, et al: Junctional tachycardia in in-fants and children after open heart surgery for congenital heart disease. Am J Cardiol 1987; 59:1216–1218.

116. Young ML, Mehta MB, Martinez RM, et al: Combined alpha-adrenergic blockade and radiofrequency ablation to treat junctional ectopic tachycardia successfully without atrioventricular block. Am J Cardiol 1993; 71:883–885.

117. Bash SE, Shah JJ, Albers WH, et al: Hypothermia for the treatment of post-surgical greatly accelerated junctional ectopic tachycardia. J Am Coll Cardiol 1987; 10:1095–1099.

118. Waldo AL, Krongrad E, Kupersmith J, et al: Ventricular paired pacing to control rapid ventricular heart rate following open heart surgery. Observations on ectopic automaticity: Report of a case in a four-month old patient. Circulation 1976; 53:176–181.

119. Zeigler VL: Postoperative rhythm disturbances. Crit Care Nurs Clin North Am 1994; 6:227–235.

120. Kugler JD: Sinus node dysfunction. In Gillette PC, Garson A Jr. (eds.): Pediatric Arrhythmias: Electrophysiology and Pacing. Philadelphia: WB Saunders Company; 1990:250–300.

121. Yabek SM, Jarmakani JM: Sinus node dysfunction in children, adolescents, and young adults. Pediatrics 1978; 61:593–598.

122. Kurer CC, Tanner CS, Vetter VL: Electrophysiologic findings after Fontan repair of single ventricle. J Am Coll Cardiol 1991; 17:174–181.

123. Kugler JD, Yabek SM: Sick sinus syndrome: Clinical features and non-invasive evaluation. In Yabek SM, Gillette PC, Kugler JD (eds.): The Sinus Node in Pediatrics. New York: Churchill Livingstone; 1984:48–66.

124. Kramer H, Rammos S, Krogman O, et al: Cardiac rhythm after Mustard repair and after arterial switch operation for complete transposition. Int J Cardiol 1991; 32:5–12.

125. Lien WP, Chang F, Chen C: The sick sinus syndrome: Natural history of dysfunction of the sinoatrial node. Chest 1977; 72:628–634.

126. Alpert MA, Flaker GC: Arrhythmias associated with sinus node dysfunction. Pathogenesis, recognition, and management. JAMA 1983; 250:2160–2166.

127. Menozzi C, Brignole M, Alboni P, et al: The natural course of untreated sick sinus syndrome and identification of the variables predictive of unfavorable outcome. Am J Cardiol 1998; 82:1205–1209.

128. Rubenstein JJ, Schulman CL, Yurchak PM, et al: Clinical spectrum of the sick sinus syndrome. Circulation 1972; 46:5–13.

129. Bharati S, Lev M: Sequelae of atriotomy and ventriculotomy on the endocardium, conduction system and coronary arteries. Am J Cardiol 1982; 50:580–587.

130. Bharati S, Molthan ME, Veasy LG, et al: Conduction system in two cases of sudden death two years after the Mustard procedure. J Thorac Cardiovasc Surg 1979; 77:101–108.

131. El-Said G, Rosenberg HS, Mullins CE, et al: Dysrhythmias after Mustard's operation for transposition of the great arteries. Am J Cardiol 1972; 30:526–532.

132. Campbell R, Dick M, Byrum C, et al: Serial electrophysiologic observation after Mustard repair. Circulation 1982; 66:316. Abstract.

133. Gillette PC, Kugler JD, Garson A, et al: Mechanisms of cardiac arrhythmias after the Mustard operation for transposition of the great arteries. Am J Cardiol 1980; 45:1225–1230.

134. Vetter VL, Tanner CS, Horowitz LN: Electrophysiologic consequences of the Mustard repair of d-transposition of the great arteries. J Am Coll Cardiol 1987; 10:1265–1273.

135. Weber SH, Hellenbrand WE, Kleinman CS, et al: Predictors of rhythm disturbances and subsequent morbidity after the Fontan operation. Am J Cardiol 1989; 64:762–767.

136. Driscoll DJ, Offord KP, Feldt RH, et al: Five to fifteen year follow-up after Fontan operation. Circulation 1992; 85:469–496.

137. Yabek SM, Swensson RE, Jarmakani JM: Electrocardiographic recognition of sinus node dysfunction in children and young adults. Circulation 1977; 56:235–239.

138. Martin AB, Kugler JD: Sinus node dysfunction. In Gillette PC, Garson A Jr. (eds.): Clinical Pediatric Arrhythmias. 2nd ed. Philadelphia: WB Saunders Company; 1999:51–62.

139. Flinn CJ, Wolff GS, Campbell RM, et al: Natural history of supraventricular rhythms in 182 children following the Mustard operation: A collaborative multi-center study. J Am Coll Cardiol 1983; 1:613. Abstract.

140. Hesslein PS, Gutgesell HP, Gillette PC, et al: Exercise assessment of sino-atrial node function following the Mustard operation. Am Heart J 1982; 103:351–357.

141. Gregatoros G, Cheitlin MD, Conill A, et al: ACC/AHA guidelines for implantation of cardiac pacemakers and antiarrhythmia devices. J Am Coll Cardiol 1998; 31:1175–1209.

142. Nakamura F, Nadas A: Complete heart block in infants and children. N Engl J Med 1964; 270:1261–1268.

143. Pinsky WW, Gillette PC, Garson A Jr., et al: Diagnosis, management, and long term results of patients with congenital complete atrioventricular block. Pediatrics 1982; 69:728–733.

144. Van der Merwe PL, Weymar HW, Torrington M, et al: Progressive familial heart block (type I). A follow-up study after 10 years. S Afr Med J 1988; 73:275–276.

145. Scott WA, Dick M: Two-to-one (2:1) atrioventricular block in infants with congenital long QT syndrome. Am J Cardiol 1987; 60:1409–1410.

146. Michaelsson M, Jonzon A, Riesenfeld T: Isolated congenital complete atrioventricular block in adult life: A prospective study. Circulation 1995; 91:442–449.

147. Siren MK, Julkunen H, Kaaja R, et al: Role of HLA in congenital heart block: Susceptibility alleles in children. Lupus 1999; 8:60–67.

148. Goble MM, Dick M, McCune J, et al: Atrioventricular conduction in children of women with systemic lupus erythematosus. Am J Cardiol 1993; 71:94–98.

149. Byron JP, Hiegert R, Cope J, et al: Autoimmune-associated congenital heart block: Demographics, mortality, morbidity, and recurrence rates obtained from a national neonatal lupus registry. J Am Coll Cardiol 1998; 31:1658–1666.

150. Menon A, Silverman E, Gow RM, et al: Chronotropic competence of the sinus node in congenital complete heart block. Am J Cardiol 1998; 82:119–121.

151. Fukushige J, Takahashi N, Igarashi H, et al: Perinatal management of congenital complete atrioventricular block: A report of nine cases. Acta Paediatr Jpn 1998; 40:337–340.

152. Groves AM, Allan LD, Rosenthal E: Outcome of isolated congenital complete heart block diagnosed in utero. Heart 1996; 75:190–194.

153. Molthan ME, Miller RA, Hastreiter AR, et al: Congenital heart block with fatal Adams-Stokes attacks in childhood. Pediatrics 1962; 30:32–41.

154. Kertesz NJ, Friedman RA, Colan SD, et al: Left ventricular mechanics and geometry in patients with congenital complete atrioventricular block. Circulation 1997; 96:3430–3435.

155. Winkler RB, Freed MD, Nadas AS: Exercise-induced ventricular ectopy in children and young adults with complete heart block. Am Heart J 1980; 99:87–92.

156. Michaelsson M, Riesenfeld T, Jonzon A: Natural history of congenital complete atrioventricular block. Pacing Clin Electrophysiol 1997; 20:2098–2101.

157. Bonatti V, Agnetti A, Squarcia U: Early and late postoperative heart block in pediatric patients submitted to open-heart surgery for congenital heart disease. Pediatria Medicae Chirugica 1998; 20:181–186.

158. Kugler JD, Danford DA, Deal BJ, et al: Radiofrequency ablation for tachyarrhythmias in children and adolescents. N Engl J Med 1994; 330:1481–1487.
159. Schultz TE: Heart block after induction of anesthesia. AANA J 1999; 67:326–328.
160. Folino AF, Buja GF, Martini B, et al: Prolonged cardiac arrest and complete AV block during upright tilt test in young patients with syncope of unknown origin—prognostic and therapeutic implications. Eur Heart J 1992; 13:1416–1421.
161. Freed MD, Rosenthal AR: Complete heart block after heart catheterization: A rare complication. Pediatrics 1973; 51:935–938.
162. Serwer GA, Dorostkar PC, LeRoy SS: Pediatric pacing and defibrillation usage. In Ellenbogen KA, Kay GN, Wilkoff BL (eds.): Clinical Cardiac Pacing and Defibrillation. 2nd ed. Philadelphia: WB Saunders Company; 2000:953–989.
163. Weindling SN, Saul JP, Gamble WJ, et al: Duration of complete atrioventricular block after congenital heart disease surgery. Am J Cardiol 1998; 82:525–527.
164. Hurwitz RA, Riemenschneider TA, Moss AJ: Chronic postoperative heart block in children. Am J Cardiol 1968; 21:185–189.
165. Driscoll DJ, Gillette PC, Hallman GL, et al: Management of surgical complete atrioventricular block. Am J Cardiol 1979; 43:1175–1180.
166. Lillihei CW, Sellers R, Bonnabeau R, et al: Chronic postsurgical complete heart block. J Thorac Cardiovasc Surg 1973; 46:436–456.
167. Moss AJ, Klyman G, Emmanouilides GC: Late onset complete heart block: Newly recognized sequela of cardiac surgery. Am J Cardiol 1972; 30:884–887.
168. Squarcia U, Merideth J, McGoon DC, et al: Prognosis of transient atrioventricular conduction disturbances complicating open heart surgery for congenital heart defects. Am J Cardiol 1971; 28:648–652.
169. Thompson RJ, Gustafson KE: Correlates of psychosocial adjustment. In Adaptation to Chronic Illness. Washington DC: American Psychological Association; 1996:87–113.
170. Lavigne JV, Faier-Routman J: Correlates of psychosocial adjustment to pediatric physical disorders: A meta-analytic review and comparison with existing models. J Dev Behav Pediatrics 1993; 14:117–123.
171. Alpern D, Uzark K, Dick M: Psychosocial responses to children with cardiac pacemakers. J Pediatr 1989; 114:494–501.
172. Pless IB, Roghmann KJ: Chronic illness and its consequences: Observations based on three epidemiologic surveys. J Pediatr 1971; 79:351–359.
173. Wallander JL, Hubert NC, Varni JW: Child and maternal temperament characteristics, goodness of fit, and adjustment in physically handicapped children. J Clin Child Psychol 1988; 17:336–344.
174. Compas BE, Worshan NL, Ey S: Conceptual and developmental issues in children's coping with stress. In La Greca AM, Siegal LJ, Wallander JL, Walker CE (eds.): Stress and Coping in Child Health. New York: Guilford Press; 1992:7–24.
175. Hamlett KW, Pellegrini DS, Katz KS: Childhood chronic illness as a family stressor. J Pediatr Psychol 1992; 17:33–47.
176. Blechman EA, Delamater AM: Family communication and type 1 diabetes. A window on the social environment of chronically ill children. In Cole RE, Reiss D (eds.): How do Families Cope with Chronic Illness? Hillsdale, NJ: Lawrence Erlbaum; 1993:1–24.
177. DeMaso DR, Campis LK, Wypij D, et al: The impact of maternal perceptions and medical severity on the adjustment of children with congenital heart disease. J Pediatr Psychol 1991; 16:137–149.
178. Lyons-Ruth K, Zoll D, Conell D, et al: The depressed mother and her one year old infant. Environment, interaction, attachment and infant development. In

Field T, Tronick E (eds.): Maternal Depression and Infant Disturbance. San Francisco: Jossey-Bass; 1986:61–82.

179. Satin W, La Greca AM, Zigo MA, et al: Diabetes in adolescence: Effects of multifamily group intervention and parent simulation of diabetes. J Pediatr Psychol 1989; 14:259–275.

180. Varni JW, Katz ER, Coelgrove R, et al: The impact of social skills training on the adjustment of children with newly diagnosed cancer. J Pediatr Psychol 1993; 18:251–267.

181. Yarcheski A, Scoleveno MA, Mahon N: Social support and well-being in adolescents. The mediating role of hopefulness. Nurs Res 1994; 43:288–292.

Chapter 3

Ventricular Arrhythmias

Vicki L. Zeigler, RN, MSN and Paul C. Gillette, MD

Ventricular arrhythmias are far less common in children than are supraventricular arrhythmias. Similar to the adult population, ventricular arrhythmias in children result from reentry or enhanced automaticity, originating from a site below the bifurcation of the bundle of His.[1] Select ventricular arrhythmias in children are considered benign and require no treatment, while others may require more aggressive management. The diagnosis and resultant treatment depend on the type of ventricular arrhythmia, the arrhythmia mechanism, the patient's unique clinical situation, the hemodynamic consequences of the arrhythmia, and the relative risk of sudden death as a result of the arrhythmia.[1]

Ventricular arrhythmias in children can occur in anatomically normal hearts with primary electrical disease such as the long QT syndrome (LQTS) and Brugada syndrome, with associated disease processes such as viral myocarditis, cardiac tumors, arrhythmogenic right ventricular dysplasia (ARVD), and cardiomyopathy, or following surgery for congenital heart disease (CHD). Ischemia-induced ventricular arrhythmias are relatively rare in the pediatric population, but can be associated with specific disease states in children, e.g., hypertrophic cardiomyopathy, Kawasaki disease, and select congenital coronary defects.[2]

The most common cause of significant ventricular arrhythmias in children is permanent damage to the myocardial tissue after surgery for CHD. This generally occurs due to an incision made into the ventricles, but can also be a result of structural defects that cause an increase in left or right ventricular pressures. Fifteen percent of patients with congenital cardiac defects develop chronic postoperative arrhythmias and 5% to 10% experience sudden death.[3]

This chapter discusses the clinical presentation of children with ventricular arrhythmias, electrocardiographic (ECG) characteristics of ven-

From Zeigler VL, Gillette PC: *Practical Management of Pediatric Cardiac Arrhythmias.*
Armonk, NY: Futura Publishing Co., Inc.; ©2001.

tricular arrhythmias in children, what constitutes benign ventricular arrhythmias, specific disease states that result in ventricular arrhythmias, the implications for clinicians when caring for children who have ventricular arrhythmias (and their families), and, finally, patient and family considerations. Since the various treatment modalities are discussed in further detail in other chapters of this book, they are only briefly alluded to here.

Clinical Presentation and Electrocardiographic Characteristics of Ventricular Arrhythmias

Premature Ventricular Contractions

Clinical Presentation

In the pediatric population, premature ventricular contractions (PVCs) commonly result in an irregular pulse. In children with no known cardiovascular disease, 24-hour ambulatory monitoring has shown 18% of newborns and up to 50% of adolescents to have PVCs, whereas routine ECG monitoring has revealed PVCs in 0.8% and 2.2% of these patients, respectively.[4,5] In comparison, in children with postoperative CHD (specifically those who have undergone tetralogy of Fallot repair), the incidence is 8% on routine ECG and 46% on 24-hour ambulatory monitor.[6]

There are many ways in which a child may present with PVCs. Typically, an irregular beat is detected during auscultation and the PVCs are confirmed by routine ECG. Older children who are able to describe the sensation of PVCs may complain of feeling "funny beats" or "skipped beats" in their stomachs or chests.[7] These same children are usually able to keep up with their peers in play and exercise. Children with PVCs rarely complain of lightheadedness, dizziness, or syncope. There are usually no overt symptoms in the infant and younger child.

Electrocardiographic Characteristics

There are several common terms used to describe PVCs (Table 1).

Table 1
Terminology Commonly Used to Describe
Premature Ventricular Contractions

Term	Definition
Uniform	Having one QRS morphology
Multiform	Having more than one QRS morphology
Couplet	Two PVCs in a row

Table 1
Terminology Commonly Used to Describe
Premature Ventricular Contractions (*cont.*)

Term	Definition
Triplet	Three PVCs in a row
Bigeminy	Every other beat is a PVC
Trigeminy	Every third beat is a PVC
Quadrigeminy	Every fourth beat is a PVC
Interpolated	The PVC occurs in the middle of two sinus beats, with no interruption of the sinus cycle length and no compensatory pause.
Compensatory pause	A pause after a PVC that is longer than the expected sinus interval. It occurs because the sinus P wave after the PVC is blocked.
Fusion beat	A contraction that occurs when two intrinsic beats coming from two different sites merge. In the event of a PVC, the QRS complex is caused partially by the PVC and partially by the sinus impulse through the normal conduction pathway. It has electrocardiographic characteristics of both a normal beat and the PVC. The QRS is wider than normal, but not quite as wide as a usual PVC.
Sinus capture beat	A QRS that causes an irregularity in an episode of ventricular tachycardia because it is generated by conduction from the sinus node. The beat may have a normal QRS morphology or look like a fusion beat.
Monomorphic	Having one morphology
Polymorphic	Having more than one morphology
Torsades de pointes	Polymorphic ventricular tachycardia generally associated with LQTS; the QRS complexes have the appearance of "twisting" around a center axis.
T Wave Alternans	A repetitive change in T wave morphology occurring in every other complex

LQTS = long QT syndrome; PVC = premature ventricular contraction.

The basic ECG characteristics of PVCs include the following:

Rate	The sinus rate is normal for age and is usually regular but is intermittently interrupted by the PVC (Fig. 1); this results in an irregular and fluctuating heart rate.

Rhythm	The basic R-R interval is regular but is intermittently interrupted by the PVC. The R-R interval preceding the PVC is short due to the "prematurity" of the QRS complex and often the R-R interval after the PVC is longer due to a compensatory pause (Fig. 2).
P wave	The premature QRS complex is not preceded by a conducted P wave, although in certain instances the PVC may coincidentally be preceded by a nonconducted sinus P wave (Fig. 3).
PR interval	Not applicable because atrioventricular (AV) conduction is not involved.
QRS complex	The QRS duration is prolonged (>0.08 second in infants and >0.09 second in the child older than 3 years) (Fig. 4).

Silka and Garson[8] have defined five ECG criteria for PVCs that are summarized below: 1) the "premature" QRS is based on the underlying rhythm but has been defined as one that occurs ≤80 ms prior to the next anticipated regular beat[9]; 2) the QRS morphology must be different from that of the normal or regular QRS complex; although the QRS complex of the PVC is not always "wide" in children, it is different in morphology from the normal QRS complexes; 3) the QRS complex is usually (though not

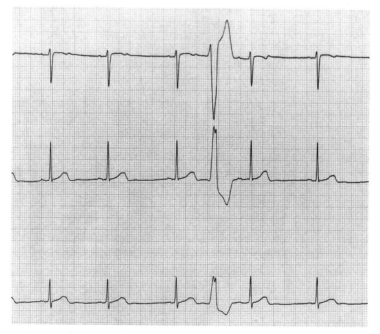

Figure 1. Surface ECG leads V$_1$, II, and V$_6$ exhibiting normal sinus rhythm with a single, interpolated premature ventricular contraction (PVC). The PVC occurs in the middle of the sinus cycle length and does not conduct in a retrograde fashion as evidenced by the next P wave occurring at the next anticipated interval.

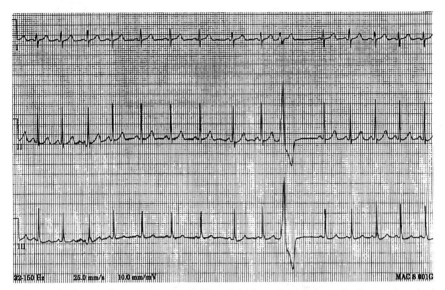

Figure 2. Surface ECG leads I, II, and III exhibiting normal sinus rhythm and a single premature ventricular contraction (PVC). The increase in QRS duration of the PVC when compared with the sinus QRS is classic of PVC description.

always) prolonged in duration (e.g., >80 ms in infants and >90 ms in children older than 3 years); 4) the ST segment and T wave have abnormalities with a T wave vector that is discordant to the QRS complex; and 5) there is no premature atrial depolarization preceding the PVC.[8]

Ventricular Tachycardia

Clinical Presentation

The clinical presentation of the child with ventricular tachycardia (VT) varies from patient to patient. The infant may remain totally asymptomatic with the only indication being a rapid heart rate, generally greater than 220 beats per minute (bpm), or exhibit symptoms such as pallor, poor feeding, tachypnea, lethargy, and, in extreme cases, mottling, cyanosis, or both. In rare cases, the infant may present in unexplained sudden cardiac arrest. Older children with VT may complain of palpitations, dizziness, near-syncope, or syncope. They rarely complain of exercise intolerance or chest pain.

In general, the pediatric patients most likely to experience more serious symptoms from their VT include infants, patients with LQTS, and those patients who have previously undergone surgery for CHD. Additionally, patients with any form of structural heart disease, whether operated or unoperated, may experience more hemodynamic compromise than their counterparts with anatomically normal hearts.

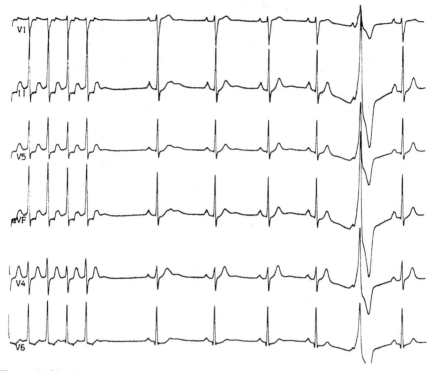

Figure 3. Six simultaneous surface ECG leads in a patient with supraventricular tachycardia (SVT) and premature ventricular contractions (PVCs). At the beginning of the ECG rhythm strip, there are four beats of SVT that spontaneously convert to normal sinus rhythm. After four beats of sinus rhythm, a PVC occurs after the inscription of a sinus P wave. The P wave proximity to the QRS complex is such that AV conduction could not have occurred from the P wave to the QRS, making it somewhat incidental. The QRS duration and the morphology of the QRS meet the criteria for a PVC despite the incidental P wave preceding it.

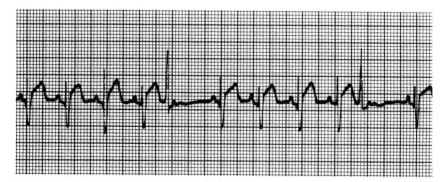

Figure 4. Surface ECG lead II rhythm strip recording from a patient after repair of tetralogy of Fallot. The basic rhythm is normal sinus rhythm with right bundle branch block. Two premature ventricular contractions occur with narrow or equal QRS duration but with very different morphologies. In children, there are no rigid criteria for QRS duration as a determinant for ventricular differentiation, rather the difference in QRS morphology and relationship to the P wave are critical in this case.

Electrocardiographic Characteristics

VT is defined as more than three consecutive PVCs in a row, generally with a rate greater than 120 bpm.[8] Since the QRS duration may not be prolonged, the morphology of the QRS complex, i.e., the difference between it and the normal QRS complex, is even more important.

The basic ECG characteristics of VT include the following:

Rate	The ventricular rate is generally greater than 120 bpm or at least 10% greater than the previous sinus rhythm rate (Fig. 5).
Rhythm	The R-R interval is usually regular, but may be irregular if there are sinus "capture" beats.
P wave	The P wave may appear in one of three different scenarios: 1) it may be seen after some or all of the QRS complexes with a constant RP interval in the presence of retrograde conduction; 2) it may not be visible at all; or 3) it may exhibit a rate less than the QRS rate with AV dissociation.
PR interval	Not applicable.
QRS complex	Usually prolonged: infants, 0.06 to 0.11 second, children greater than 3 years, greater than 0.09 second; QRS morphology is different from that of sinus rhythm and is usually, but not always, prolonged in duration. The QRS morphology is generally consistent with single PVCs.

Silka and Garson[8] have defined criteria that "favor" the diagnosis of VT in children. These are summarized below: 1) AV dissociation is present in the majority of children; 2) 1:1 retrograde ventriculoatrial conduction may be present, i.e., a P wave follows each QRS complex; 3) intermittent fusion or sinus capture beats may occur; and 4) the rates in infants can range between 167 and 500 bpm,[10] although it is unusual for children to have a sustained rate of greater than 250 bpm.

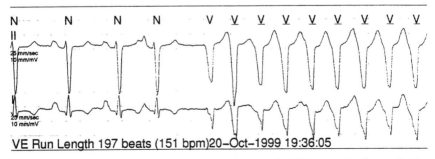

Figure 5. Onset of monomorphic ventricular tachycardia (VT) recorded from a 24-hour ambulatory monitor. The third beat from the left is a premature beat, which is followed by a pause ending with a ventricular escape beat. The escape beat is then followed by a run of VT.

Ventricular Fibrillation

Clinical Presentation

Ventricular fibrillation (VF) is rare in the pediatric population. In earlier reports, VF was identified as the terminal rhythm in only 6% of chronically ill patients under the age of 18 years.[11] More recently, it has been identified in nearly 20% of patients under the age of 18 years as the initial cardiac rhythm during attempted resuscitation.[12] This increase in the reported incidence of VF is thought to be due to improvements in emergency response systems. In contrast to the aforementioned patients, the child with VF presents in full cardiac arrest. There is complete loss of consciousness, absence of respirations, and no palpable pulses.

Electrocardiographic Characteristics

VF is a state of uncoordinated ventricular depolarizations that results in no effective cardiac output (Fig. 6). The basic ECG characteristics of VF include the following:

Rate	None
Rhythm	None
P wave	Not visible
PR interval	Not applicable
QRS complex	Unidentifiable; variable amplitude, rapid and irregular waveforms

Silka and Garson[8] warn that the ECG morphology of VF is similar to that observed when an ECG electrode has lost contact with the patient's skin; therefore, if VF is suspected, one should first quickly assess breathlessness and pulselessness of the patient prior to initiating cardiopulmonary resuscitation.

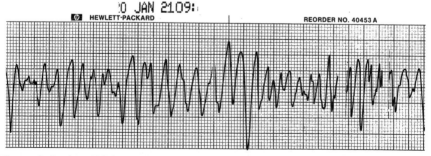

Figure 6. Surface ECG recording of ventricular fibrillation. Note the complete lack of baseline and variation in amplitude.

Benign Ventricular Arrhythmias

Premature Ventricular Contractions

PVCs can result from hypoxia, hypovolemia, electrolyte abnormalities, or irritation from intracardiac monitoring or pacing catheters, or it can be idiopathic in nature. Additionally, medications such as isoproterenol, digoxin, and imipramine have been known to contribute to the development of PVCs.[13] Although the aforementioned instances are not always considered benign, once the metabolic imbalance has been corrected or the cardiac irritant removed or discontinued, the ectopy generally subsides. Recent studies have suggested that although some children are denoted to have "benign PVCs," care should be taken to evaluate any repolarization changes that may be indicative of underlying substrate abnormalities.[14]

A thorough evaluation is warranted in children who present with PVCs without any of the aforementioned conditions and with an anatomically and otherwise electrically normal heart. This evaluation, initially done by 24-hour ambulatory monitor, is performed to ascertain the percentage of PVCs (compared with normal beats) over a 24-hour period, the PVC morphologies (Figs. 7 and 8), and the PVC frequency (i.e., bigeminy, trigeminy, etc.) (Fig. 9). In order to be considered benign, the PVCs should be uniform in morphology, should suppress with exercise, should produce no significant hemodynamic effects, and should not be associated with any identifiable heart disease. Research has documented that although these patients continue to have PVCs a decade later, they experience no adverse sequelae.[4] Some centers may even perform annual 24-hour ambulatory monitoring to ensure that the incidence and/or characteristics of the ectopy have not changed over time.

Accelerated Idioventricular Rhythm

Accelerated idioventricular rhythm, a variant of VT, is characterized by a regular, wide QRS complex, with a rate consistent with that of the preceding sinus rhythm[15,16] (Fig. 10). It terminates with the resumption of sinus rhythm and may exhibit AV dissociation. The presence of accelerated idioventricular rhythm may appear on surface ECG as a "slow" VT. MacLellan-Tobert and Porter[17] studied 12 patients with the diagnosis of accelerated idioventricular rhythm, in order to determine whether this arrhythmia should be considered benign. The following criteria were used by the authors to define accelerated idioventricular rhythm: 1) wide QRS complex; 2) regular rhythm; 3) rate within 10% of preceding sinus rate; 4) termination into sinus rhythm versus VF; and 5) if observed, the presence of fusion beats.

Nine of the 12 patients in this study had structurally normal hearts, while three were postoperative for CHD.[17] Seven patients received

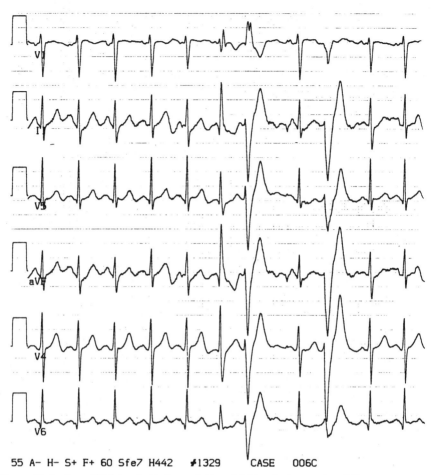

Figure 7. Surface ECG leads V_1 through V_6 exhibiting fusion and multiform premature ventricular contractions (PVCs). The basic rhythm is sinus tachycardia at the end of an exercise stress test. The sixth beat is a fusion beat between the sinus beat and the PVC as shown by the shorter PR interval and different appearance of the QRS complex. The seventh beat is a PVC, and in conjunction with beat 6 forms a couplet. Beat 9 is a multiform PVC, since the morphology of the QRS complex is different from the previous PVC. Lead V_1 most accurately depicts these findings in this particular patient.

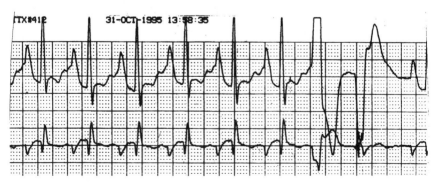

Figure 8. Surface ECG leads II and V_1 exhibiting a ventricular couplet. The two different PVC morphologies are quite obvious in both leads.

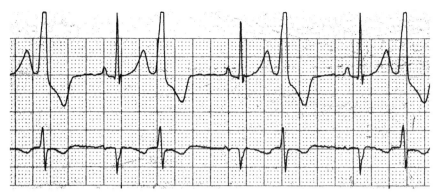

Figure 9. Surface ECG recording of premature ventricular contractions (PVCs) in a bigeminal pattern in which every other beat is a PVC.

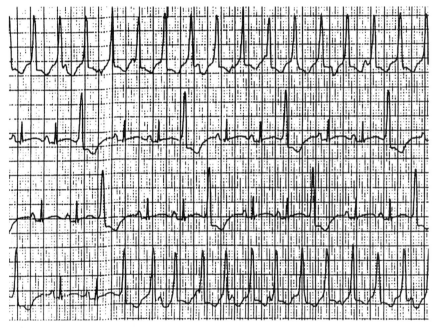

Figure 10. Accelerated ventricular rhythm. Accelerated idioventricular rhythm from a newborn exhibiting a wide QRS complex rhythm with AV dissociation. The rate of the ventricular rhythm is 140 to 150 bpm compared with a sinus rate of 120 bpm. Reproduced from Silka MJ, Garson A Jr.: Ventricular arrhythmias. In Gillette PC, Garson A Jr. (eds.): Clinical Pediatric Arrhythmias. 2nd ed. Philadelphia: WB Saunders Company; 1999:127, with permission.

medications that failed to impact the ventricular arrhythmia. All patients were alive and asymptomatic at the time of last follow-up, although two patients had short arrhythmia episodes on 24-hour ambulatory monitor. The authors concluded that the patients with accelerated idioventricular rhythm with normal cardiac evaluations have excellent long-term outcomes with no activity restrictions. Caution must be used when differentiating between accelerated idioventricular rhythm and VT. Echocardiography is pivotal in ascertaining the presence of structural cardiovascular disease. The authors of this study recommend further evaluation in the presence of ventricular dilation or depressed ventricular function, but no further follow-up in patients diagnosed with benign accelerated idioventricular rhythm unless palpitations, presyncope, or syncope occur, at which time 24-hour ambulatory monitoring should be pursued. Once again, some centers routinely perform annual 24-hour ambulatory monitoring to document the stability of or any changes in the child's rhythm over time.

Disease States Associated with Ventricular Arrhythmias in Children

There are several disease states, for lack of better terminology, that are associated with and are the underlying etiology of ventricular rhythm disturbances in the young. These conditions can occur in children with anatomically normal hearts or in those with structurally abnormal hearts. In the structurally normal heart, the disease states include the congenital form of LQTS, the Brugada syndrome, and idiopathic VT. Those that occur in the abnormal heart include postoperative CHD, cardiomyopathy (hypertrophic, dilated, and restrictive), viral myocarditis, ARVD, and myocardial tumors.

Primary Electrical Disease

Long QT Syndrome

A heart may be totally normal, both mechanically and hemodynamically, and have serious electrical imbalances. One such electrical imbalance is LQTS, which is due to altered repolarization and can be caused by congenital defects of sodium and potassium channels, electrolyte imbalances, or certain pharmacologic agents. The following discussion is limited to the congenital form of LQTS.

The congenital form of LQTS has been defined as a genetically determined abnormality of ventricular repolarization that results in cardiac instability that can lead to potentially life-threatening arrhythmias and/or sudden death. It was originally characterized by Jervell and Lange-Nielsen in 1957 as a syndrome involving congenital deafness, prolonged QT/torsades de pointes, syncope/sudden death, and autosomal recessive transmission.[18] In 1963, Romano et al.[19] and in 1964, Ward[20] described the characteristics of prolonged QT/torsades de pointes, syncope/sudden death, and an autosomal dominant inheritance pattern. All authors reported that event triggers, such as emotional stress and/or physical exertion/distress, played an important role in the precipitation of episodes.

More recently, it has become known that the sodium and potassium ion channel abnormalities seen in patients with LQTS are caused by abnormal proteins coded by mutated genes.[21] There are several different genes responsible, both dominant and recessive, with linkage to chromosome 11 (LQT1), chromosome 7 (LQT2), chromosome 3 (LQT3), and chromosome 4 (LQT4).[21–24] This rudimentary understanding of genotype/phenotype relationships has led to a better understanding of the affected ion channels which in turn has redirected our efforts at more effective treatments.[25] For example, patients with some sodium channel defect forms of LQTS are now very effectively treated with the sodium channel blocker, mexiletine.

It is important to note that not all patients with prolonged QT intervals have LQTS and, perhaps more importantly, not all patients with LQTS have a prolonged QT interval at rest. Approximately 50% of patients with LQTS have hereditary transmission and the mortality in untreated individuals approaches 60% within 10 years of their initial syncopal episode.[26] Children are frequently misdiagnosed with benign syncope or seizure disorders.[27,28]

Clinical Presentation

The diagnosis of LQTS relies on a group of clinical and ECG manifestations. The clinical presentation of patients with LQTS is varied and can include the following: syncope (associated with noise, stress, and/or exercise), presyncope, palpitations, seizures, ventricular arrhythmias, cardiac arrest, and sudden death. Associated findings include congenital AV block, congenital deafness (rare), syndactyly (rare), and a family history of LQTS or sudden death.

Electrocardiographic Characteristics

ECG criteria for LQTS include, but are not limited to, a prolonged corrected QT interval (QTc), variations in T wave morphology, bradycardia, and ventricular arrhythmias (Fig. 11). The QT interval is measured from the beginning of the QRS complex to the end of the T wave. A high-quality 12-lead ECG with minimal filtering, i.e., 0.1 to 100 Hz, is necessary for accurate measurements, thus making 24-hour ambulatory monitors, transport monitors, and standard hospital monitors relatively ineffective in this regard. One of the most difficult aspects of QT measurement is determining the terminal portion of the T wave, as well as whether to include a "second hump" or U wave in the measurement (Fig. 12). In general, if the U wave is ≥50% of the height of the T wave, it should be included in the measurement.

Once the QT interval is measured, it must be corrected for heart rate. This is done using Bazett's formula of QTc = QT interval divided by the square root of the preceding R-R interval measured in seconds.[29] The QT interval is best measured in surface ECG lead II. A QTc of 0.44 seconds (or

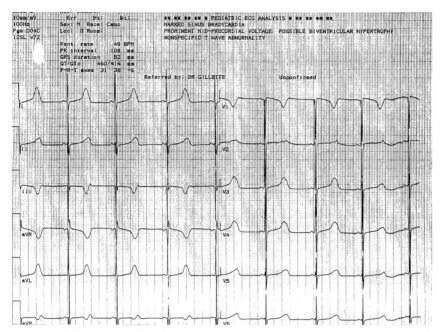

Figure 11. Initial 12-lead ECG from a patient with long QT syndrome and sinus brady-cardia. Note that the computer algorithm failed to detect the prolonged corrected QT interval. This patient experienced sudden death during excitement despite being treated with β-blockers and a permanent cardiac pacemaker.

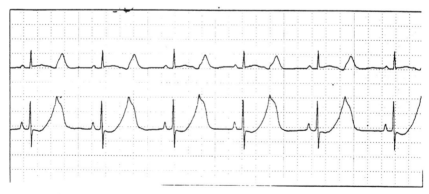

Figure 12. Simultaneously recorded surface ECG leads taken from a 24-hour ambulatory monitor in a patient with long QT syndrome. The second part of the T or U wave is very large, as is often the case in these particular patients. There is 2:1 AV block in this patient due to delayed repolarization of the ventricular myocardium. The blocked P waves are the sharp and pointed portion of the large T waves seen best in the lower lead.

440 ms) or greater is considered prolonged. Modern ECG machines will often automatically calculate ECG intervals using predetermined criteria (Fig. 13). The machine will place annotation marks on the points that it has used to calculate these intervals. One should always use caution in accepting these measurements at face value; thus, the accuracy of the

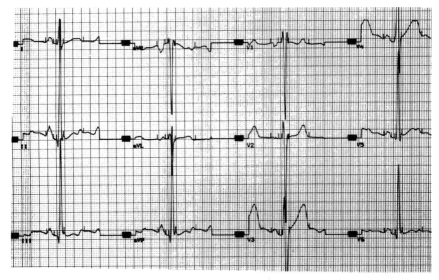

Figure 13. Twelve-lead surface ECG with "annotation marks" depicting measurements of the PR, QRS, and QT intervals in a patient with a normal sinus rhythm. This computerized system measures the QT interval while ignoring the small "U" waves. Using this system, the earliest Q wave is compared to the last T wave offset in any given lead. The corrected QT interval is then calculated based on the R-R interval.

annotation marks should always be evaluated to ensure that they have been placed correctly (Fig. 14). A hand measurement should always be made to verify the accuracy of the computer-generated value.

Another ECG characteristic helpful in the diagnosis of LQTS is the T wave morphology. The following are T wave characteristics that may be

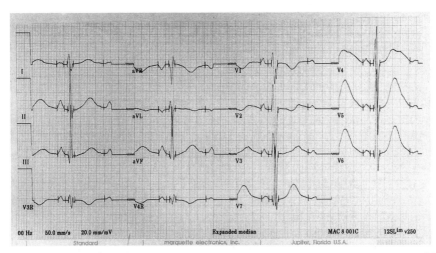

Figure 14. Fifteen-lead surface ECG with "annotation marks" in a patient with long QT syndrome. Note the abnormal T waves in the left precordial leads. The computerized program accurately annotates the T wave offset.

seen in patients with LQTS: notched T waves; T wave alternans; low-amplitude, delayed T waves; broad-based, prolonged T waves; biphasic T waves; and a normal T wave after a prolonged ST segment. Additional ECG criteria include sinus bradycardia and AV block, the latter of which is frequently 2:1 AV block. Ventricular arrhythmias that may be seen include PVCs, VT, torsades de pointes, and VF. Torsades de pointes is a form of polymorphic VT that is generally associated with a prolonged QT interval (Fig. 15); its name comes from its appearance in that the QRS complexes are "twisting" around a center axis.[30]

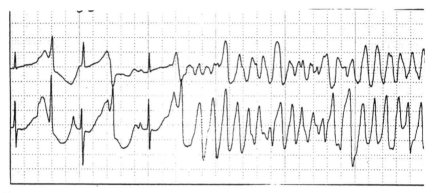

Figure 15. Twenty-four-hour ambulatory ECG recording of torsades de pointes. There is variation in the T wave morphology at the beginning of the recording with a very long QT interval. Torsades de pointes is depicted as a rhythmic change from larger to smaller to larger QRS complexes with a rapid ventricular rate.

Adjunct Diagnostic Tools

Other diagnostic tools include exercise stress testing, ambulatory monitoring, detailed patient and family history, and occasionally, catecholamine infusions. Exercise stress testing may reveal the following: lack of QT shortening with exercise, failure to achieve maximal heart rate response, exaggerated QT prolongation during recovery (1 minute), T wave alternans, and ventricular arrhythmias. Although 24-hour ambulatory monitoring should not be used for the initial diagnosis of LQTS, it can be used to assess for bradycardia or AV block, T wave abnormalities, and ventricular arrhythmias. Catecholamine infusions can be helpful in identifying those patients with LQTS who exhibit a normal QT interval on resting ECG. In patients without LQTS, the administration of catecholamines results in QT shortening with faster heart rates. Those patients with covert LQTS will exhibit the opposite of what is considered normal, i.e., QT prolongation.

The importance of recognizing LQTS can be appreciated when one considers the sudden death that may occur if it is not diagnosed and treated properly. A careful family history is extremely helpful in most cases, and should include questions about sudden death, seizures, pre-syncope, or syncope, especially in younger relatives.[31] Since symptoms may be related to exercise, noise, or anger, specific questions should be asked that address these issues. The compilation of a family pedigree can potentially provide a pattern of suspicious situations and can help trace transmission of the disease.

Management Strategies

Once the diagnosis of LQTS is made, the specific treatment modality is dependent on the presenting symptoms and family history and varies from patient to patient. Treatment modalities include medical therapy (with β-blockers, mexiletine, or phenytoin), permanent cardiac devices (pacemakers and/or implantable cardioverter defibrillators [ICDs]), left stellate ganglionectomy, and activity and medicine restrictions. Other management issues include cardiopulmonary resuscitation training for family members, automatic external defibrillators (AEDs), screening of other family members, and genetic counseling. These issues are discussed further in the section on patient and family considerations

Brugada Syndrome

The Brugada syndrome is a newly recognized syndrome of altered re-polarization, characterized on surface ECG by a right bundle branch block pattern with ST segment elevation in leads V_1 and V_3[32] (Fig. 16). It occurs in patients with structurally normal hearts and, like LQTS, can result in syncope and/or sudden death in otherwise healthy patients. It is geneti-cally determined, is thought to be transmitted through an autosomal dom-inant pattern,[32] and results in an abnormality of the sodium channel.

The first known patient with Brugada syndrome was a 3-year-old Pol-ish boy who had experienced multiple syncopal episodes and multiple re-suscitations by his father and had a sibling who died unexpectedly at 2 years of age with a very similar ECG.[33] The sibling also had several episodes of aborted sudden death and an abnormal resting ECG; however, at the time of her death she was being treated with amiodarone and a ven-tricular pacemaker.

At this time, it is difficult to ascertain the incidence of Brugada syn-drome, but it may account for 4% to 12% of unexpected sudden deaths.[33] It appears at present that the syndrome is more prevalent in males than fe-males and seems to have a higher incidence in southeast Asia, suggestive of a genetic predetermination to the disease.[33] Similar to LQTS, Brugada syndrome is thought to be a defect in the encoding of genes that form that cardiac action potential, specifically, the sodium channel *SCN5A*.[34] These genetic mutations can result in total loss of function of the sodium channel to acceleration of the sodium channel's recovery from inactivation.

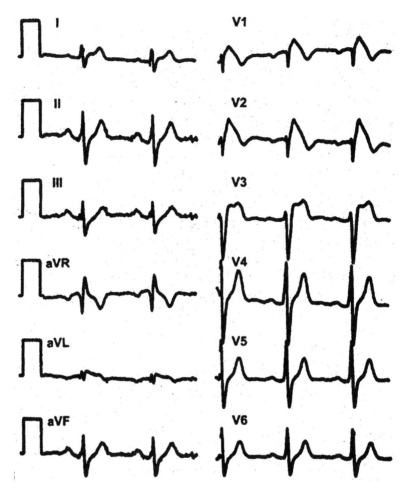

Figure 16. Typical surface ECG pattern seen in patients with Brugada syndrome, including the appearance of a right bundle branch block pattern in lead V_1 and ST segment elevation in leads V_1 to V_3. There is also slight prolongation of the PR interval. Reproduced from Antzelevitch C, Brugada P, Brugada J, et al: The Brugada Syndrome. In Camm AJ (ed.): Clinical Approaches to Tachyarrhythmias. Vol. 10. Armonk, NY: Futura Publishing Company, Inc.; 1999:3, with permission.

Clinical Presentation

Unfortunately in patients with Brugada syndrome, the only presenting symptom may be sudden death.[35] Other potential manifestations include an abnormal resting ECG, syncope, and/or ventricular arrhythmias. The syncopal and sudden death episodes in these patients are the result of rapid, polymorphic VT or VF. These episodes are spontaneous and without prodrome. There may be a history of resuscitated sudden death episodes as well as a family history of sudden cardiac death.

Electrocardiographic Characteristics

The typical ECG of patients with Brugada syndrome exhibits a pattern of right bundle branch block and ST segment elevation. The most common ventricular arrhythmia exhibited by these patients is polymorphic VT or VF.

Management Strategies

The prognosis of patients with Brugada syndrome who go undiagnosed and/or untreated is extremely poor. The difficulty in treating these patents becomes difficult to justify when there are no symptoms. Symptomatic patients are definitely at risk for sudden death, and since antiarrhythmic drugs cannot prevent sudden death,[35] the most definitive treatment is placement of an ICD.

Idiopathic Ventricular Tachycardia

There are two additional clinically identifiable types of VT that occur in children and young adults with anatomically normal hearts. They are both relatively benign in that they are not often associated with sudden death and they are both sensitive to the calcium channel blocker, verapamil. One of these is known as right ventricular outflow tract (RVOT) tachycardia and the other as left ventricular septal (or left posterior fascicular) tachycardia.[36]

RVOT tachycardia is due to an automatic (or ectopic) focus located in the RVOT or to delayed afterdepolarizations.[37] It is a paroxysmal type of tachycardia that, like other ectopic/automatic focus tachycardias, cannot be initiated or terminated by pacing maneuvers. It is sensitive to the agent isoproterenol. Left ventricular septal tachycardia tends to be more sustained than RVOT tachycardia and, although unclear at this time, the mechanism is thought to be reentry.

Clinical Presentation

Patients with either of these types of idiopathic VT may present with the tachycardia itself or with single, uniform PVCs. In most cases, the patient will complain of palpitations and/or sensations of a rapid heartbeat, but he or she rarely suffers hemodynamic compromise.

Electrocardiographic Characteristics

RVOT tachycardia is characterized on surface ECG by a left bundle branch block pattern with an inferior axis (Fig. 17). There may be short, nonsustained runs of tachycardia, single, uniform PVCs, or sustained

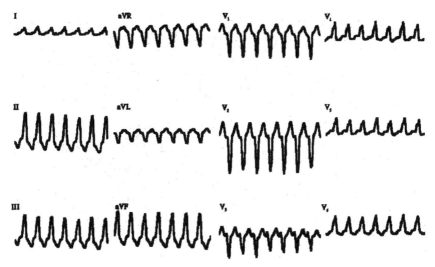

Figure 17. Twelve-lead ECG recording of right ventricular outflow tract tachycardia. Note the left bundle branch block, inferior axis ECG morphology with negative complexes in lead V_1. Reproduced from Bourke JP, Doig JC: Ventricular Tachyarrhythmias in the Normal Heart. In Camm AJ (ed.): Clinical Approaches to Tachyarrhythmias. Vol. 8. Armonk, NY: Futura Publishing Company, Inc.; 1998:13, with permission.

tachycardia. Left ventricular septal tachycardia, on the other hand, is characterized on surface ECG by a right bundle branch block pattern and left anterior hemiblock (Fig. 18).

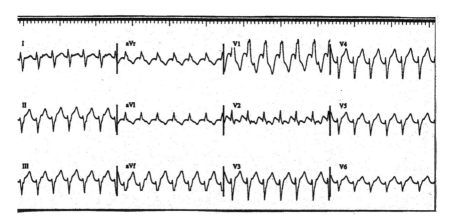

Figure 18. Twelve-lead surface ECG of idiopathic left ventricular tachycardia ("fascicular"/verapamil-sensitive). The more common form of the tachycardia has a right bundle branch block, left axis deviation morphology, and the rarer form has a right bundle branch block, right axis deviation pattern. Note the relatively narrow QRS, typically less than 150 ms. Reproduced from Bourke JP, Doig JC: Ventricular Tachyarrhythmias in the Normal Heart. In Camm AJ (ed.): Clinical Approaches to Tachyarrhythmias. Vol. 8. Armonk, NY: Futura Publishing Company, Inc.; 1998:25, with permission.

Management Strategies

As previously mentioned, both of these types of VT are sensitive to verapamil, making it the pharmacologic agent of choice in these patients.[38] Alternatively, each of these tachycardias may be amenable to radiofrequency catheter ablation (RFCA).[39,40]

Structurally Abnormal Hearts

Postoperative Congenital Heart Disease

Ventricular arrhythmias can occur in patients with unoperated CHD (e.g., mitral valve prolapse and aortic stenosis), but have been extensively studied and reported on in those patients who have undergone surgery for congenital heart defects.[41] As previously mentioned, 15% of patients with congenital cardiac defects will develop chronic ventricular arrhythmias and 5% to 10% will experience sudden death.[3] Specific congenital heart defects that result in an increased risk of postoperative arrhythmias, both ventricular and supraventricular, are listed in Table 2.

Ventricular arrhythmias in children with postoperative CHD generally occur in patients who have undergone ventriculotomies, myocardial resection, or other surgeries that may result in subsequent scarring of the myocardium. The underlying causes of these rhythm disturbances include chronic volume or pressure overload, incomplete myocardial preservation at the time of surgery, residual postoperative defects, and fibrosis at the site of ventriculotomy.[42,43] The most studied of the congenital defects is tetralogy of Fallot.[6,44–47] Risk factors for arrhythmia development include greater length of follow-up after repair, older age at repair, elevated right ventricular systolic or diastolic pressures, and/or left ventricular dysfunction.[6]

Table 2
Incidence of Postoperative Arrhythmias in Congenital Heart Defects

Type of Defect	Incidence (%)
Dextrotransposition of the great arteries following intraatrial repair	50–85
Tetralogy of Fallot	30–60
Fontan repair	25–40
Aortic and subaortic stenosis	10
Ventricular septal defect	10
Atrioventricular canal defect	10
Secundum atrial septal defect	9
Total anomalous pulmonary venous return	0

Reprinted with permission from Vetter VL: What every pediatrician needs to know about arrhythmias in children who have had cardiac surgery. Ped Ann 1991; 20:378–385.

Clinical Presentation

PVCs in a postoperative patient may be discovered by routine noninvasive follow-up such as a surface ECG on a regularly scheduled outpatient visit or on a routine 24-hour ambulatory monitor. The presence of PVCs on a resting ECG is somewhat ominous, as this is probably indicative of their relative frequency. It has been estimated that greater than 10 PVCs per minute on 24-hour ambulatory monitor is associated with a bad prognosis in a patient who has previously undergone surgery for tetralogy of Fallot.[48] Multiform PVCs, couplets, and nonsustained or sustained VT are also less than optimal clinical findings.

The association of a wider than usual right bundle branch block has been associated with ventricular arrhythmias, sudden death, and inducibility of VT/VF on electrophysiology study.[49,50] Gatzoulis and colleagues[49] reported, in an older series of English patients with repaired tetralogy of Fallot, that a QRS duration greater than 180 ms was an important predictor of sudden death and ventricular arrhythmias. More recently, Balaji and colleagues[50] noted that a QRS duration greater than 160 ms correlated with ventricular arrhythmia induction during routine postoperative electrophysiology testing. In both studies, the QRS duration was related to sequelae and ventricular dysfunction, thus confirming the importance of performing routine 12-lead ECG in these patients and in others with different defects as well.

As previously mentioned, some postoperative patients with ventricular arrhythmias may be completely asymptomatic, while others may experience palpitations, presyncope, syncope, and/or sudden death. Symptoms may be more pronounced in patients who experience a sustained VT than in those who present with PVCs. Obviously, those with VF will present with syncope and/or sudden death.

Electrocardiographic Characteristics

The ECG characteristics of ventricular arrhythmias in patients after surgery for CHD vary from patient to patient. The PVCs may assume a right, left, or intermittent bundle branch block morphology depending on their site of origin. Both monomorphic and polymorphic tachycardias occur in postoperative patients.

Adjunct Diagnostic Tools

Use of the signal-averaged ECG to detect late potentials in postoperative patients has not proven very useful in this patient population, probably in part because so many of the patients have right bundle branch block, which skews the interpretation.

Routine 24-hour ambulatory monitoring every 2 to 3 years is useful in following postoperative patients with the potential for ventricular arrhythmias. The frequency of ventricular events and their complexity can be assessed, along with their hemodynamic and ECG data, to predict problems during follow-up. Changes over time and/or in response to treatment can also be documented.

Exercise stress testing has been helpful in detecting ventricular arrhythmias after repair of tetralogy of Fallot; however, the disappearance of PVCs during exercise testing does not suggest (or predict) that the patient is not at risk for VT or sudden death.[51] This is distinctly different from the patient with an anatomically normal heart.[4] Exacerbation of PVCs during exercise stress testing is probably an important negative prognostic sign.

Transtelephonic monitoring can be used when the arrhythmia is transient and cannot be documented by routine ECG or 24-hour ambulatory monitor. Specific devices that have been found to be most helpful are those with memory and/or looping capabilities.

Intracardiac electrophysiology studies are reported to have mixed results when used in patients after surgery for tetralogy of Fallot. In a previously reported series, a negative electrophysiology study predicted 100% freedom from sudden death in 100 postoperative tetralogy of Fallot patients.[50] Two patients later developed sustained monomorphic VT which was well tolerated. One large multicenter study of the efficacy of electrophysiology study in postoperative tetralogy of Fallot patients found it to be not useful in predicting sudden death. The stimulation protocols used in this study were extremely variable and may have affected the results.[45]

Management Strategies

Not all ventricular arrhythmias in the postoperative CHD patient require treatment, e.g., single, infrequent, monomorphic PVCs. Since there is always a risk of sudden death after CHD surgery, a high index of suspicion must be used in deciding if and when treatment is necessary. Treatment for ventricular arrhythmias after surgery for CHD can be pharmacologic, nonpharmacologic, or a combination. In each patient being considered for treatment, consideration should be given to whether interventional or surgical procedures may help suppress the arrhythmia by improving overall hemodynamics.

Pharmacologic therapy is a double-edged sword in postoperative CHD patients. Phenytoin and mexilitine have both proven to be effective and safe in patients after surgery for CHD. Both are Class Ib antiarrhythmic agents that do not prolong the QRS or QT interval. They suppress abnormal automaticity and delayed afterdepolarizations and improve conduction through diseased tissue. Garson and colleagues[48] and Moak and collegues[52] have shown the efficacy of these drugs in postoperative tetralogy of Fallot patients. James et al[53] failed to find efficacy with quinidine. Amiodarone can also be used safely in patients after surgery for CHD.[54,55] Careful monitoring of patients receiving antiarrhythmic agents must be done to assess exacerbation of bradyarrhythmias or potential proarrhythmia. Flecainide can be used with caution in postoperative patients, with use of both noninvasive and invasive monitoring.[56] β-Blockers, including sotalol, which is classified as a Class III agent but also has β-blocking properties, could theoretically lead to significant depression of sinus node function and/or ventricular contractility.

Nonpharmacologic treatment consists of hemodynamic enhancement by catheter intervention or surgery, catheter ablation, permanent pacemakers, and ICDs. The severity of the residual defect or sequelae in addition to the likelihood of improvement and the degree of arrhythmia must be considered when determining the best treatment option for a specific patient.

Permanent pacemakers are only used to treat ventricular arrhythmias when bradycardia is also present. Catheter ablation has been successful in some postoperative patients with reentry circuits in the right ventricle. These patients generally have multiple reentry circuits, and in a very abnormal right ventricle, new circuits are likely to develop, making catheter ablation a less than optimal treatment modality. New noncontact mapping systems are likely to improve results in this group of patients.

ICDs are useful in postoperative patients whose tachyarrhythmias cannot be successfully treated with drugs or catheter ablation.[57] Overdrive pacing has been successfully used to treat monomorphic VT; however, the availability of defibrillation is always necessary in the event that overdrive pacing is proarrhythmic. ICDs may also be used in postoperative patients who have VF that cannot be induced at electrophysiology study or in cases in which antiarrhythmic drugs fail to suppress the arrhythmia. The exact role of ICDs in the management of ventricular arrhythmias in postoperative CHD patients is still evolving. The indications will change not only due to improved understanding of the natural history of such arrhythmias but also due to the performance and size of the devices.

With use of the above approach, most sudden death in postoperative CHD patients can be prevented and morbidity due to ventricular arrhythmias minimized. Specific defects (other than tetralogy of Fallot) in which close surveillance and a high index of suspicion are necessary include truncus arteriosus, double-outlet right ventricle, ventricular septal defect with pulmonary hypertension, transposition of the great arteries, and repaired endocardial cushion defects.

Diseases of the Myocardium

Abnormalities of the myocardium are an important cause of ventricular arrhythmias in children. The cardiomyopathies can be subdivided into dilated, hypertrophic, restrictive, and localized. They may be acute, subacute, or chronic in nature and can be genetic, idiopathic, or viral in etiology. The primary cardiomyopathies, i.e., dilated, hypertrophic, and restrictive are discussed here, whereas viral myocarditis, a localized abnormality of the myocardium, is discussed in a later section of this chapter.

Cardiomyopathies

Dilated cardiomyopathy causes the patient to exhibit the signs and symptoms of congestive heart failure (CHF); hence the use of the term "congestive cardiomyopathy." One (usually the left) or both ventricles are dilated and hypocontractile to varying degrees, resulting in systolic dysfunction. Hypertrophic cardiomyopathy, also known as hypertrophic obstructive cardiomyopathy and, formerly, idiopathic hypertrophic subaortic stenosis, results in left ventricular hypertrophy with usually preserved systolic function but resultant left ventricular outflow obstruction, diastolic dysfunction, arrhythmias, and sudden death. Restrictive cardiomyopathy results in markedly dilated atria with generally normal ventricular size and systolic function but an impairment in diastolic filling, and thus produces symptoms related to pulmonary and right-sided systemic venous congestion.

Dilated and hypertrophic cardiomyopathies are familial and are most commonly transmitted via an autosomal dominance inheritance pattern.[58–60] Restrictive cardiomyopathy is relatively uncommon in children and accounts for only 5% of pediatric cardiomyopathies.[61] By far, the form of cardiomyopathy most associated with ventricular arrhythmias and sudden death in children is hypertrophic cardiomyopathy.

Hypertrophic cardiomyopathy is accountable for less than 1% of sudden deaths in the pediatric and young adult population, with the most common age group being from 15 to 35 years.[62] Recently, the role of ventricular arrhythmias (versus myocardial ischemia) in the sudden death of these patients has been questioned.[63] The Pediatric Electrophysiology Society evaluated these risk factors in 135 patients and found the following on 24-hour ambulatory monitor: 31% had PVCs (isolated), 14% had multiform PVCs or couplets, and 7% had VT.[64] There was a 13% incidence of sudden death in a 7-year follow-up period, but the primary risk factor was family history rather than ventricular arrhythmia documentation or hemodynamic variables. Although the presence of ventricular arrhythmias in these patients may not be predictive of sudden death, their presence must be acknowledged and subsequent treatment pursued.

Twenty-four-hour ambulatory monitoring in patients with dilated cardiomyopathy has shown a 10% to 30% incidence of VT in these patients[65–67]; however, the cause of sudden death may be bradycardia (progressing to asystole) rather than VT or fibrillation.[68] Since the ventricular arrhythmias in these patients may be more related to worsening ventricular dysfunction, efforts to improve hemodynamics may result in a decreased incidence of ventricular ectopy.

Clinical Presentation

Since restrictive cardiomyopathy is less common in the pediatric population, the discussion on clinical presentation of patients with cardiomyopathy is limited to the hypertrophic and dilated forms. The clinical presentation of the child with dilated cardiomyopathy varies from patient to patient. Symptoms include the signs and symptoms of CHF, decreased exercise tolerance and dyspnea with exertion in older children, tachypnea with feeding in infants, palpitations, presyncope, syncope, tachycardia, paleness, cyanosis, decreased peripheral perfusion, and ventricular arrhythmias. The physical examination in patients with dilated cardiomyopathy may reveal diminished breath sounds, muffled heart sounds, a gallop rhythm, and a long systolic murmur. The heart is generally enlarged on chest roentgenogram.

The clinical presentation of patients with hypertrophic cardiomyopathy is similar to that of those with dilated cardiomyopathy, although some of these patients may be asymptomatic. The symptoms may include chest pain, palpitations, tachypnea, tachycardia, poor feeding, presyncope, syncope, ventricular arrhythmias, and sudden death (often after exercise). Infants may present with CHF, while older children are more prone to sudden death. The physical examination in patients with hypertrophic cardiomyopathy can be normal in some cases, but often an overactive precordium is noted upon auscultation, as is a short systolic murmur. Cardiomegaly may or may not be noted on chest roentgenogram.

Electrocardiographic Characteristics

Many ECG abnormalities are found in patients with the various cardiomyopathies. There may be P wave or QRS indicators of atrial or ventricular dilation, hypertrophy, or scarring. T wave changes or ST segment changes may also indicate myocardial disorders or ischemia. Arrhythmias seen in cardiomyopathy include atrial or ventricular premature beats or tachycardia. Polymorphic, nonsustained tachycardia is the most common type of VT seen in this subset of patients.

Adjunct Diagnostic Tools

The diagnosis of cardiomyopathy is primarily made by careful, quantitative echocardiography. Even mild dilation of the left or right ventricular end-diastolic dimension in a patient with a ventricular arrhythmia may indicate underlying myocardial pathology. Cardiac catheterization with angiography, electrophysiology testing, and myocardial biopsy are often needed in these patients to clarify etiology and severity as well as to formulate a treatment plan. An astute assessment of the patient's family history should also be included to ascertain the incidence of sudden death in family members in order to then assess the patient's relative risk.

Management Strategies

The treatment plan for patients with cardiomyopathies is often multi-faceted. Attention must be paid to myocardial function and afterload reduction without increasing myocardial irritability. Electrolyte balance is important in these patients, since hypokalemia may worsen ventricular arrhythmias. Ventricular arrhythmias should be treated in patients with moderate myocardial dysfunction, syncope, or VT. Care must be taken to avoid pharmacologic agents that may produce proarrhythmia, such as Class Ia or Ic antiarrhythmic drugs. Also, agents that depress myocardial function should only be used in patients whose myocardium can tolerate them. Mexiletine has been effective in treating some of these patients, but amiodarone has by far been the most effective with the fewest cardiac side effects.[69] In patients with hypertrophic cardiomyopathy, medical, surgical, and pacing therapies have been met with varied success.[70–72] Permanent dual chamber pacing has been successful in these patients. With pacing of the right ventricle, paradoxical movement of the interventricular septum ensues which increases the dimensions of blood flow velocity through the left ventricular outflow tract. This in turn decreases anterior motion of the mitral valve during systole and diminishes mitral regurgitation.[73] Implantable dual chamber cardioverter defibrillators can accomplish this same goal in these patients while also providing defibrillation in the presence of life-threatening ventricular arrhythmias.[74,75] Finally, cardiac transplantation may be a final option for patients with severe cardiomyopathy.[62]

Viral Myocarditis

Although myocarditis can be caused by a variety of pathogens, i.e., bacteria, fungus, protozoa, parasites, it is usually associated with a viral illness in children. Myocarditis is an inflammatory process of the heart muscle that can lead to temporary or permanent damage to myocardial structure and/or cell function. It is characterized by inflammatory infiltrate of the myocardium with necrosis and/or degeneration of adjacent myocytes not typical of the ischemic changes associated with coronary artery disease.[76] Adenovirus and Coxsackie virus are the most frequent viral etiologies for viral myocarditis. Why they lead to myocarditis in some but not all affected patients remains unclear at this time. The myocarditis itself is due to an immune response.

Clinical Presentation

The clinical presentation of children with viral myocarditis varies from patient to patient. Many patients are asymptomatic depending on whether the illness is in the acute or subacute phase. Most children will have a history of a bacterial or viral illness, and parents may note that the child seems lethargic. Other presenting symptoms include fever, tachycardia, arrhythmias (mostly PVCs), and if the myocarditis is severe, the signs and symptoms of CHF. Most patients that present with arrhythmias will exhibit ventricular ectopy, but in severe cases, may exhibit atrial tachyarrhythmias and bradyarrhythmias as well.[77]

Electrocardiographic Characteristics

In most cases, the resting ECG is normal except for arrhythmias, although ST changes may be present. The most common arrhythmia seen in these patients is PVCs. Even though the predominant arrhythmia in these patients is ventricular, patients with severe forms of the disease may exhibit tachyarrhythmias and bradyarrhythmias, including complete AV block.

Adjunct Diagnostic Tools

The echocardiogram is useful in these patients to determine ventricular size and function as well as to rule out any other cardiovascular structural abnormalities and to evaluate valve function. The most definitive diagnostic tool in these patients is the endomyocardial biopsy and subsequent microscopic analysis of the specimen.[78]

Management Strategies

The treatment of acute or subacute viral myocarditis is controversial. The use of corticosteroids is favored by some, but has not been proven in a double blind study. Depending on the presenting arrhythmia, supportive measures may only need to be temporary until the underlying substrate is treated. Although immunosuppressive therapy may result in improved histologic findings by repeat endomyocardial biopsy, it does not always result in an improvement in the ventricular arrhythmia.[79] Other studies suggest that despite the resolution of inflammation in those treated with corticosteroids but who continue to have ventricular ectopy, antiarrhythmic drug therapy may be required on a long-term basis.[80] Whether aggressive treatment of subacute myocarditis will prevent later dilated cardiomyopathy is not known. Newer therapies in addition to or instead of corticosteroids may also be considered, including the use of intravenous (IV) immune globulin.

Arrhythmogenic Right Ventricular Dysplasia

ARVD is a genetically determined disease that causes fatty replacement of the right ventricular musculature and results in arrhythmias and often sudden death. It is characterized by regional or diffuse right ventricular contraction abnormalities and a left bundle branch block QRS morphology during tachycardia episodes. It may be responsible for up to

33% of VTs in young patients with apparently normal hearts[8] and is believed to be one cause of unexplained sudden death during exertion.[81] The degree of impairment of the right ventricle can range from no functional impairment to severe impairment. The arrhythmias seen in these patients originate from the dysplastic areas of the right ventricle.

The incidence of ARVD in the general population is difficult to assess, but accounts for 29% of sudden deaths in young people in northern Italy.[81] Denfield and colleagues[62] speculate that ARVD may account for 24% to 30% of patients who present with idiopathic right VT. The disease is being recognized with increasing frequency in the United States, but the exact prevalence is still unknown. It is a familial disease[82–85] and has been genetically mapped to chromosome 14.[86,87]

Clinical Presentation

The clinical presentation of patients with ARVD varies and includes such symptoms as syncope, palpitations, PVCs, VT (often associated with exercise), and, unfortunately, sudden death.[81,85] In general, the physical examination is normal, but it may be abnormal with such associated findings as diastolic filling sounds and prominence of the left anterior thorax.[88] An irregular rhythm, due to PVCs, is often noted by peripheral pulse palpation or auscultation. Right ventricular failure is rare.

Electrocardiographic Characteristics

The PVCs and VT associated with ARVD are thought to originate in 1 of 3 areas of the right ventricle (termed the "triangle of dysplasia"),[88] leading to multiple left bundle branch block QRS morphologies during tachycardia. Additionally, T wave inversion in the anterior precordial leads during sinus rhythm and postexcitation waves at the ST segment can be characteristic of ARVD.[8] The T wave inversion, which is highly suggestive of ARVD in adults, may be overlooked in some children as it may be a normal finding in children less than 12 years of age.[89]

Adjunct Diagnostic Tools

In addition to the surface ECG, other diagnostic tools may be helpful in identifying patients with ARVD. If there is no right ventricular failure, the chest roentgenogram should be normal. Exercise stress testing may be helpful in those with exercise-induced tachycardia, but differentiation between tachycardia associated with ARVD versus that seen in patients with idiopathic RVOT is critical due to the more ominous prognosis associated with ARVD.

Echocardiography can be a useful tool in diagnosing ARVD in the presence of right ventricular dysfunction, but it is not often definitive.

Magnetic resonance imaging (MRI) can be helpful, but cardiac angiography is probably the most definitive diagnostic tool in which the hallmark of the disease, systolic bulging of the right ventricular free wall, can be delineated (Fig. 19). Additionally, cardiac catheterization can be used to assess overall hemodynamics, while endomyocardial biopsy can be used to ascertain classic pathologic changes. Electrophysiology testing should be undertaken to assess the hemodynamic consequences of the tachycardia, to determine the exact location of the arrhythmogenic substrate, and to evaluate the efficacy of various treatment modalities.

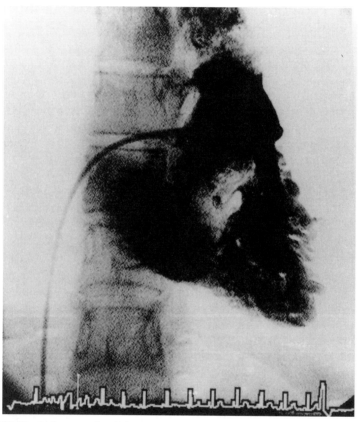

Figure 19. Posterior-anterior right ventricular angiogram in a patient with arrhythmogenic right ventricular dysplasia as evidenced by the heavy trabeculation of the right ventricle. Two "bulges" are seen in the right ventricular outflow tract, one medial and one lateral in position.

Management Strategies

The major management goal for patients with ARVD is to control the ventricular arrhythmia and attempt to prevent sudden cardiac death. Antiarrhythmic drugs including β-blockers, sotalol, amiodarone, and others can be used in these patients.[90] In patients with moderate to severe ventricular arrhythmias, treatment may include catheter ablation, ICDs,[91,92] and cardiac transplantation.

Cardiac Tumors

Noncancerous cardiac tumors can cause incessant VT in the pediatric population.[93] These tumors are known as rhabdomyomas, myocardial hamartomas or Purkinje cell tumors, and histiocytic/oncocytic tumors. Most of the patients with cardiac tumors present in infancy, but this disease entity can be seen in children up to 5 years of age.[94] Five percent to 10% of infants presenting with VT will have rhabdomyomas and tuberous sclerosis, while histiocytic or oncocytic tumors in children are extremely rare.[8] Another cardiac tumor seen in young children is the myocardial hamartoma or Purkinje cell tumor, which can be found on the epicardium or endocardium and can be multifocal. The tissue of this tumor is white to gray in color and the cells have been described as being only a few layers in thickness, similar in appearance to embryonic Purkinje cells.[93]

Clinical Presentation

The clinical presentation of children with cardiac tumors varies depending on the type of tumor and associated disease, infringement of the tumor on other intracardiac structures, and the hemodynamic effects of the ventricular arrhythmia. Because the VT associated with cardiac tumors is incessant in nature (defined as >10% of the time, but more likely >90% of the time), the presenting symptoms usually consist of CHF or cardiac arrest. The patients presenting with cardiac arrest may do so as a result of inappropriate drug treatment of what was initially thought to be supraventricular tachycardia (SVT). Some of these patients may be less symptomatic or even asymptomatic in rare cases. Due to the young age at presentation, these patients may exhibit nonspecific symptoms related to their arrhythmia but can present with symptoms common in infants with SVT, including poor feeding, pallor, lethargy, decreased peripheral pulses, and increased respiratory effort.

Electrocardiographic Characteristics

The ECG characteristics of VT in the young secondary to cardiac tumors include variable ventricular rates that may range from slightly faster than normal to up to 400 bpm.[95] Additionally, the QRS duration is wider than the QRS duration in normal sinus rhythm, but not always wider than normal for age. AV dissociation may or may not be present and/or discernable, especially in the presence of rapid ventricular rates.

Adjunct Diagnostic Tools

In this subgroup of patients, 24-hour ambulatory monitoring is helpful to ascertain tachycardia rates, morphologies, and duration of tachycardia episodes. It can also be used to evaluate treatment efficacy. Echocardiograms may or may not be helpful depending on the size of the tumor as well as its infringement on intracardiac structures. MRI has been found to delineate some tumors that echocardiography cannot. T2 weighted images were the most useful in these authors' experience. In contrast, there are tumors not detected by MRI that were visible during surgical intervention. Transesophageal pacing may be helpful in determining if AV dissociation or retrograde conduction is present. Invasive electrophysiology testing is primarily used in this subset of patients with ventricular arrhythmias to localize the site of the arrhythmogenic substrate.

Management Strategies

Historically, surgical treatment was the preferred method of treatment in infants and young children with refractory VT secondary to myocardial tumors.[95] The initial attempts at surgical intervention were successful but, with newer and better pharmacologic agents, medical therapy is now being used with increasing frequency.[94] Antiarrhythmic medications used to treat incessant VT secondary to cardiac tumors include amiodarone, flecainide, propranolol, and propafenone.[94,96,97] Surgery is generally reserved for those who are medically refractory and whose symptoms are deemed life-threatening. Interestingly, the natural history of some of these tumors is to regress in size over the years, eventually requiring no treatment. Because the arrhythmia is likely to subside over time and most of these patients are infants, RFCA is rarely performed.

Implications for Clinicians

Nurses and other clinicians involved in the care of children and young adults with ventricular arrhythmias must have a basic knowledge of arrhythmia mechanisms in children as well as of the disease entities associated with the particular arrhythmogenic substrate. It is not always necessary to be able to identify the specific arrhythmia, but it is critical that the caregiver be able to assess the hemodynamic effect that the arrhythmia is having (or not having) on the patient. This section reviews the general clinical implications for children with PVCs, VT, and VF, and is followed by more disease-specific implications in the section on patient and family considerations.

Premature Ventricular Contractions

Most patients with PVCs are hemodynamically stable, yet the clinician should constantly monitor the ECG for any changes in the patient's baseline status. These changes include increases in the frequency of PVC occurrence, changes in PVC morphology, progression from single PVCs to more in succession (i.e., couplets, triplets, or VT), and any changes in the patient's hemodynamic response to the ventricular arrhythmia. Additionally, any changes in the patient's level of consciousness, vital signs, color, respiratory status, and/or peripheral pulses should be documented and communicated to the patient's physician, as should any of the previously mentioned arrhythmia changes.

The clinician should also be cognizant of any other potential causes of ventricular ectopy, such as central venous lines or pacing catheters, electrolyte imbalances, and certain pharmacologic agents. If the patient experiencing PVCs requires IV line placement, patency of that line and site characteristics should be continuously assessed. In patients with CHD, an air filter should be placed on all IV lines to alleviate the risk of air embolism.

Clinicians caring for patients with PVCs must be knowledgeable regarding the potential treatment modalities for these patients. If pharmacologic agents are to be used, the nurse should be aware of the drug's mechanism of action, dosage, duration of action, potential adverse effects, any known drug interactions, and reversal agents (if available) (see chapters 4 and 5). Patient and family education is pivotal in the care of patients with PVCs. This education should involve information regarding the arrhythmia itself, any nursing or medical procedures that the child must undergo, and any treatment modalities that are being considered. All explanations should be brief, simple, repeated often, and in terms that each individual patient and his or her family can understand.

Ventricular Tachycardia

VT in young patients can be a difficult problem and can result in hemodynamic compromise. Again, any changes in the tachycardia, i.e., changes in QRS morphology, heart rate, or frequency, should be documented and immediately reported to the child's physician. A continuous assessment of the child should include any changes in level of consciousness, decreased peripheral pulses, hypotension, pallor, cyanosis, mottling, tachypnea, nasal retractions, and the use of accessory muscles with respiration. Any hint of hemodynamic compromise should be immediately communicated to the child's attending physician.

The clinician should maintain and continuously assess any lines used for peripheral or central venous access, including patency and entry/exit site characteristics, especially when administering medications that may cause vein irritation. Air filters should be placed on all patients with suspected or known CHD to alleviate the risk of air embolism.

The clinician should be knowledgeable regarding all treatment modalities, including the principles of cardioversion and defibrillation[98,99] in the event that assistance is needed with these maneuvers. If administering antiarrhythmic drugs, the nurse should be aware of that agent's mechanism of action, dosage, duration of action, potential adverse effects, any known drug interactions, and reversal agents (if available). Many of these agents have cardiac side effects that can worsen the child's condition. β-Blockers are known to depress myocardial contractility, while sodium channel blockers are associated with proarrhythmia. The child's response to the antiarrhythmic agent being administered should be evaluated and documented, including both therapeutic and adverse effects.

Ventricular Fibrillation

Although rare in the pediatric population, VF is a cardiac emergency that if not quickly corrected ends in the patient's demise. Because the morphology of VF is similar to that of an ECG electrode that is not making good skin contact, it is pivotal that the nurse assess the patient, not the ECG monitor. Prior to initiating any treatment, the nurse should assess the patient's airway, breathing, and circulation. Once breathlessness and pulselessness have been established, cardiopulmonary resuscitation should be initiated. Other emergency measures include establishing IV or intraosseous access, assistance with defibrillation, administration of emergency medications, and airway management.

Patient and Family Considerations

The impact of ventricular arrhythmias on the patient and family can be quite devastating, depending on the specific arrhythmia, the underlying etiology, the treatment modality used for the arrhythmia, and the family's ability to understand and cope with the diagnosis and subsequent plan of care. The specific considerations for the patient and family are discussed in the same manner as the implications for clinicians. General considerations are reviewed for PVCs, VT, and VF, and are followed by more specific information related to the specific disease processes associated with ventricular arrhythmias.

Premature Ventricular Contractions

Abnormal findings associated with the heart, benign or otherwise, can provoke anxiety in the calmest of individuals. At initial presentation, the child and family may be extremely anxious, with many questions that may not immediately have answers. One of the most important services that health care professionals can provide is patient and family education.

The first step is to determine what the patient and family already know (or don't know) about the child's condition. Once a baseline knowledge assessment is made, a plan of care can be developed. Because of the overwhelming anxiety of having a "heart problem," the ability to retain information is often fleeting at best. The best patient education is that which is provided in a simple, brief, and repetitive manner. Any written information that can be provided is extremely helpful, since the patient and family can refer to this at a later date, hopefully when their anxiety level has decreased.

In most cases, the child diagnosed with PVCs will require further follow-up by a pediatric cardiovascular specialist. In the case of benign PVCs, parents should be encouraged to treat their child normally and to not place unnecessary activity restrictions on the child. It is often hard for these families to "let go" of their anxiety once presented with essentially a normal cardiovascular evaluation. Reinforcement of the child's normalcy by the cardiovascular caregivers is important in alleviating some of this anxiety.

The differential diagnosis of PVCs associated with a specific disease entity has a different impact on the patient and family. In cases where the etiology requires further assessment, the child may be required to undergo additional testing. These tests may include 24-hour ambulatory monitoring, MRI, cardiac catheterization, electrophysiology testing, and/or endomyocardial biopsy. Explanations of these procedures as well as what to expect in the hospital environment should be given to the child in age-appropriate language and parental information provided as simply or in as much detail as the family requires. The patients and families that come in contact with cardiovascular caregivers have a variety of educational backgrounds and knowledge levels that must be taken into account when planning care and providing patient and family education.

Ventricular Tachycardia

In caring for patients with VT, patient and family education as well as psychosocial support is a crucial component of the overall plan of care. The arrhythmia should be explained to the child in age-appropriate language and to the family, based on a previous assessment of their baseline knowledge level. Anything that the child must undergo, nursing interventions, medical procedures, or medicine administration, should be explained to the patient and family prior to its implementation. Once again, brief and simple information that is repeated often will help the family retain information and will also provide an opportunity for them to ask questions.

The nurse caring for these patients and their families plays an important role in helping the family to understand and hopefully cope with the child's illness. Simply taking time to sit down and talk with them regarding their feelings about the child and the impact on the family is extremely helpful. When their fears and concerns are identified, coping strategies can be delineated and if other resources are deemed necessary (i.e., clergy, social services, child life, psychiatry), they can be pursued. A written "plan" can be very helpful to these families, especially those with children who are newly diagnosed, and should include the child's diagnosis, medications, signs and symptoms requiring notification of the child's cardiologist, and any activity restrictions imposed on the child. This "plan" can be shared with others who participate in the child's care, including primary care providers, dentists, teachers, school nurses, and even emergency medical services.

Ventricular Fibrillation

VF, secondary to its lethal nature, can provoke the most emotional reaction from the patient's family. At this time, as much support as possible should be afforded to these families, including clergy, social services, and/or psychiatric services. Because many of these families are angry that their child has fibrillated, they may need to be encouraged to ventilate their feelings. During the attempted resuscitation, the nurse should provide ongoing information to the patient's family. This should be done at regular intervals and in a private and quiet environment away from other families.

If the child is successfully resuscitated, he/she may also need to ventilate. Many patients are unable to remember what happened, while on the other hand, the parents can hardly stop talking about it. This is often distressing to the patient but, at the same time, healthy for the parent. If the child seems upset or bothered by his or her parents constantly "reliving" the event, it might be better if they discussed their feelings outside of the child's presence. In some instances, the patient and/or family may require counseling by a professional trained in psychology or psychiatry.

If the child cannot be resuscitated, the family will experience a huge emotional crisis. They may exhibit extreme shock, disbelief that this happened to them and their child, and guilt that they are somehow responsible. Other responses include anticipatory grief, denial, withdrawal, and/or avoidance.[100] In the event that the child dies, the nurse should allow the parents an opportunity to be with their child at the bedside. Emotional support is pivotal at this time and can range from just being silently present to providing a quiet place for the family to telephone relatives and assisting with initiating funeral arrangements.

Primary Electrical Diseases

The primary electrical diseases previously discussed include LQTS, Brugada syndrome, and idiopathic VT. Since Brugada syndrome is a newly recognized disease and very little is known about event triggers and patient and family precautions, this discussion is limited to the patient and family considerations associated with LQTS and idiopathic VT.

Long QT Syndrome

Once the diagnosis of LQTS is made, there is much to be accomplished in regard to patient and family education. Because there are still many things about LQTS that are unknown, this task can be somewhat difficult. Once again, available information regarding the disease itself should be provided to the patient in age-appropriate language and to the family in simple terms that they are able to understand. Repeating the information often and providing any written material on the disease and/or treatments can be quite helpful.

Since the treatment modalities are varied depending on the presenting symptoms and family history, the patient and family education should be tailored to the specific treatment(s). The child receiving antiarrhythmic drugs should be informed of the drug's intended action, any potential adverse effects, and what to do if a dose is inadvertently missed. The importance of taking the medication should be stressed to both the patient and family. The authors prefer the use of name brand antiarrhythmic medications versus generic ones and parents are told to notify their cardiologist if the pharmacist attempts to substitute generic for name brand. In most cases, the agents are very similar in constitution, but there are variations because the generic brands are not always as rigorously tested for bioavailability and absorption. Any written material that may be helpful is a useful adjunct (Table 3).

Patients who receive implantable devices as a treatment modality have specific needs prior to, during, and after device implantation. Once again, the nurse should provide ongoing information to the patient and family regarding the work-up prior to the device implantation, what to expect during the procedure and subsequent hospitalization, the recuperation period, and ongoing needs and issues that occur once the child has been discharged from the hospital. More in-depth information regarding these issues can be found in chapters 7 and 8.

If there are other children in the family, appointments should be made for them to undergo initial screening for LQTS. The parents should also be screened, and if they are planning on expanding their family, genetic counseling should be encouraged. In many institutions, genetic studies are being undertaken to screen as many relatives as possible in order to further delineate the pathology, etiology, and genetic basis of LQTS.

Since LQTS is associated with life-threatening arrhythmias, it is part of the authors' protocol to have at least the parents trained in basic life support (i.e., cardiopulmonary resuscitation). This can be done in the hospital environment if the child is hospitalized for treatment or through community-based programs through the local chapter of the American Heart Association.

The need for early defibrillation has prompted the use of AEDs in the general population.[101,102] Many parents of children with LQTS are now asking if this is an appropriate device for them to have in the event that

Table 3
Written Instructions for Patients Receiving Mexiletine

Name of medication: Your child's dose:	MEXILETINE (Mexitil) _____ _____
What it does:	Mexiletine helps to decrease or stop episodes of irregular or fast heart beats in the lower chambers of the heart.
What you need to know:	Mexiletine is usually taken three times a day. It is best to give this medication at the same time each day. It is not necessary to wake your child to give this medication. Instead, space the doses apart evenly during your child's waking hours. *If your child does not swallow capsules, or your child's dose is not the exact amount that is in one capsule, you will need to make a liquid form of the capsule. Your nurse will teach you how to make a liquid form if this is needed or will contact your pharmacy. A blood test is usually done at your regular check-up with the heart doctor to tell whether the Mexiletine dose your child is taking is still right for him or her.
Things to watch for:	Headaches, dizziness, and stomach upset are side effects of Mexiletine. It is best to take this medicine with some type of food. This food could be a cracker or applesauce. It may cause your child to have a stomachache if taken on an empty stomach. If your child passes out while taking this medicine, please notify your heart doctor immediately.
What to do if you miss a dose:	If is has been more than 3 hours since the scheduled time, wait until the next dose. If it has been less than 3 hours, give the medicine.

*GET YOUR PRESCRIPTION REFILLED 1 WEEK BEFORE IT RUNS OUT. ALSO, ASK FOR A NEW PRESCRIPTION AT YOUR VISITS.

*KEEP THIS AND ALL MEDICINES OUT OF THE REACH OF CHILDREN

*CONSULT YOUR PHYSICIAN BEFORE BECOMING PREGNANT WHEN TAKING ANY MEDICINE.

If you have any questions, please call:

Your Pediatric Cardiologist or
Your Cardiology Nurse, _____ or
Your Primary Care Provider, _____.

their child experiences a life-threatening arrhythmia. Currently, AEDs are indicated for use in children over 8 years of age[103] and are manufactured by a variety of vendors. Some insurance companies or third party payers will pay for the device with a physician's order if it is deemed medically necessary. The decision to procure one of these devices for home use should be discussed by the patient/family with the child's pediatric cardiologist/electrophysiologist.

One of the hardest things that the nurse caring for patients with LQTS must do is reinforce the prescribed activity restrictions. This is very difficult in young, sports-minded teenagers who may become very angry and defiant when told that they are no longer able to participate in competitive athletics. Reinforcement and an explanation in laymen's terms of why this is so important should be implemented.

The family must be made aware of certain drugs that patients with LQTS should avoid. Since the list seems to get longer every day, clinicians caring for patients with LQTS must remain abreast of any new developments in order to pass this information along to patients and families. Two organizations, the Sudden Arrhythmia Death Syndromes (SADS) Foundation and the Cardiac Arrhythmias Research and Education (CARE) Foundation, provide updated lists and will supply them free of charge to healthcare providers and patients and their families. Because any of these agents could likely result in a negative outcome, it is important that all personnel involved in the care of the patient with LQTS be informed. This includes primary care providers, dentists, and other practitioners who are likely to prescribe medication for these patients. Because several of the agents can be obtained without a prescription, it is critical that the parents remain cognizant of the medications to avoid. Alternative medications should be discussed with the child's cardiologist. The current list of medications that patients with LQTS should avoid can be found in Tables 4 and 5. The family should be encouraged to share this list with their primary care provider, dentist, and any other health care practitioner who becomes involved in the child's care.

Support groups for patients with LQTS can be very helpful. For a patient who is newly diagnosed, talking to another patient of the same age may be helpful. Support network meetings in which the entire family is involved have proven very helpful, because not only can the parents, patient, and siblings get individual support, but the families can get more medical information about the disease itself. Many patients now rely on the Internet to obtain information and to communicate with other patients. As health care professionals, we must ensure that our patients get correct information about the disease, specific treatment options, and current research.

Although support groups and support network meetings are sufficient for most families, some patients (and their families) will need to be referred for professional psychological counseling. It is extremely important that cardiovascular health care providers stress to the patient and

Table 4
Drugs to Avoid in Patients with Long QT Syndrome

Drug (brand names)	Drug Class (clinical usage)
Amiodarone (Cordarone)	Antiarrhythmic (heart rhythm)
Amitriptyline (Elavil, Endep)	Antidepressant (depression, pain, others)
*Amoxapine (Asendin)	Antidepressant (depression, pain, others)
Ampicillin (Omnipen, Principen, Polycillin)	Antibiotic
Astemizole (Hismanal)	Antihistamine (allergy)
Bepridil (Vascor)	Antianginal (heart pain)
Chlorpromazine (Thorazine)	Mental illness and nausea/vomiting
Cisapride (Propulsid)	Stimulates intestinal motility
Clarithropmycin (Biaxin)	Antibiotic
*Clemastine (Tavist)	Antihistamine
Clomipramine (Anafranil)	Mental illness
Desipramine (Norpramin)	Antidepressant (depression and others)
Diphenhydramine (Benadryl)	Antihistamine
Disopyramide (Norpace)	Antiarrhythmic (heart rhythm)
Doxepin (Sinequan, Zonalon)	Antidepressant (depression, pain, others)
Erythromycin (Akne-Mycin, E.E.S., EryDerm, Erygel, Ery-Tab, Erythrocin, Erythromycin Base Filmtab, Erythro-statin Ilotycin, PCE, Staticin)	Antibiotic and intestinal stimulant
*Flecainide (Tambocor)	Antiarrhythmic (heart rhythm)
Fludrocortisone (Florinef)	Maintain blood pressure/retain sodium
*Fluphenazine (Prolixin)	Mental illness, Parkinson's disease
Haloperidol (Haldol)	Mental illness, agitation
Ibutilide (Corvert)	Antiarrhythmic (heart rhythm)
Imipramine (Tofranil)	Antidepressant (depression, pain, others)

Table 4
Drugs to Avoid in Patients with Long QT Syndrome (*cont.*)

Drug (brand names)	Drug Class (clinical usage)
Indapamide (Lozol)	Diuretic (stimulates water and salt loss)
*Ipecac	Stimulates vomiting in poisoning
Maprotiline (Ludiomil)	Antidepressant (depression)
*Moricizine (Ethmozine)	Antiarrhythmic (heart rhythm)
Nortriptyline (Pamelor)	Antidepressant (depression and others)
Pentamidine (Pentacarinat, Pentam, NebuPent)	Anti-infective (pneumonia and others)
*Perphenazine (Trilafon)	Mental illness
Pimozide (Orap)	Tourette's syndrome, seizures
Probucol (Lorelco)	Lowers cholesterol
Procainamide (Procan, Procanbid, Pronestyl)	Antiarrhythmic (heart rhythm)
Prochlorperazine (Compazine)	Nausea
*Protriptyline (Vivactil)	Antidepressant (depression)
Quinidine (Cardioquin, Duraquin, Quinidex, Quinaglute)	Antiarrhythmic (heart rhythm)
*Ipecac Risperidone (Risperdal)	Mental illness
Sotalol (Betapace)	Antiarrhythmic (heart rhythm)
Tamoxifin (Nolvadex)	Breast cancer treatment
Terfenadine (Seldane)	Antihistamine (allergy)
Thioridazine (Mellaril)	Mental illness
Thiothixene (Navane)	Mental illness
*Tocainide (Tonocard)	Antiarrhythmic
*Trifluoperazine (Stelazine)	Mental illness
Trimethoprim sulfamethoxazole (Bactrim, Septra)	Antibiotic

*There are only limited data to suggest the drug's ability to prolong QT or induce torsades de pointes. Reproduced from SADS Heart to Hearth. Sudden Arrhythmia Death Syndromes Foundation. Salt Lake City, UT 1999, with permission.

Table 5
Additional Drugs to be Avoided in Patients
with the Long QT Syndrome

The following drugs have the potential to stimulate the sympathetic nervous system and therefore should be avoided in patients with the long QT syndrome. If they must be given, careful monitoring is essential.

Asthma/allergy medications	Asthma medications
Ephedrine (Adrenaline, Bronchaid, Epifin, Epinal, Epipen, Epitrate, Eppy/N, Medihaler, Epi, S-2) Isoproterenol (Isuprel, Medihaler-Iso)	Albuterol (Proventil, Ventolin, Ventolin Rotahaler or syrup, Volmax Xopenex) Metaproterenol (Alupent, Metaprel, Metaproterenol) Salmeterol (Serevent) Terbutaline (Brethaire, Brethine, Brethine-SC, Bricanyl)
Decongestants Phenylephrine (Neosynephrine) Phenylpropanolamine (Acutrim, Dexatrim, Phenoxine, Phenyldrine, Propagest, Phindecon) Pseudoephredrine (Novafed, Pedia-Care Decongestant, Sudafed)	**Diet pills** Fenfluramine (Pondimin) Phentermine (Adipex, Fastin, Ionamin, Obenix, Obephen, Obermine, Obestin, T-diet) Sibutramine (Meridia)
Drugs to prevent low blood pressure Midodrine (ProAmatine) Norepinephrine (Levophed)	**Medication to prevent premature labor** Ritodrine (Yotopar)

Reproduced from SADS Heart to Hearth. Sudden Arrhythmia Death Syndromes Foundation. Salt Lake City, UT 1999.

families that referral to these services is only a "phone call away" and that it is "okay" to use these services. In some cases, patients and families just need an objective listener who is not directly involved in their care. This opportunity can be used to express fear, anxiety, and even anger about their diagnosis and any treatments. This type of therapy is as important to the overall well being of the child and his or her family, as the child's medical care and should be initiated when their usual coping abilities have become ineffective.

Idiopathic Ventricular Tachycardia

Although idiopathic VT is still a somewhat frightening diagnosis for patients and families, children with this condition have a fairly positive prognosis. The treatment options of antiarrhythmic medication or RFCA make palliation and cure more likely. These patients and their families should also be encouraged to ventilate their feelings regarding their diagnosis and subsequent treatment plans. More specific patient and family considerations can be found in chapters 5 and 6.

Structurally Abnormal Hearts and Diseases of the Myocardium

The patient and family considerations for patients with structurally abnormal hearts vary according to the specific underlying disease etiology. The specific disease states include postoperative CHD, cardiomyopathies, viral myocarditis, ARVD, and cardiac tumors.

Postoperative Congenital Heart Disease

Many patients who have undergone surgery for CHD are quite shocked when an arrhythmia is discovered. Chronic illness is known for its negative effects on the child and family, especially in the adolescent and young adult age group.[104–106] These patients may become sad, depressed, or angry, especially when faced with the need for more treatments and potential hospitalizations. Once again, these patients should be encouraged to ventilate their feelings. They should be allowed to make as many decisions as possible regarding their care, and should be paired with other patients their age with similar conditions for support. Additionally, these patients and their families should be encouraged to pursue any available support groups.

Since many of the patients with ventricular arrhythmias after surgery for CHD are adolescents and young adults, the issues and challenges that they must endure are immense. Such issues include, but are not limited to, parental overprotectiveness, physical growth and activity limitations, interpersonal relationships, repeat hospitalizations and procedures, sexuality and reproductive issues, employability, and insurability.[107]

Cardiomyopathies

The family of a child diagnosed with ventricular arrhythmias and cardiomyopathy is usually devastated upon hearing the initial diagnosis, secondary to the poor prognosis associated with the disease. In most cases, they are in a state of shock and retain very little of what is initially told to them. Written information regarding the disease and simple, brief, and repeated explanations can be helpful to these families at this time. Any emotional/psychological support that is available should also be provided at this time.

Many of these families will begin a long journey of treatment modalities associated with the diagnosis of cardiomyopathy. While many may be palliated with medical therapy, there are severe or progressive cases that may require ICD implantation and/or cardiac transplantation. In some cases, an ICD is implanted as a "bridge" to transplantation. It is important for these families to know that although an ICD can prevent sudden cardiac death, it is not a cure. Similarly, although cardiac transplantation may improve quality of life and increase longevity, it is not without its problems and consequences either. As cardiovascular health care providers, it is our duty to correctly inform these patients and their families of the "realities" of these various treatment options.

Once again, for any patient experiencing difficulty coping with his or her disease process and/or treatment options, referral to psychiatric services may become necessary. As pediatric cardiovascular clinicians, we are able to provide a great deal of support, but occasionally this is not enough. It is important to make the family aware of the services available to them and to encourage them to call if they determine (or suspect) that their child may be having difficulty coping.

Specific information regarding ICD implantation issues can be found in chapter 8. If the child is referred for cardiac transplantation, the cardiovascular team should meet with the patient and family (perhaps first with the parents and then with them and the child) to discuss the usual progression of events. It is important that a realistic version of the sequence of events be presented in understandable terms, from what they should expect during the transplant evaluation phase to the usually long wait for a suitable donor and, importantly, to the intense and continuous aftercare following the transplantation. Once the decision has been made to place the child on the transplant list, further patient and family considerations, including education, should be made by the nurse transplant coordinator at the institution where the transplant will take place.

Viral Myocarditis

Because of the silent nature of myocarditis, it is sometimes difficult for affected patients and families to realize the importance of adhering to the treatment plan, especially if the child was fairly healthy at presentation. Education of the patient and family is critical regarding any and all medications, especially when corticosteroids are used on a tapering schedule. It is also important to inform parents of the potential adverse effects of immunosuppressive therapy, e.g., increased appetite, depression, facial swelling. If long-term therapy is required, writing the medication schedule on a calendar may help to ensure proper dosage changes.

If the child requires antiarrhythmic drug therapy, information given to the parents should be reviewed with the child and family with written material as an adjunct. Such information should include the drug's intended action, any potential adverse effects, what to do if a dose is inadvertently omitted, and specific things that require physician notification.

Arrhythmogenic Right Ventricular Dysplasia

The patient and family considerations of patients with ARVD vary with the specific treatment modality that is chosen. The specific method chosen is generally secondary to the degree of involvement and the extent of associated ventricular arrhythmias. Because of recent findings of a genetic linkage, genetic testing and evaluation of other family members may become more prevalent in the future. Information regarding the patient and family considerations for the treatment options of antiarrhythmic drugs, catheter ablation, and ICD implantation can be found in their respective chapters in this text. The patient and family considerations associated with cardiac transplantation can be found in the previous subsection on cardiomyopathies in this chapter.

Cardiac Tumors

The patient and family considerations associated with the diagnosis of cardiac tumors is slightly different in that the mention of the word "tumor" is frightful in and of itself. First and foremost, the family should be informed that the tumor is not a cancer-causing tumor and will not "metastasize" like cancerous tumors often do.

Depending on the child's presenting symptomatology and infringement of the tumor on cardiac structures, the treatment plan will need to be individualized for each patient. Regardless of the specific treatment modality chosen, information should be provided to the family simply, briefly, and repeatedly. If the child is initially admitted to the intensive care unit, the specifics of the environment should be explained to the patient and family.

The various treatment options should be reiterated to the patient and family, and any questions clarified. Since antiarrhythmic drugs are often successful in treating the arrhythmia, it should be stressed that surgery may not be necessary. If surgery should become necessary, the child and family should be educated regarding the open heart surgery process, including preoperative, perioperative, and postoperative specifics.

It is important to stress to patients with this diagnosis and to their families that the tumor may not always be visible using conventional diagnostic techniques (i.e., echocardiography) and that over time, the natural history of the tumor is to regress and the arrhythmia subside. This will eventually obviate the need for a lifetime of antiarrhythmic drug therapy. Similar to other patients with ventricular arrhythmias, psychological and emotional support is pivotal during this difficult time and should be ongoing throughout the child's follow-up.

In summary, caring for children with ventricular arrhythmias can be quite challenging for cardiovascular health care professionals. The advances in determining the etiology and often genetic basis for many of the disease states associated with ventricular arrhythmias have skyrocketed over the past decade and will continue to do so in the new millennium. This better understanding of disease etiology has led to the development and use of newer and better treatment modalities for these patients leading to decreased mortality and improved quality of life in this patient population.

References

1. Garson A Jr.: Ventricular arrhythmias. In Gillette PC, Garson A Jr. (eds.): Pediatric Arrhythmias: Electrophysiology and Pacing. Philadelphia: WB Saunders Company; 1990:427–500.

2. Johnsrude CL, Towbin JA, Cecchin F, et al: Postinfarction ventricular arrhythmias in children. Am Heart J 1995; 129:1171–1177.
3. Vetter VL: What every pediatrician needs to know about arrhythmias in children who have had cardiac surgery. Pediatr Ann 1991; 20:378–385.
4. Jacobsen JR, Garson A Jr., Gillette PC, et al: Premature ventricular contractions in normal children. J Pediatr 1978; 92:36–38.
5. Nagashima M, Tsushima M, Ogawa A, et al: Cardiac arrhythmias in healthy children revealed by 24-hour ambulatory monitoring. Pediatr Cardiol 1987; 8:103–108.
6. Garson A Jr.: Ventricular arrhythmias after repair of congenital heart disease: Who needs treatment? Cardiol Young 1991; 1:177–181.
7. Zeigler VL: Ventricular rhythms. In Paul S, Hebra JD (eds.): The Nurse's Guide to Cardiac Rhythm Interpretation: Implications for Patient Care. Philadelphia: WB Saunders Company; 1998:221–234.
8. Silka MJ, Garson A Jr.: Ventricular arrhythmias. In Gillette PC, Garson A Jr. (eds.): Clinical Pediatric Arrhythmias. 2nd ed. Philadelphia: WB Saunders Company; 1999:121–145.
9. Yabek SM: Ventricular arrhythmias in children with an apparently normal heart. J Pediatr 1991; 119:1–11.
10. Davis AM, Gow RM, McCrindle BW, et al: Clinical spectrum, therapeutic management and follow-up of ventricular tachycardia in infants and young children. Am Heart J 1996; 131:186–191.
11. Walsh CK, Krongrad E: Terminal cardiac electrical activity in pediatric patients. Am J Cardiol 1983; 51:557–561.
12. Mogayzel C, Quan L, Graves JR, et al: Out of hospital ventricular fibrillation in children and adolescents: Causes and outcomes. Ann Emerg Med 1995; 25:484–491.
13. Garson A Jr., Gillette PC, McNamara DG: A Guide to Pediatric Cardiac Dysrhythmias. New York: Grune & Stratton; 1980.
14. Miga DE, Case CL, Gillette PC: High prevalence of repolarization abnormalities in children with simple ventricular ectopy. Clin Cardiol 1996; 19:726–728.
15. Sclarovsky S, Strasberg B, Martonovich G, et al: Ventricular rhythms with intermediate rates in acute myocardial infarction. Chest 1978; 74:180–182.
16. Nakagawa M, Hamaoka K, Okano S, et al: Multiform accelerated idioventricular rhythm (AIVR) in a child with acute myocarditis. Clin Cardiol 1988; 11:853–855.
17. MacLellan-Tobert SG, Porter CJ: Accelerated idioventricular rhythms: A benign arrhythmia in childhood. Pediatrics 1995; 96:122–125.
18. Jervell A, Lange-Nielsen F: Congenital deaf-mutism, functional heart disease with prolongation of the QT and sudden death. Am Heart J 1957; 54:59–68.
19. Romano C, Gemme G, Pongiglione R: Artmie cardiache rare dell 'eta pediatrica. Clin Pediatr 1963; 45:658–683.
20. Ward OC: A new familial cardiac syndrome in children. J Irish Med Assoc 1964; 54:103–106.
21. Keating M, Atkinson D, Dunn C, et al: Linkage of a cardiac arrhythmia, the long QT syndrome, and the Harvey ras-1 gene. Science 1991; 252:704–706.
22. Jiang C, Atkinson D, Towbin JA, et al: Two long QT syndrome loci map to chromosomes 3 and 7 with evidence for further heterogenicity. Nat Genet 1994; 8:141–147.
23. Schott JJ, Charpentier F, Peltier S, et al: Mapping of a gene for long QT syndrome to chromosome 4q 25–27. Am J Hum Genet 1995; 57:1114–1122.
24. Wang Q, Shen J, Splawski I, et al: SCN5A mutations associated with an inherited cardiac arrhythmia, long QT syndrome. Cell 1995; 80:805–811.
25. Schwartz PJ, Priori SG, Locati EH, et al: Long QT syndrome patients with mutations of the SCN5A and HERG genes have differential responses to

sodium channel blockade and to increases in heart rate. Implications for gene-specific therapy. Circulation 1995; 92:3381–3386.

26. Schwartz PJ: Idiopathic long QT syndrome: Progress and questions. Am Heart J 1985; 109:399–411.

27. Horn CA, Beekman RH, Dick M II, et al: The congenital long QT syndrome. An unusual cause of childhood seizures. Am J Dis Child 1986; 140:659–661.

28. Pacia SV, Devinsky O, Luciano DJ, et al: The prolonged QT syndrome presenting as epilepsy: A report of two cases and literature review. Neurology 1994; 44:1408–1410.

29. Bazett HC: An analysis of the time relations of electrocardiograms. Heart 1918; 7:353–370.

30. Hayes DL, Maue-Dickson W, Stanton MS: Dictionary of Cardiac Pacing Electrophysiology and Arrhythmias. Miami Lakes: Peritus Corp; 1993.

31. Singh B, al Shahwan SA, Habbah MA, et al: Idiopathic long QT syndrome: Asking the right question. Lancet 1993; 341:741–742.

32. Brugada P, Brugada J: Right bundle branch block, persistent ST segment elevation and sudden cardiac death: A distinct clinical and electrocardiographic syndrome. J Am Coll Cardiol 1992; 20:1391–1396.

33. Antzelevitch C, Brugada P, Brugada J, et al: The Brugada Syndrome. In Camm AJ (ed.): Clinical Approaches to Tachyarrhythmias. Vol. 10. Armonk, NY: Futura Publishing Company, Inc.; 1999:1–93.

34. Chen O, Kirsch GE, Zhang D, et al: Genetic basis and molecular mechanisms for idiopathic ventricular fibrillation. Nature 1998; 392:293–296.

35. Brugada J, Brugada R, Brugada P: Right bundle branch block and ST segment elevation in leads V_1-V_3: A marker for sudden death in patients with no demonstrable structural heart disease. Circulation 1998; 97:457–460.

36. Proclemer A, Ciani R, Feruglio GA: Right ventricular tachycardia with left bundle branch block and inferior axis morphology: Clinical and arrhythmological characteristics in 15 patients. Pacing Clin Electrophysiol 1989; 12:977–989.

37. Nakagawa H, Mukai J, Nagata K, et al: Early afterdepolarizations in a patient with idiopathic monomorphic right ventricular tachycardia. Pacing Clin Electrophysiol 1993; 16:2067–2072.

38. Gill JS, Blaszyk K, Ward ED, et al: Verapamil for the suppression of idiopathic ventricular tachycardia of left bundle branch block-like morphology. Am Heart J 1993; 126:1126–1133.

39. O'Connor BK, Case CL, Sokoloski MC, et al: Radiofrequency catheter ablation of right ventricular outflow tract tachycardia in children and adolescents. J Am Coll Cardiol 1996; 27:869–874.

40. Silka MJ, Kron J: Radiofrequency catheter ablation for idiopathic right ventricular tachycardia: First, last, or only therapy—who decides? (editorial; comment) J Am Coll Cardiol 1996; 27:875–876.

41. Altman CA, Vick GN III, Perry JC, et al: Ventricular tachycardia after repair of congenital heart disease. Prog Pediatr Cardiol 1995; 4:229–236.

42. Sullivan JD, Presbitero P, Gooch VM, et al: Is ventricular arrhythmia in repaired tetralogy of Fallot an effect of operation or a consequence of the cause of the disease? A prospective study. Br Heart J 1987; 58:40–44.

43. Deanfield JE, Anderson RH, Hallidie-Smith KA: Late sudden-death after repair of tetralogy of Fallot. A clinicopathologic study. Circulation 1983; 67:626–631.

44. Gillette PC, Yeoman MA, Mullins CE, et al: Sudden death after repair of tetralogy of Fallot. Circulation 1977; 56:566–571.

45. Chandar JS, Wolff GS, Garson A, et al: Ventricular arrhythmias in postoperative tetralogy of Fallot. Am J Cardiol 1990; 65:655–661.

46. Vaksman G, Fournier A, Davignon A, et al: Frequency and prognosis of arrhythmias after operative "correction" of tetralogy of Fallot. Am J Cardiol 1990; 66:346–349.

47. Cullen S, Celemajer DS, Franklin RC, et al: Prognostic significance of ventricular arrhythmia after repair of tetralogy of Fallot: A 12 year prospective study. J Am Coll Cardiol 1994; 23:1151–1155.
48. Garson A Jr, Kugler JD, Gillette PC, et al: Control of late postoperative ventricular arrhythmias with phenytoin in young patients. Am J Cardiol 1980; 46:290–294.
49. Gatzoulis MA, Till JA, Redington AN: Depolarization-repolarization inhomogeneity after repair of tetralogy of Fallot: The substrate for malignant ventricular tachycardia? Circulation 1997; 95:401–404.
50. Balaji S, Lau Y, Case C, et al: QRS prolongation is associated with inducible ventricular tachycardia after repair of tetralogy of Fallot. Am J Cardiol 1997; 80:160–163.
51. James FW, Kaplan S, Schwartz DC, et al: Response to exercise in patients after total surgical correction of tetralogy of Fallot. Circulation 1976; 54:671–679.
52. Moak J, Gillette PC, Garson A Jr.: Mexiletine: An alternative to Dilantin in pediatric ventricular arrhythmias. Circulation 1984; 70(suppl 2):207.
53. James FW, Kaplan S, Chou TC: Unexpected cardiac arrest in patients after surgical correction of tetralogy of Fallot. Circulation 1975; 52:691–695.
54. Gillette PC, Zeigler V, Ross BA, et al: Amiodarone in children. Clin Prog Electrophysiol Pacing 1986; 4:328–330.
55. Guccione P, Paul T, Garson A Jr.: Long-term follow-up of amiodarone therapy in the young: Continued efficacy, unimpaired growth, moderate side effects. J Am Coll Cardiol 1990; 15:1118–1124.
56. Zeigler V, Gillette PC, Ross BA, et al: Flecainide for supraventricular and ventricular arrhythmias in children and young adults. Am J Cardiol 1988; 62:818–820.
57. Silka MJ, Kron J, Dunnigan A, et al: Sudden cardiac death and the use of implantable cardioverter-defibrillators in pediatric patients. The Pediatric Electrophysiology Society. Circulation 1993; 87:800–807.
58. Berko BA, Swift M: X-linked dilated cardiomyopathy. N Engl J Med 1987; 316:1186–1191.
59. Towbin JA, Hejmancik JF, Brink P, et al: X-linked dilated cardiomyopathy: Molecular genetic evidence of linkage to the Duchenne muscular dystrophy (dystrophin) gene at the Xp21 locus. Circulation 1993; 87:1854–1865.
60. Clark CE, Henry WO, Epstein SE: Familial prevalence and genetic transmission of idiopathic hypertrophic subaortic stenosis. N Engl J Med 1973; 289:709–714.
61. Lewis AB: Clinical profile and outcome of restrictive cardiomyopathy in children. Am Heart J 1992; 123:1589–1593.
62. Denfield SW, Gajarski RJ, Towbin JA: Cardiomyopathies. In Garson A Jr., Bricker JT, Fisher DJ, Neish SR (eds.): The Science and Practice of Pediatric Cardiology. 2nd ed. Baltimore: Williams & Wilkins; 1998:1851–1883.
63. Fananapazir L, Epstein SE: Hemodynamic and electrophysiologic evaluation of patients with hypertrophic cardiomyopathy surviving cardiac arrest. Am J Cardiol 1991; 67:280–287.
64. Hordof A, Keuhl K, Vetter V, et al: Risk factors for sudden death in patients with hypertrophic obstructive cardiomyopathy. Circulation 1988; 78:II595. Abstract.
65. Friedman RA, Moak JP, Garson A Jr.: Clinical course of idiopathic dilated cardiomyopathy in children. J Am Coll Cardiol 1991; 18:152–156.
66. Chen C, Naori S, Balfour J, et al: Clinical profile of congestive cardiomyopathy in children. J Am Coll Cardiol 1990; 15:189–193.
67. Burch M, Sidden SA, Cleremajer DS, et al: Dilated cardiomyopathy in children: Determinants of outcome. Br Heart J 1994; 72:246–250.
68. Luu ML, Stevenson WG, Stevenson LW, et al: Diverse mechanisms of unexpected cardiac arrest in advanced heart failure. Circulation 1989; 80:1675–1680.

69. McKenna WJ, Oakley CM, Krikler DM, et al: Improved survival with amiodarone in patients with hypertrophic cardiomyopathy and ventricular tachycardia. Br Heart J 1995; 53:412–416.
70. Tendera M, Wycisk A, Schneeweiss A, et al: Effect of sotalol on arrhythmias and exercise tolerance in patients with hypertrophic cardiomyopathy. Cardiology 1993; 82:335–342.
71. Theodoro DA, Danielson GK, Feldt RH, et al: Hypertrophic obstructive cardiomyopathy in pediatric patients: Results of surgical treatment. J Thorac Cardiovasc Surg 1996; 112:1589–1599.
72. Fananapazir L, McAreavey D: Hypertrophic cardiomyopathy: Evaluation and treatment of patients at high risk for sudden death. Pacing Clin Electrophysiol 1997; 20:478–501.
73. Fananapazir L, Epstein ND, Curiel RV, et al: Long-term results of dual chamber (DDD) pacing in obstructive hypertrophic cardiomyopathy. Evidence for progressive symptomatic and hemodynamic improvement and reduction of left ventricular hypertrophy. Circulation 1994; 90:2731–2742.
74. Kaminer SJ, Pickoff AS, Dunnigan A, et al: Cardiomyopathy and the use of implanted cardio-defibrillators in children. Pacing Clin Electrophysiol 1990; 13:593–597.
75. Talard P, Lèvy S, Bonal J, et al: Sudden death as a presenting symptom of hypertrophic cardiomyopathy: Treatment with an implantable cardioverter defibrillator. Pacing Clin Electrophysiol 1996; 19:1264–1267.
76. Aretz HT, Billingham ME, Edwards WD, et al: Myocarditis: A histopathologic definition and classification. Am J Cardiovasc Pathol 1986; 1:3–14.
77. Straumanis JP, Wiles HB, Case CL: Resolution of atrial standstill in a child with myocarditis. Pacing Clin Electrophysiol 1993; 16:2196–2201.
78. Lurie PR: Endomyocardial biopsies in cardiomyopathies of childhood. Prog Pediatr Cardiol 1992; 1:71–81.
79. Balaji S, Wiles HB, Sens MA, et al: Immunosuppressive treatment for myocarditis and borderline myocarditis in children with ventricular ectopic rhythm. Br Heart J 1994; 72:354–359.
80. Friedman RA, Kearney DL, Moak JP, et al: Persistence of ventricular arrhythmia after resolution of occult myocarditis in children and young adults. J Am Coll Cardiol 1994; 24:780–783.
81. Thiene G, Nava A, Corrado D, et al: Right ventricular cardiomyopathy and sudden death in young people. N Engl J Med 1988; 318:129–133.
82. Ruder MA, Winston SA, Davis JC, et al: Arrhythmogenic right ventricular dysplasia in a family. Am J Cardiol 1985; 56:799–800.
83. Rakovec P, Rossi L, Fontaine G, et al: Familial arrhythmogenic right ventricular disease. Am J Cardiol 1986; 58:377–378.
84. Laurent M, Descaves C, Biron Y, et al: Familial form of arrhythmogenic right ventricular dysplasia. Am Heart J 1987; 113:827–829.
85. Solenthaler M, Ritter M, Candinas R, et al: Arrhythmogenic right ventricular dysplasia in identical twins. J Am Coll Cardiol 1994; 74:303–304.
86. Rampazzo A, Nava A, Danieli GA, et al: The gene for arrhythmogenic right ventricular cardiomyopathy maps to chromosome 14 q 23–q 24. Hum Mol Genet 1994; 3:959–962.
87. Severini GM, Krajinovic M, Pinamonti B, et al: A new focus for arrhythmogenic right ventricular dysplasia on the long arm of chromosome 14. Genomics 1996; 31:193–200.
88. Marcus FI, Fontain GH, Guiraudon G, et al: Right ventricular dysplasia: A report of 24 adult cases. Circulation 1982; 65:384–398.
89. Davignon A, Rautaharjup P, Boisselle E, et al: Normal ECG standards for infants and children. Pediatr Cardiol 1979; 1:123–152.
90. Wichter T, Borggrefe M, Haverkamp W, et al: Efficacy of antiarrhythmic drugs in patients with arrhythmogenic right ventricular disease. Results in patients

with inducible and noninducible ventricular tachycardia. Circulation 1992; 86:29–37.

91. Fontaine G, Frank R, Rougier I, et al: Electrode catheter ablation of resistant ventricular tachycardia in arrhythmogenic right ventricular dysplasia: Experience of 15 patients with a mean follow-up of 45 months. Heart Vessels 1990; 5:172–187.

92. Kullo IJ, Edwards WD, Seward JB: Right ventricular dysplasia: The Mayo Clinic experience. Mayo Clin Proc 1995; 70:541–548.

93. Ludomirsky A: Cardiac tumors. In Garson A Jr., Bricker JT, Fisher DJ, Neish SR (eds.): The Science and Practice of Pediatric Cardiology. 2nd ed. Baltimore: Williams & Wilkins; 1998:1885–1893.

94. Zeigler VL, Gillette PC, Crawford FA Jr., et al: New approaches to treatment of incessant ventricular tachycardia in the very young. J Am Coll Cardiol 1990; 16:681–685.

95. Garson A Jr., Smith RT Jr., Moak JP, et al: Incessant ventricular tachycardia in infants: Myocardial hamartomas and surgical cure. J Am Coll Cardiol 1987; 10:619–626.

96. Villain E, Bonnet D, Kachaner J, et al: Tachycardies ventriculaires incessantes idiopathiques du nourrisson. Arch Mal Couer Vaiss 1990; 83:665–671.

97. Wren C: Ventricular arrhythmias. In Wren C, Campbell RWF (eds.): Paediatric Cardiac Arrhythmias. Oxford: Oxford University Press; 1996:127–156.

98. Suddaby EC, Riker IL: Defibrillation and cardioversion in children. Pediatr Nurs 1991; 17:477–481.

99. American Heart Association and American Academy of Pediatrics: Textbook of Pediatric Advanced Life Support. Dallas: American Heart Association; 1988:66–67.

100. Miles MS, Warner JB: The dying child in the intensive care unit. In Hazinski MF (ed.): Nursing Care of the Critically Ill Child. 2nd ed. St. Louis: Mosby-Yearbook, Inc.; 1992:101–116.

101. Newman MM: Early defibrillation: Making waves across America: The critical moment when resuscitation depends on rapid defibrillation. J Emerg Med 1997; (suppl):S5-S8.

102. Mancini ME, Richards N, Kaye W: Saving lives with automated external defibrillators. Nursing 1997; 101:42–43.

103. Emergency Cardiac Care Committee and Subcommittees AHA: Guidelines for cardiopulmonary resuscitation and emergency cardiac care. IV. Pediatric advanced life support. JAMA 1992; 268:2262–2275.

104. Harkins A: Chronic Illness. In Betz C, Hunsberger M, Wright S (eds.): Family-Centered Nursing Care of Children. Philadelphia: WB Saunders Company; 1994:651–688.

105. Tong E, Sparacino PSA: Special management issues for adolescents and young adults with congenital heart disease. Crit Care Nurs Clin North Am 1994; 6:199–214.

106. Zeigler VL: Care of adolescents and young adults with arrhythmias. Prog Cardiovasc Nurs 1995; 10:13–21.

107. Garson SL: Psychological aspects of heart disease in childhood. In Garson A Jr., Bricker JT, Fisher DJ, Neish SR (eds.): The Science and Practice of Pediatric Cardiology. 2nd ed. Baltimore: Williams & Wilkins; 1999:2929–2937.

Chapter 4

Immediate Arrhythmia Management

Barbara J. Knick, RN, CVT and J. Phillip Saul, MD

In the pediatric population, the initial or immediate management of arrhythmias is generally determined by the patient's overall hemodynamic status and the mechanism of the presenting arrhythmia. In most cases, the arrhythmia mechanism can be easily determined, but in some cases immediate intervention may be required in order to delineate further treatment strategies. For the most part, children with cardiac arrhythmias present with symptoms that are less than life threatening. In the case of direct hemodynamic compromise or concern that the arrhythmia may rapidly result in clinical deterioration, immediate action may be required. This action may be definitive, i.e., it may restore normal sinus rhythm, or it may be palliative, e.g., atrial pacing may be used to provide 2:1 atrioventricular (AV) block in order to control the patient's ventricular rate.

The critical component in determining whether immediate intervention is warranted and what type of intervention is to be chosen is the individual patient assessment. Children may exhibit various signs and symptoms of the effects of the cardiac arrhythmia on their overall hemodynamic status. These signs and symptoms include palpitations, neck pulsations, shortness of breath, nasal flaring, use of accessory muscles, pallor, mottling, cyanosis, poor feeding, lethargy, decreased peripheral pulses, dizziness, syncope, hypotension, and, rarely, cardiac arrest. The specific management technique chosen for a specific patient should be based on the child's symptomatology, although in certain cases it may also be based somewhat on the child's age as well as the clinician's assessment of the patient's overall hemodynamic status.

For the purposes of this chapter, a "stable" (or compensated) cardiac arrhythmia is defined as one that does not result in hemodynamic com-

From Zeigler VL, Gillette PC: *Practical Management of Pediatric Cardiac Arrhythmias.* Armonk, NY: Futura Publishing Co., Inc.; ©2001.

promise, i.e., the child is alert, has normal vital signs for age and health status (except heart rate), and exhibits signs of good cardiac output, such as brisk capillary refill and palpable and strong peripheral pulses. An "unstable" (or decompensated) cardiac arrhythmia is defined as one that produces decreased cardiac output as evidenced by decreased peripheral pulses, increased respiratory effort, color changes, prolonged capillary refill, hypotension, and/or changes in the child's level of consciousness (LOC).

This chapter delineates the various maneuvers, procedures, and treatment modalities used to initially treat or acutely manage a child's cardiac arrhythmia. These treatment modalities include simple vagal maneuvers, pharmacologic therapies, temporary pacing modalities, electrical cardioversion and defibrillation, and automatic external defibrillation. Since some of the treatment modalities are alluded to in other chapters as they relate to specific arrhythmia mechanisms, this chapter focuses on the specific management techniques. Each treatment modality is defined, its mechanism of action delineated, the amenable arrhythmias specified, and the implications for clinicians as well as patient and family considerations reviewed.

Vagal Maneuvers

Vagal maneuvers are generally used in children with hemodynamically stable supraventricular tachycardias (SVTs) that incorporate the AV node as part of their circuit. In Ludomirsky and Garson's review of 346 pediatric patients with SVT,[1] the success rate of vagal maneuvers was found to be 62%, with age being a significant variable in that success rate. Vagal maneuvers are used as an initial treatment modality because of the their simplicity and relative noninvasiveness. Vagal maneuvers work by inducing a negative dromotropic effect through the AV node. Vagal maneuvers used in children include the diving reflex, the Valsalva maneuver, pressure on the solar plexus for infants and toddlers, and carotid massage for school-aged and older children. Ocular pressure is not used in children because of the risk of serious eye injury including retinal detachment. Other similar noninvasive, vagal-like maneuvers that can be used in children with stable SVT include deep inspiration with brief breath holding, drinking ice water, performing a momentary hand stand, and the induction of a gag or cough. Although the specific vagal maneuvers are discussed separately, the implications for clinicians and patient and family considerations apply to all of them.

Diving Reflex

One of the most common vagal maneuvers used in the pediatric population is the diving reflex. It will induce an all-or-none response in that it will either terminate the tachycardia or it will not. Ludomirsky and Garson[1] state that the diving reflex is most effective in small infants and can be accomplished in one of two ways depending on the age of the child.

In the neonate or infant, a bag of ice is placed over the child's mouth and nose for 10 to 30 seconds. In the older child, the face is immersed into ice cold water for approximately the same amount of time. To avoid skin injury, ice should never be directly applied to the face of an infant.

Mechanism of Action

The diving reflex is present at birth and produces strong efferent stimulation of the vagus nerve and sympathetic withdrawal in response to afferent stimulation of the trigeminal nerve in the cheeks, nasal bridge, and forehead. The face of the infant is exposed or the child's face is immersed in extremely cold ice water and a strong reflex vagal activation occurs. The vagus nerve releases acetylcholine, which slows conduction and lengthens the refractory period of the AV node tissue, causing one of the tachycardia beats to be "blocked" and interrupting the reentry circuit.

Amenable Arrhythmias

Cardiac arrhythmias that are amenable to the diving reflex include any stable SVT that requires the AV node as part of its circuit. Specific arrhythmias include SVT associated with an accessory pathway (including manifest and concealed Wolff-Parkinson-White [WPW]), the permanent form of junctional reciprocating tachycardia (PJRT), Lown-Ganong-Levine (LGL) tachycardia, AV nodal reentry tachycardia (AVNRT), and tachycardias due to a Mahaim fiber. Since atrial flutter, other intraatrial reentry tachycardias (IARTs), and ectopic/automatic foci do not require the AV node for tachycardia perpetuation, the diving reflex is rarely effective with these specific substrates.

Valsalva Maneuver

The Valsalva maneuver is defined as a voluntary forced exhalation against a closed glottis,[2] and is similar to "bearing down" as if having a bowel movement. It can be used in older children, who can cooperate by following commands, and is a simple, noninvasive treatment modality for reentrant SVTs that incorporate the AV node as part of their circuit. The child is instructed to either bear down or blow against a thumb placed over closed lips.

Mechanism of Action

The Valsalva maneuver has four phases: 1) at onset, initial ejection of blood from the thorax briefly increases aortic pressure; 2) forced collapse of the thoracic veins, leading to reduced systemic venous return, decreased cardiac output, and a progressive drop in aortic pressure; 3) at release, immediate recoil of blood to the thorax, briefly reducing aortic pressure; and

4) restoration of "dammed-up" systemic venous return, increasing cardiac output and aortic blood pressure to levels higher than those prior to the maneuver. During phase 2, there is reflex sympathetic activation, which increases the SVT rate slightly but constricts peripheral arteries such that the pressure increase in phase 4 is even larger. Reflex vagal activation occurs slightly in phase 2 and dramatically in phase 4, particularly when arterial pressure rebounds significantly above baseline. Thus, tachycardias are most likely to terminate 5 to 10 seconds after the Valsalva release, when arterial pressure and reflex vagal activation peak. The reflex vagal output to the heart causes the release of acetylcholine, which slows the heart rate and lengthens the refractory period of the AV node. This in turn blocks one of the tachycardia beats, which interrupts the reentry circuit.

Amenable Arrhythmias

Arrhythmias that are amenable to the Valsalva maneuver are the same as those listed under the diving reflex. The specific arrhythmias include SVT due to an accessory connection (including concealed and manifest WPW, PJRT, and LGL), AVNRT, and tachycardia associated with Mahaim fibers. Once again, because atrial flutter, other IARTs, and ectopic/automatic focus tachycardias do not use the AV node as part of their circuits, this maneuver will not likely result in tachycardia termination in these patients.

Carotid Massage

Carotid massage is yet another vagal maneuver that can be used for the immediate management of supraventricular tachyarrhythmias that incorporate the AV node within their circuit. It is important to note that only one carotid sinus is massaged at a time for approximately 5 to 10 seconds, to avoid too marked a reduction in cerebral blood flow.

Mechanism of Action

Unilateral carotid massage is used to increase carotid sinus outflow to the brain, mimicking an increase in carotid pressure and inducing reflex vagal nervous outflow. Once again, acetylcholine release leads to slowing of the heart rate and an increase in AV node refractoriness. This then results in a "blocked" tachycardia beat, which interrupts the reentry circuit.

Amenable Arrhythmias

Cardiac arrhythmias that are amenable to carotid massage include any stable SVT that incorporates the AV node as part of its circuit. Specific arrhythmias include SVT associated with an accessory pathway (including manifest and concealed WPW) and AVNRT. Tachycardia associated with PJRT, LGL, and Mahaim fibers may also be amenable to carotid massage. Since atrial flutter, other IARTs, and ectopic/automatic foci do not require the AV node for tachycardia perpetuation, carotid massage is rarely effective with these specific substrates.

Implications for Clinicians

Although vagal maneuvers are relatively benign treatment modalities, the clinician should be aware of certain adverse sequelae. Patients may experience rebound bradycardia and/or a long pause (asystole) after prolonged episodes of tachycardia, especially patients with an impaired sinus node or those already receiving antiarrhythmic drugs that may suppress normal sinus and AV node function. It is advisable that preparations be made in advance for at least temporary transcutaneous pacing prior to initiating the vagal maneuvers in select pediatric patients. Once again, when performing carotid massage, it is extremely important to massage only one side at a time.

If vagal maneuvers are being used in older children, the clinician should explain the procedure to the child in order to gain trust and cooperation. If the clinician provides this information and is truthful, the child will be more likely to assist rather than resist the maneuvers' implementation. Since most of the child's anxiety is due to fear of the unknown, this instruction and support will be much valued by the child as well as the child's family.

Patient and Family Considerations

The diving reflex is often attempted for the initial conversion of SVT in neonates and infants. Since this may be the first time that the parents/family have been told their child has a cardiac arrhythmia, it can be particularly stressful. Parental support and education are key at this time. It is important to explain the procedure in terms that the parents can understand with reassurance that the procedure will not harm their child, but may indeed alleviate the need for more invasive maneuvers if it is successful.

The Valsalva maneuver is generally used in older children who can follow commands, such as "bearing down" as if having a bowel movement. An explanation in age-appropriate language should be given to the child prior to actually performing the maneuver. This is also an excellent opportunity for the parents to "listen in" and understand the purpose of the procedure also. In many institutions, patients and parents are instructed to use this technique at home for recurrent episodes. Patient and family education in this regard should include explanation of when to use the maneuver, how many times to use the maneuver, and what to do in the event that the maneuver does not work.

Carotid massage may be used in nearly any age group but is probably the least frequently used of the vagal maneuvers in children. Regardless of which specific vagal maneuver is used, it is important to explain to patients and their families that other treatment modalities are available in the event that these techniques are not successful in terminating the child's arrhythmia.

Pharmacologic Therapy

Certain pharmacologic agents can be very helpful in the immediate management of both bradyarrhythmias and tachyarrhythmias. The agents that are discussed are all intravenous (IV) agents, although some of them may also be available in the oral formulation. They are discussed in alphabetical order and include adenosine, amiodarone, atropine, bretylium, digoxin immune Fab (Digibind), digoxin, esmolol, ibutilide, isoproterenol, lidocaine, phenytoin, and procainamide. The medications are discussed in the format previously used, including mechanism of action, amenable arrhythmias, and implications for clinicians. Patient and family considerations are discussed for the pharmacologic agents as a whole. Additional information regarding the specific agents, i.e., dosage, onset of action, potential adverse effects, drug interactions, cardiovascular contraindications, and general comments, can be found in Appendix 4–1.

Adenosine

Adenosine, a purine nucleoside that is present in each of the cells within the human body, can be used both therapeutically to terminate specific reentrant tachyarrhythmias and diagnostically to delineate specific arrhythmogenic substrates.[3,4] Since its approval by the US Food and Drug Administration (FDA) in 1989, the use of adenosine has virtually eliminated the use of IV verapamil for SVT in children, and it is not associated with verapamil's potential for severe adverse hemodynamic effects.[5,6] This is primarily due to its extremely short half-life variably quoted as 0.5 to 5.0 seconds[7,8] to 10 to 30 seconds,[9] but probably closest to the former.

Mechanism of Action

The electrophysiologic effects of adenosine are directly related to its cellular effects, specifically 1) the shortening of the action potential secondary to activation of outward potassium current,[10] and 2) a reduction in impulse formation in the sinus and AV nodes and a slowing of conduction to the point of block through the AV node, which interrupts the reentry circuit of SVTs that require the AV node for perpetuation. In patients with automatic atrial tachycardias, atrial flutter, or other IARTs, the administration of adenosine will result in temporary AV block, but generally will not affect or terminate the arrhythmia since the AV node is not required for tachycardia perpetuation (Fig. 1). Such an effect is often diagnostic by

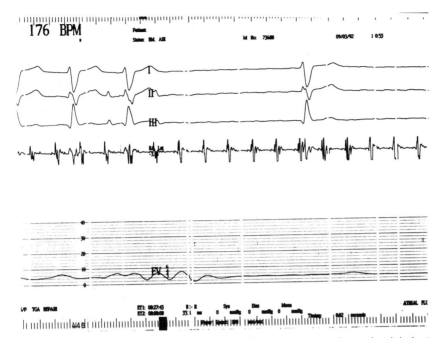

Figure 1. Surface ECG leads I, II, and III and a bipolar transesophageal atrial electrogram recording of a patient experiencing atrial flutter. Adenosine is administered, resulting in transient atrioventricular block with continuation of the atrial flutter as noted on the atrial electrogram. In this postoperative congenital heart disease patient, the very small flutter waves on the surface ECG make it appear that the tachycardia has been terminated demonstrating the usefulness of both adenosine and transesophageal atrial electrogram recording in diagnosing the arrhythmia.

demonstrating that either the atrial or ventricular tachycardia (VT) continues unabated during transient AV block.

Amenable Arrhythmias

Due to its direct effects on AV nodal conduction, adenosine is only likely to terminate SVT that incorporates the AV node as part of its circuit (Fig. 2). Specific arrhythmias include SVT due to an accessory connection, either manifest or concealed, and AVNRT. It will NOT usually terminate the following arrhythmias: atrial ectopic tachycardia (AET), atrial flutter or other intraatrial reentry circuits, atrial fibrillation, or VT; however, its use in these patients can be diagnostic and will generally result in temporary AV block. In patients with subtle WPW, adenosine will decrease AV node conduction while enhancing antegrade conduction over the accessory pathway, helping to identify ventricular preexcitation, i.e., the presence of a delta wave. VTs are generally unresponsive to adenosine administration with the exception of some right ventricular outflow tract tachycardias.[11]

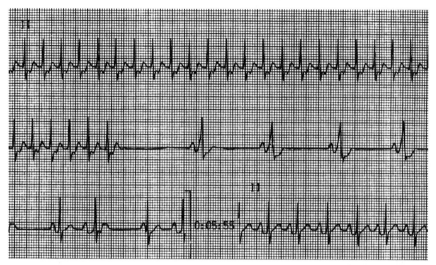

Figure 2. Continuous lead II ECG recording in a patient with supraventricular tachycardia. Adenosine is administered with termination of the reentrant tachycardia followed by a sinus pause and subsequent normal sinus rhythm with Wolff-Parkinson-White (WPW) and intermittent preexcitation. The latter part of the third strip exhibits normal sinus rhythm *without* WPW.

Implications for Clinicians

The specific IV route of administration varies based on availability of venous access. In some cases, the establishment of IV access alone will terminate the arrhythmia by initiating a vagal response to pain. Adenosine can be given peripherally or through a central venous line in a port as close to the patient as possible, and is immediately followed by a relatively large (10 cc) and rapidly administered saline flush. The one route that is contraindicated in the pediatric population is through an umbilical artery catheter.[6] This particular route is often used for access in preterm and term neonates. When given intraarterially, adenosine must traverse both the systemic and pulmonary circulations prior to reaching the myocardium via the coronary arteries. Consequently, it is likely to be already metabolized by the time it reaches the sinus and AV nodes, rendering it completely ineffective.

Prior to administering adenosine, the clinician should obtain certain information from the patient and family. First and foremost is the presence of any and all allergies, particularly any known hypersensitivity to adenosine. Second, the clinician should inquire about any history of asthma, since adenosine can cause bronchial constriction, which aggravates symptoms in asthmatic patients. If adenosine is to be administered in patients with asthma, adequate precautions should be taken prior to the drug's administration. Third, since caffeine makes adenosine less effective, information regarding the child's caffeine intake or the use of caffeinelike agents such as theophylline prior to adenosine administration can be helpful in determining the drug's dose and potential efficacy.

Continuous electrocardiographic (ECG) monitoring is required during adenosine administration and should be in the immediate proximity of the patient, not in a remote location such as a centralized telemetry monitor. The clinician caring for the patient receiving IV adenosine should be prepared for transient asystole, since this extremely short asystole episode almost always seems longer than it really is. Precautions, such as the ability to provide temporary pacing, must be taken in advance to prepare for prolonged bradycardia and/or asystole.

Since adenosine works very rapidly, most children will not require sedation for its administration. Older children are likely to experience some of the more common adverse effects of adenosine administration, so the clinician should explain these to the older patient prior to medication administration. These effects, which include chest pressure, facial flushing, palpitations, and shortness of breath, should be explained to the patient in age-appropriate language with an emphasis on the fact that they are only temporary. This may provoke some anxiety in the patient who has never received adenosine before, but will reassure him or her that these feelings are "normal" and are related to the drug versus the arrhythmia.

Amiodarone

IV amiodarone, a potent Class III antiarrhythmic agent, can be used safely and effectively for the treatment of resistant atrial and ventricular arrhythmias in children.[12-14] Although amiodarone has many electrophysiologic effects, its major mode of action is that it prolongs refractoriness in most cardiac tissue. In addition, the current IV formulation, which includes the polysaccharide Tween 80, is a potent vasodilator.

Mechanism of Action

Amiodarone has a multitude of cellular electrophysiologic effects. It acts directly on the myocardium to delay repolarization and increase action potential duration. Amiodarone's delayed repolarization effects are due to an inhibition of outward potassium current, which results in prolongation of refractoriness in all cardiac tissues. Amiodarone also directly depresses sinus and AV node automaticity and slows conduction in the atria, AV node, His-Purkinje system, and ventricles. Although classified as a Class III antiarrhythmic agent, amiodarone is also a weak sodium channel blocker, a noncompetitive inhibitor of α- and β-receptors, and a possessor of both vagolytic and calcium channel blocking properties; thus, it possesses characteristics of all four classes of Vaughan Williams' antiarrhythmic activity.

Amenable Arrhythmias

Due to its potent electrophysiologic effects, IV amiodarone has been successful in controlling a variety of supraventricular and ventricular tachyarrhythmias. Specific arrhythmias include chaotic atrial tachycardia, AET, both congenital and postoperative junctional ectopic tachycardia (JET), postoperative VT, and VT secondary to myocardial tumors.[12–14] Although seldom necessary, it can be used to treat incessant SVT resulting from an accessory connection (with manifest or concealed WPW), AVNRT (rarely), and VT in the absence of structural heart disease.

Implications for Clinicians

In the majority of instances, the child receiving IV amiodarone will be in the intensive care unit (ICU). The patient should have continuous ECG monitoring in a lead that P waves are easily identifiable (once the tachycardia has been terminated) in order to periodically assess the PR interval. Additionally, oxygen saturation should be continuously monitored during IV amiodarone administration. Since the most common adverse effect associated with IV amiodarone use is hypotension, continuous blood pressure monitoring must be observed, preferably by arterial pressure measurement. The use of external automated blood pressure monitors is less ideal because of their propensity to become inaccurate in the presence of hypotensive states and the limited frequency of measurements.

The nurse caring for the patient receiving IV amiodarone has many responsibilities. First and foremost is to be as knowledgeable about the drug as possible. Amiodarone, in its oral and IV forms, has many potential adverse effects, which are listed in Appendix 4–1. IV amiodarone should be mixed in 5% dextrose solution or normal saline for administration to avoid precipitation. Continuous amiodarone infusions should be administered using an infusion pump.

Amiodarone should be used with caution in postoperative congenital heart disease (CHD) patients, especially those with known or suspected sinus and/or AV node dysfunction. In these patients, a temporary pacemaker should be available at the patient's bedside. In patients with permanent cardiac pacemakers, IV amiodarone administration has no known effects on cardiac pacing thresholds.

The clinician should be cognizant of any other medications that the patient may be receiving that may have an interaction with amiodarone. The most discussed pharmacologic interaction is that of digoxin and amiodarone. Concomitant administration of these two agents has been noted to cause a 25% to 100% rise in serum digoxin concentrations.[15] Prior to amiodarone administration, the digoxin dose should be decreased by 33% to 50% in order to avoid digoxin toxicity. Coadministration of amiodarone and other antiarrhythmic agents can also result in increased serum concentrations of those agents, including the sodium channel blockers, procainamide, flecainide, quinidine, and phenytoin. Use of concomitant calcium and/or β-blockers, because of similar electrophysiologic effects, may exacerbate sinus and AV node dysfunction. Last, the coadministration of amiodarone and warfarin may result in increases in prothrombin time measurements and international normalized ratio (INR) values.

Atropine

Atropine sulfate is an anticholinergic agent that is primarily used in patients with symptomatic bradycardia that does not respond to conventional patient stimulation, or sinus bradycardia induced by drugs or toxic substances. It is a parasympatholytic agent that typically improves bradycardia that occurs at a site above the ventricles. It also possesses bronchodilator effects.

Mechanism of Action

Atropine blocks muscarinic receptors to antagonize the action of acetylcholine in a dose-dependent manner; however, it does not block acetylcholine's actions at the nicotinic neuromuscular junction. The increase in heart rate occurs due to atropine's vagolytic effect, as it blocks the effects of acetylcholine at the level of the sinus node. Since most patients have some vagal tone, administration of atropine increases sinus rate and increases conduction velocity in the AV node. Atropine also enhances automaticity in atrial and junctional tissue, but rarely in the ventricular escape pacemaker.

Amenable Arrhythmias

Atropine can be useful in patients with symptomatic bradycardia (i.e., with signs and symptoms of poor systemic perfusion), symptomatic bradycardia with AV block, vagally mediated bradycardia, and asystole. Specific arrhythmias include bradycardia from any structure that has vagal innervation, including sinus and junctional bradycardia. Although second-degree AV block of the Wenckebach variety (Type I) is often reversed by atropine, Type II second-degree AV block or complete AV block is often not reversed with atropine. It may increase the ventricular rate in some cases. Suprahisian block may respond to atropine, but infrahisian block distal to the bundle of His is usually unaffected.

Implications for Clinicians

When administering atropine, it is important to give a large enough dose to produce a vagolytic action since lower doses (<0.01 mg/kg) can result in a paradoxical decrease in heart rate through atropine's parasympathomimetic effect. The American Heart Association/American Academy of Pediatrics[16] recommend 0.02 mg/kg with a minimum of 0.1 mg repeated at 5-minute intervals with continuous ECG monitoring. The maximum cumulative dose is 1.0 mg. Additionally, atropine is relatively long acting, with a half-life of 45 minutes to 1 hour, so the clinician must remain cognizant when explaining the potential adverse effects to patients who are old enough to understand them.

The most common adverse effects of atropine that the clinician should be aware of, in order to appropriately monitor for and to inform the patient of, are tachycardia, dry mouth, dilated pupils, and flushed/dry skin. Careful blood pressure monitoring, either by frequent cuff pressure or indwelling arterial line when available, should accompany atropine administration, since this drug can cause both hypertension and hypotension. It should also be noted that atropine can exacerbate SVT by enhancing AV nodal conduction and, hence, increasing the rate.

Bretylium

Bretylium tosylate is a Class III antiarrhythmic drug that was first approved by the FDA in 1978 for treating ventricular arrhythmias. Since the availability and widespread use of IV amiodarone, the use of bretylium is on the decline; this has led to speculation that it may eventually no longer be manufactured. It has little inhibitory effect on nodal or conduction tissue, but rather is concentrated in the terminal sympathetic neurons, where it affects norepinephrine release and reuptake.[9] Although there are no published data regarding its use in the pediatric population, it is occasionally used in the resuscitative setting for resistant polymorphic or monomorphic ventricular tachyarrhythmias.[15]

Mechanism of Action

Bretylium works by causing an initial release of stored norepinephrine with subsequent further release and prevention of reuptake. This initial release in norepinephrine causes a transient increase in blood pressure and heart rate followed in minutes by a decrease in both with no change in cardiac output. The electrophysiologic effects of bretylium include an increase in action potential duration and refractoriness without slowing conduction velocity or membrane responsiveness. It has no direct effect on automaticity. Bretylium use in children is based on adult studies, in which it has been effective in making ventricular fibrillation (VF) more responsive to defibrillation.[17,18]

Amenable Arrhythmias

Bretylium is generally used in children as a last resort after multiple unsuccessful or transiently successful defibrillation attempts and IV lidocaine have failed. Specific arrhythmias that may respond to bretylium administration include VT and VF.

Implications for Clinicians

The clinician caring for the patient receiving bretylium should be aware of certain specifics regarding the agent's effects. The antifibrillatory effects of IV bretylium occur within minutes of administration, while the electrophysiologic effects such as VT suppression take considerably longer and last 30 to 120 minutes.[15] Bretylium is known to cause significant hypotension, which can be managed with judicious volume replacement. Due to its significant hypotensive effects, the drug should be diluted in 5% dextrose and also administered more slowly in patients with hemodynamically stable VT, to avoid nausea and vomiting.

Digibind

Digibind was approved by the FDA in 1986 and is an agent that is used specifically for digoxin toxicity and its associated arrhythmias. The reversal that accompanies its administration is rapid and rarely accompanied by adverse effects. The medication itself is derived from digoxin-specific antibodies obtained from immunized sheep.

Mechanism of Action

Digibind works by binding to molecules of digoxin and digitoxin (its metabolite) rendering them unavailable for binding at the site of action on the cells. In other words, it binds to the serum digoxin, basically rendering it inactive.[19] One known adverse effect, hypokalemia, may develop as sodium pump activity is regained and potassium is transferred from blood to muscle.[20]

Amenable Arrhythmias

It is recommended that Digibind only be used in patients whose arrhythmia is known to be caused by digoxin toxicity and in those who are hemodynamically compromised secondary to this arrhythmia. Specific arrhythmias related to digoxin toxicity include VT, VF, progressive bradycardia, and/or second- or third-degree AV block not responsive to atropine.

Implications for Clinicians

The dose calculation for Digibind is somewhat complicated and can be calculated using one of two formulas. First, the estimated total body load (TOTAL LOAD) in milligrams is calculated based on 1) the digoxin plasma concentration or 2) the amount of digoxin ingested, and is shown as follows:

1) TOTAL LOAD (mg)

$$= \frac{\text{Plasma concentration (ng/mL)} \times 5.6 \times \text{weight (in kg)}}{1000}$$

or

2) TOTAL LOAD (mg) = ingested digoxin amount (mg) $\times$ 0.8

After the estimated total body load of digoxin is calculated, the Digibind dose is calculated as follows:

Digibind dose (mg) = TOTAL LOAD (from above) $\times$66.7

Digibind is administered over 30 minutes with a 0.22-micron filter. For imminent cardiac arrest, it can be administered as a bolus by adding 4 mL of sterile water to each vial and mixing gently. The mixture should be used promptly or it may be diluted with normal saline to a convenient volume. Clinical improvement should be seen in at least 30 minutes, since the response to Digibind is nearly immediate. Repeat dosing is often necessary, as the arrhythmia may recur as tissue-bound digoxin is released into the plasma. A decrease in the patient's digoxin serum concentration will not be readily seen because the digoxin is still present in the serum but is prevented from getting to the cells by the Digibind. It is recommended that no digoxin serum concentrations be obtained for 6 to 8 hours after initial Digibind administration.

Patients receiving Digibind should undergo continuous ECG and blood pressure monitoring as well as continuous percutaneous oxygen saturation measurement. Electrolyte imbalances, such as hypokalemia, hypercalcemia, and hypomagnesemia, should be corrected as soon as possible to optimize the effects of the Digibind, since any of these conditions can be a factor predisposing the patient to digoxin toxicity. In patients with bradyarrhythmias secondary to digoxin toxicity, temporary cardiac pacing may be necessary to provide cardiovascular support while coordinating efforts to administer Digibind. In patients who were receiving digoxin for congestive heart failure (CHF), the clinician should continuously assess during the first hour after Digibind administration for the return of the signs and symptoms of CHF.

Digoxin

Digoxin, a cardiac glycoside approved by the FDA in 1952, is not classified as an antiarrhythmic drug, although it possesses distinct electrophysiologic properties. It is used primarily to enhance myocardial function while decreasing myocardial oxygen consumption.

Mechanism of Action

Digoxin has both indirect and direct properties that result in its electrophysiologic effects. Indirectly, digoxin's electrophysiologic effects include hyperpolarization, shortening of atrial action potentials, and increases in AV nodal refractoriness. Directly, digoxin binds to the sodium/potassium adenosine triphosphatase transport complex, thereby inhibiting the outward flux of sodium ions. At higher concentrations, this direct action could result in enhanced ventricular automaticity, which is why it is not used for the termination of ventricular arrhythmias.

Amenable Arrhythmias

Digoxin is used to terminate reentrant arrhythmias that incorporate the AV node as part of their circuit. These arrhythmias include SVT associated with an accessory pathway without antegrade conduction (i.e., concealed WPW), PJRT, LGL, and AVNRT. Because it may shorten, lengthen, or result in no change in the antegrade refractory period of accessory pathways, its use in patients with WPW remains controversial.[21,22] Digoxin is also used in patients with atrial flutter, atrial fibrillation, and other IARTs to rarely terminate the arrhythmia, and more commonly to produce AV block with a resultant decrease in the ventricular rate. Digoxin is also used in patients with postoperative JET, mostly for improvement in myocardial function, although occasionally it may cause arrhythmia termination.

Implications for Clinicians

Because digoxin is one of the most common drugs prone to dosage error, it is preferred that two people independently calculate the dosage for any given patient. Once the dosage has been determined, the physician's order should be written as a total dose and a volume dose on all orders. For example, an acceptable initial digoxin order for a child weighing 20 kg at a dose of 15 μg/kg using the pediatric injectable preparation of 100 μg/mL is as follows: Give 300 μg/3 mL of 100 μg/mL IV over 5 to 10 minutes now. The injectable form of digoxin is also available as 250 μg/mL, so the clinician MUST know the concentration when verifying the amount to administer. If there is ever any question regarding the dosage or preparation, the clinician should make every effort to clarify the issue prior to administering the medication.

Patients receiving IV digoxin should undergo continuous ECG monitoring. The clinician should constantly assess the child for nausea, vomiting, and/or drowsiness, as these are the primary extracardiac symptoms indicating toxicity in infants and children. Cardiac rhythm disturbances, such as second- or third-degree AV block, are the most common signs of cardiac toxicity. It is generally not necessary to obtain digoxin serum concentrations during IV administration, unless signs and symptoms of toxicity are noted.

Esmolol

Esmolol hydrochloride, approved by the FDA in 1986, is a Class II, ultra short-acting, nonselective β-adrenergic blocker. Its ultrashort half-life is due to its rapid conversion into inactive metabolites by blood esterases. Esmolol has virtually replaced the use of IV propranolol in the pediatric population because it has a very short duration of action. In addition to its electrophysiologic effects, esmolol increases systemic vascular resistance and decreases myocardial contractility leading to decreased myocardial oxygen consumption.

Mechanism of Action

The mechanism of action of esmolol is the blockade of sympathetic stimulation that is mediated by β_1-adrenergic receptors in the heart and vascular smooth muscle. Esmolol's electrophysiologic actions occur predominantly at the level of the sinus and AV nodes, with the specific actions of increasing the sinus cycle length, increasing sinus node recovery times, and slowing AV nodal conduction. This negative chronotropic effect should result in a decrease in heart rate and blood pressure, but will also result in decreased myocardial contractility.

Amenable Arrhythmias

Esmolol can be used to treat a variety of tachyarrhythmias in children, especially those that occur after surgery for CHD.[23,24] Arrhythmias that are amenable to esmolol therapy include reentrant SVTs such as those associated with WPW, concealed WPW, PJRT, LGL, AVNRT, JET (rarely), atrial flutter, other intraatrial tachycardias, and VT.

Implications for Clinicians

Because esmolol has a negative inotropic effect and can depress ventricular function, it should be avoided in patients with overt heart failure, and used with extreme caution in patients with known or suspected decreased ventricular function. Prior to esmolol administration, a baseline evaluation of ventricular function should be performed using echocardiography. Children receiving IV esmolol are generally in a critical care unit or catheterization laboratory with continuous ECG and blood pressure monitoring. Due to the fact that 50% of patients experience hypotension during esmolol bolus therapy, an indwelling arterial monitoring catheter for blood pressure evaluation is preferred. The incidence of drug-induced hypotension is increased in smaller children and those with single ventricle physiology,[15] warranting somewhat slower administration in these patients. The effects of esmolol can be reversed with isoproterenol, norepinephrine, dopamine, and dobutamine.[25]

Esmolol is best administered by an infusion control device in D_5W, normal saline, or Ringer's lactate solutions. It is compatible with potassium chloride but is not compatible with sodium bicarbonate, diazepam, furosemide, or thiopental sodium. Clinicians caring for patients receiving IV esmolol should continuously evaluate the IV site for patency and early signs of infiltration, since extravasation of esmolol can lead to skin necrosis. Concentrations of greater than 10 mg/mL should not be used, as higher concentrations can result in more severe vein irritation and phlebitis.[26]

Ibutilide

Ibutilide, a Class III antiarrhythmic drug, was approved by the FDA in 1995 for the immediate treatment of atrial flutter and atrial fibrillation in adults. Its application to the pediatric population is somewhat limited at this time, as there have been no studies published describing safe use in children. Because it is more successful at terminating atrial flutter than atrial fibrillation, ibutilide may be particularly useful in pediatric patients with atrial reentrant tachycardia after repair of CHD; however, an approximately 5% incidence of torsades de pointes or VF has limited enthusiasm for its use. It may be used prior to or as an adjunct to elective cardioversion as a treatment choice in select patients in the future.[27,28]

Mechanism of Action

Although ibutilide is classified as a selective Class III antiarrhythmic agent, rather than blocking outward potassium currents, it promotes the influx of sodium through slow inward sodium channels. Ibutilide prolongs action potential duration and effective refractory periods in both atrial and ventricular myocardial cells,[29,30] with mild slowing of the sinus rate and AV node conduction.

Amenable Arrhythmias

Since pediatric usage of ibutilide is limited at this time, arrhythmias amenable to ibutilide therapy include atrial flutter and atrial fibrillation of recent onset in adults.[31] Ibutilide should be used with caution in any patient, as it is associated with serious proarrhythmia including QT prolongation, torsades de pointes, and polymorphic VT with up to 2% of patients requiring cardioversion.[30,32]

Implications for Clinicians

Patients receiving ibutilide should undergo continuous ECG monitoring during and at least 4 hours following ibutilide administration or until the corrected QT has returned to baseline. Defibrillation and external pacing capabilities should be readily available. Efforts to correct any electrolyte abnormalities, such as hypokalemia or hypomagnesemia, should be undertaken prior to ibutilide administration. Medications for the treatment of VT including magnesium sulfate should be immediately available in the event of proarrhythmia. The concomitant use of Class Ia and other Class III antiarrhythmic drugs is not recommended during ibutilide administration and for 4 hours post infusion because all of these agents prolong refractoriness. If the patient is being treated with these agents on a long-term basis, it is recommended that they be held for at least five half-lives prior to ibutilide administration.[33]

Isoproterenol

Isoproterenol is a pure β-adrenergic agonist used in the treatment of hemodynamically significant bradycardia that is due to sinus node dysfunction or AV block and that is resistant to atropine.[16] It causes an increase in heart rate, conduction velocity, and cardiac contractility, as well as producing peripheral vasodilation leading to an increase in pulse pressure.

Mechanism of Action

Isoproterenol is a positive inotrope as well as a vasodilator. It acts directly and nonselectively on β-adrenergic receptors and increases myocardial oxygen consumption. Electrophysiologically, isoproterenol shortens refractory periods, increases conduction velocity, and enhances sinus and AV node function.

Implications for Clinicians

Patients receiving isoproterenol should undergo continuous ECG and blood pressure monitoring. The intended action of isoproterenol is to increase the patient's heart rate, which is also an adverse effect that patients may complain of if they receive isoproterenol while awake. Patients receiving isoproterenol also tend to complain of headache, chest pressure/pounding, and nausea/vomiting, and should be warned about these effects prior to isoproterenol administration, especially if they are to be awake while receiving it. The American Heart Association/American Academy of Pediatrics recommend the following formula for determining the IV solution of isoproterenol to be administered by infusion pump[16]: multiply 0.6 by the child's weight in kilograms to equal the amount of drug to be added to the IV solution for a total volume of 100 mL. In order to provide 0.1 μg/kg/min, an infusion rate of 1 mL/hr is used.

Lidocaine

Lidocaine, a Class Ib antiarrhythmic drug, is a local anesthetic that is also used for the immediate management of ventricular arrhythmias.

It is classified as a sodium channel blocker that depresses spontaneous ventricular depolarization but usually does not affect sinus or AV node depolarization.

Mechanism of Action

IV lidocaine decreases depolarization, automaticity, and excitability in the ventricle during the diastolic phase by direct action on the tissues (especially the Purkinje network) without involvement of the autonomic nervous system. Specifically, it blocks the fast sodium channel and slows frequency dependence with little to no effects on structures above the bundle of His. It acts selectively on diseased or ischemic tissue, where it is thought to promote conduction block thereby interrupting certain reentry circuits. It seldom impairs AV node function or conduction. Lidocaine also significantly increases the VF threshold,[34] which theoretically should decrease the defibrillation threshold making it easier to terminate VF.

Amenable Arrhythmias

Arrhythmias that are amenable to lidocaine administration include premature ventricular contractions (PVCs) and VT. Its primary efficacy is for the suppression of PVCs in the patient at risk for recurrent VT.[35] Lidocaine's efficacy for converting hemodynamically stable VT to normal sinus rhythm is approximately 20%, which proved it less effective than procainamide in a double blind cross-over study.[36] It is also used for VF.

Implications for Clinicians

Pediatric patients generally receive IV lidocaine during cardiopulmonary resuscitation or in the critical care environment. Regardless of the environment, the ECG should be monitored constantly. On rare occasions, IV lidocaine can be proarrhythmic, and it can exacerbate supraventricular arrhythmias. If it is being administered to extinguish PVCs, their frequency on the surface ECG should be noted at periodic intervals during lidocaine infusion.

The IV infusion site should be monitored frequently for the signs and symptoms of infection as well as vein irritation. IV lidocaine is known to cause soreness at the IV infusion site. It is recommended that the continuous infusion of lidocaine contain 120 mg of lidocaine per 100 mL of D_5W[16] yielding 1200 μg/mL. In order to deliver 20 μg/kg/min, an infusion rate of 1 mg/kg/hr is used.

IV lidocaine has various effects on the child's mental status and LOC. Although serum concentrations can be measured and should be evaluated periodically, the clinician should constantly evaluate the child's LOC and mental status for somnolence, confusion, and paresthesia, which may be the first signs of an impending reaction. In severely ill patients, the first sign of toxicity may be seizures. Newborns may be especially sensitive to changes in LOC, since the half-life is slightly prolonged in these patients (3 hours versus 2 hours) compared to older children.[15]

Phenytoin

Phenytoin, a Class Ib antiarrhythmic agent approved by the FDA in 1938, is most commonly used to treat seizures in the pediatric population. It is a sodium channel blocker with local anesthetic effects similar to lidocaine. The oral form of phenytoin has been used most successfully for the treatment of chronic ventricular arrhythmias after repair of CHD.[37]

Mechanism of Action

Phenytoin inhibits the fast sodium current while shortening the action potential duration, especially in abnormally long action potentials.[38] It acts selectively on diseased or ischemic tissue and is now thought to have an effect on delayed afterdepolarizations. It is not thought to have any effect on sinus or AV node automaticity,[37] but it may be effective for reducing automaticity in nonsinus atrial cells, such as in AET.

Amenable Arrhythmias

Arrhythmias that are amenable to IV phenytoin include PVCs, VT, and AET. Although phenytoin may suppress ventricular arrhythmias in the anatomically normal heart, it seems to be more successful in patients who have had previous surgery for CHD.[37] It can also be used in the treatment of ventricular arrhythmias related to the congenital long QT syndrome.[9]

Implications for Clinicians

Because of phenytoin's propensity to be highly teratogenic, it is imperative that females of child-bearing age undergo pregnancy testing prior to its administration. The administration of IV phenytoin for ventricular arrhythmias in children should proceed as follows: a total loading dose of 15 mg/kg is given over 1 hour.[39] Because of its instability and propensity to precipitate, it is not diluted. A syringe with one twelfth of the total loading dose is given in an IV push every 5 minutes followed quickly with a saline flush. Because of this instability and propensity to precipitate when mixed with a diluent, it is recommended that IV phenytoin NOT be given as a continuous infusion when it is being used to treat ventricular arrhythmias.[39]

The clinician should be aware of the adverse effects of IV phenytoin administration. The most common adverse effect is that of hypotension, which precludes its administration in patients with severely altered hemodynamics. Patients receiving IV phenytoin for ventricular arrhythmias should undergo continuous ECG and frequent blood pressure monitoring. In cases of moderate hypotension, it is recommended that the bolus injections be stopped for 10 to 15 minutes until the patient's blood pressure increases. Phenytoin causes burning at the injection site and extravasation can result in local tissue damage. Phenytoin should be discontinued if a rash appears.

Procainamide

IV procainamide, a sodium channel blocker, is the Class Ia agent most commonly used in the pediatric population.[15] It is a potent sodium channel blocker with moderate potassium channel blocking effects and it is also an anticholinergic.

Mechanism of Action

Procainamide suppresses automaticity in both atrial and ventricular tissue, slowing conduction in the atrium, bundle of His, and ventricle. Its direct effects prolong conduction through the AV node with greater effects at faster heart rates; however, because of its anticholinergic effects, AV node conduction is usually enhanced by IV procainamide. It does not prolong the QT interval to the same extent as quinidine does.[9]

Amenable Arrhythmias

IV procainamide can be used for a variety of supraventricular and ventricular arrhythmias. Specific arrhythmias amenable to procainamide administration include SVT due to an accessory connection (such as WPW, concealed WPW, and PJRT), AVNRT, atrial flutter, other IARTs, atrial fibrillation, PVCs, and VT. In fact, in one double blind cross-over study, procainamide was much more effective than lidocaine in converting sustained monomorphic VT to sinus rhythm.[36] Because it enhances AV node conduction and may thereby increase the ventricular response to an atrial tachycardia, IV procainamide should only be given after digoxin loading in such patients with second-degree AV block.

Implications for Clinicians

The administration of IV procainamide requires that the patient undergo continuous ECG monitoring, usually in the critical care environment. The ECG should be monitored for heart rate and rhythm as well as QRS duration and QT interval. Additionally, because of the drug's proarrhythmic effect, any exacerbation of the arrhythmia being treated or any new-onset arrhythmias should be documented by obtaining a rhythm strip, and the child's physician should be notified immediately.

The major adverse effect of IV procainamide administration is that of hypotension. Consequently, it should only be administered with continuous or very frequent arterial pressure monitoring. This effect can be lessened by administering the loading dose slowly, but may require concomitant administration of volume expanders, such as colloidal infusions. The clinician should have the capability for temporary pacing in the event of bradycardia and/or AV block. Patients with existing second- or third-degree AV block without a permanent cardiac pacemaker should not receive IV procainamide without the ability for back-up temporary pacing.

Patient and Family Considerations

Patient and family education is an important component of the overall care of the child receiving pharmacologic agents for immediate arrhythmia management. This education should include the drug's intended action, the predicted onset of action, and any adverse effects associated with its use. Since many of these agents will be administered in the critical care environment, it is helpful for families to know what to expect as well as what not to expect. For example, adenosine works very rapidly, whereas IV procainamide requires a loading dose and may require several hours before an improvement in the child's arrhythmia is seen. Also, if blood drawing is necessary for measuring serum concentrations, the patient and family should be informed of this up front.

Any precautionary measures, such as having a temporary pacemaker or defibrillator at the patient's bedside, should be explained to the family in advance whenever possible. Also, families must be aware that not only does the drug affect the abnormal rhythm, but in many cases, it can negatively affect the child's normal conduction. Explanations such as these will hopefully help to ease the family's anxiety and will aid in the development of a trusting relationship between health care providers and the patient and family.

Since most of these agents are only used on an immediate/emergent basis, families will have many questions regarding more permanent options. Those caring for these children and their families should make every effort to include the family in discussions, especially when examining treatment options. These discussions should include the advantages and disadvantages of each option with rationale for why a particular option may be best for the individual child.

Temporary Pacing Modalities

Temporary pacing modalities can be used in a variety of settings with various patient scenarios in patients with bradyarrhythmias and/or tachyarrhythmias. Patients requiring temporary pacing can present with anatomically normal hearts or having had previous surgery for CHD. The specific methods discussed in this chapter include noninvasive transcutaneous pacing, transesophageal pacing, temporary transvenous pacing, and epicardial pacing using temporary pacing wires placed at the time of surgery for CHD and are summarized in Table 1. Each modality is defined,

Table 1
Temporary Pacing Modalities Used in Children

Pacing Modality	Available Modes	Advantages	Disadvantages	Comments
Transcutaneous	VVI, VOO	• Noninvasive • Rapid implementation • Relatively inexpensive when compared with other methods • Minimal training requirements needed for implementation • Can be used in hospital and prehospital settings	• Painful • Potential for impairment in skin integrity • Requires sedation if used for prolonged period	• Cannot be used in presence of cervical spine injuries or flail chest • Limited effectiveness in patients with cardiomyopathy, hyperinflated lung disease, and large pleural/pericardial effusions • Prominent muscle contractions make vital signs difficult to monitor • Have defibrillator at bedside if not contained in device
Transesophageal	AAI, AOO	• Semi-invasive technique • Used for a variety of functions compared with other modalities • Can be used on an outpatient basis • Helpful in patients with limited venous access	• Causes esophageal discomfort • May require sedation for therapeutic uses • Requires that patient be NPO	• Can be used diagnostically and therapeutically • Generally only helpful with supraventricular tachyarrhythmias

Table 1
Temporary Pacing Modalities Used in Children (cont.)

Pacing Modality	Available Modes	Advantages	Disadvantages	Comments
Transvenous	VVI, VOO (in most cases)	• Minimal patient discomfort during use • May be left in place prophylactically up to 72 hours • Most reliable method of emergency pacing • Minimal current used in most cases	• Requires skill in venipuncture and manipulating pacing electrodes • Fluoroscopy (occasionally echocardiogram) necessary to ensure satisfactory pacing catheter position • Difficult to insert during CPR • May be displaced during CPR • More serious complications when compared with other methods	• Potential complications related to venous access: ⋋ infection ⋋ bleeding ⋋ phlebitis ⋋ local trauma ⋋ thromboembolism • Potential complications related to pacing catheter: ⋋ catheter-induced arrhythmia ⋋ cardiac perforation/ tamponade • Catheter dislodgment can result in: ⋋ loss of capture ⋋ failure to sense appropriately ⋋ knotting of the catheter

| Epicardial pacing wires | AAI, AOO, VVI, VOO, DVI, DDD, DOO, DDI | • Can be used prophylactically for transient arrhythmias
• AV synchrony preserved in presence of AV block
• May obtain atrial electrogram
• More variety for pacing modes
• Not painful to the child
• Can be diagnostic and therapeutic | • Requires clinical knowledge of advanced pacemaker function (i.e., atrial synchronous pacing)
• Wires will occasionally break
• Pacing thresholds higher due to epicardial placement
• Painful and anxiety provoking to child when removed | • Atrial wires—located on patient's right
• Ventricular wires—located on patient's left
• Always wear rubber gloves when handling wires
• When not in use, store in rubber finger cot or glove and tape to child's chest
• Potential complications:
  ∧ infection
  ∧ bleeding
  ∧ microshock
  ∧ tamponade (with removal) |

AV = atrioventricular; CPR = cardiopulmonary resuscitation; NPO = nothing by mouth.

followed by mechanism of action, amenable arrhythmias, and implications for clinicians. The patient and family considerations are identified as a group at the end of this section.

Noninvasive Transcutaneous Pacing

The concept of external cardiac pacing was introduced in the early 1950s with the work of Dr. Paul Zoll.[40] Many improvements have been made since these early attempts and, currently, the availability of external pacing electrode pads in a variety of sizes has made this treatment modality more suitable for pediatric patients. Additionally, such improvements allowing alteration of pulse width, high-impedance electrodes, and circuitry that allows a more legible surface ECG tracing[41] make this mode of temporary pacing more feasible, but it is usually still painful enough to require sedation in conscious patients.

Noninvasive transcutaneous pacing is used in children to initiate rapid rhythm control in situations requiring immediate treatment.[42] Although publications associated with this treatment modality in the pediatric population are limited, it can be used quickly as an adjunct to other resuscitative measures. The advantages of noninvasive transcutaneous pacing include its safety and effectiveness as well as its ability to be implemented quickly.[43,44] Additionally, it is easily applied, is generally immediately available (when compared to other temporary pacing options), has low complication rates, and is less costly than other temporary pacing methods.[45,46] The major disadvantage of temporary transcutaneous pacing is patient discomfort and/or pain, especially in the conscious pediatric patient. Other disadvantages include alterations in skin integrity at the site of electrode placement (such as stinging, burning, and/or small cuts or abrasions), the small risk of arrhythmia induction when using the asynchronous mode of pacing, and difficulty obtaining adequate capture in patients who are extremely large or have significant transthoracic resistance to electrical stimulation.[47] Because of the high likelihood of severe skin damage in infants, transcutaneous pacing should only be performed in the most critical of circumstances and when no other options are available.

Mechanism of Action

Noninvasive transcutaneous pacing is accomplished by placing two large skin electrode pads in anterior and posterior thoracic positions over the ventricles, allowing energy to be delivered between the two pads from an attached energy source (i.e., an external pulse generator). This energy source can be a stand-alone device used solely for noninvasive transcutaneous pacing or, more commonly, a device that incorporates temporary pacing within a standard defibrillator (Fig. 3). The energy delivered between the two electrodes is a direct low-density current that is passed directly into the heart muscle through the skin and rib cage, resulting in electrical depolarization of the myocardium. Although the maximum de-

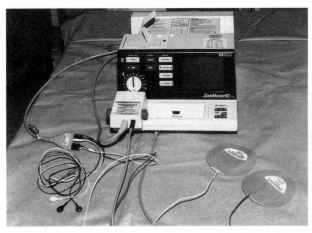

Figure 3. External defibrillator/cardioverter also capable of providing external transcutaneous pacing through the same preapplied self-adhesive electrodes.

liverable current is approximately 200 mA, only 40 to 70 mA are generally required to stimulate cardiac tissue.[48] Lower current densities secondary to long pulse widths/durations of 40 ms and large external electrodes positioned in areas with less underlying skeletal muscle now result in more tolerable adverse effects of this particular pacing modality.

Amenable Arrhythmias

Arrhythmias that are amenable to noninvasive temporary pacing include asystole, sinus arrest, sinus bradycardia, junctional bradycardia, and second- or third-degree AV block. Beland and colleagues[41] suggest other specific indications in children as follows: patients undergoing temporary epicardial pacing after surgery for CHD who experience problems (i.e., broken wires or impending exit block) from their temporary wires, pacemaker-dependent patients during routine pacing system follow-up (rare), patients with complete AV block who receive general anesthesia, patients experiencing bradycardia or AV block secondary to drug overdose, patients undergoing elective cardioversion in whom rebound bradycardia or asystole is a concern,[49] and in symptomatic patients awaiting permanent pacemaker implantation. It may also be used for patients awaiting lead revision for damaged/malfunctioning permanent pacing leads or those with pacemaker battery depletion. Noninvasive temporary pacing can also be used safely in newborns with congenital complete AV block who are awaiting permanent pacemaker implantation.[50]

Implications for Clinicians

Since most bradycardia episodes and/or cardiac arrests in children are the result of acute hypoxia and/or ventilatory problems, they will generally respond to airway support and management. In rare cases, noninvasive temporary pacing may be used in a cardiac arrest situation in which the child's LOC is irrelevant; however, in the conscious patient, sedation should be implemented with ample consideration to intubation and artificial ventilation.[51] This is especially important when using this treatment modality in infants, since the moderate amount of skeletal muscle stimulation is likely to impair the infant's spontaneous respirations.

Electrode pad size and placement are extremely important when dealing with smaller hearts. Researchers have determined that as electrode size increases, pacing threshold increases while current density decreases.[41] Taylor[45] suggests the following for electrode pad sizes in the pediatric population: the adult-sized electrode should be used in children weighing greater than 15.0 kg, the medium-sized electrode for patients weighing 5 to 15.0 kg, and the small-sized electrode for neonates weighing more than 3.0 kg. Care should be taken not to choose an electrode pad that covers the child's neck or abdomen. Prior to pad placement, the child's skin should be clean and dry. The use of alcohol or benzoin to clean the skin should be avoided because if residua is left underneath the electrode, skin burns can occur secondary to the flammable nature of these two substances. The external pacing pads are generally placed on the left subclavicular area and to the lower left sternal border. Alternatively, they may be placed on the right upper sternal border and the left ventricular apical area. In patients who require noninvasive transcutaneous pacing for prolonged periods, care must be taken to evaluate skin integrity at regular intervals, especially in smaller patients. In some neonates, small burns have been observed after only a half hour of continuous pacing, suggesting that their electrode pads should be changed a minimum of every 24 hours.[52,53] The child's skin integrity should be assessed when changing the electrode pads/patches.

Because of the discomfort and pain associated with noninvasive transcutaneous pacing, it is recommended that children receive some type of sedation agent. Certain general variables should be taken into account when choosing a particular sedative for the pediatric patient including the type of procedure (i.e., painful versus not painful), the anticipated duration of the procedure, the child's underlying medical condition, the need for narcosis and anxiolysis, and experience with alternative techniques or routes of administration.[54] Commonly used agents, such as midazolam, fentanyl, and propofol, can be effective in sedating children on a short-term basis,[55] but for children requiring prolonged noninvasive transcutaneous pacing, Taylor[45] recommends heavy sedation/general anesthesia, chemical paralysis, and artificial ventilation.

Once the appropriate electrode pads are placed and attached to the external pacemaker, proper pacemaker function must be verified. The pacing rate and output should be set as determined by the attending physician. The particular mode of pacing that results from a noninvasive transcutaneous system is either a ventricular demand (VVI) or asynchronous ventricular (VOO) pacing mode. The relatively large amount of current generated by the external pacemaker will often result in problems in evaluating the surface ECG. The pacemaker stimulus artifact (or pacemaker spike) is usually very large, leading to a decrease in the gain on the ECG monitor. This may decrease the size of the pacemaker spike but it will also decrease the size of the QRS, making it difficult to ascertain capture. Generally, the device delivering the pacemaker energy will have the most usable ECG through internal stimulus artifact suppression. If there is confusion regarding whether the pacemaker is capturing, the clinician should palpate the child's pulse. In the infant, the brachial or femoral artery is used, and in the older child, the carotid artery is used. This will provide validation that the device is indeed causing ventricular depolarization and contraction. If the pacemaker is not capturing, the clinician should turn up the pacemaker output. The child's hemodynamic status as well as underlying rhythm should also be assessed each hour while the transcutaneous pacemaker is in use.

It is critical that the clinician understand basic pacing concepts in order to determine if the device is functioning properly. The first step in being able to evaluate proper pacemaker function is identification and evaluation of the pacing mode. If the device is set to VVI or the ventricular demand mode, it should only attempt to pace when the child's heart rate is *less* than the prescribed pacing rate. For example, if the pacing rate is set at 80 pulses per minute (ppm) and the child's heart rate is 100 beats per minute (bpm), no pacing artifacts should be noted. If pacing artifacts are noted in this case, the child's native QRS complexes are not being recognized (or sensed) by the pacemaker and an adjustment in the sensitivity will be required. In the VOO or asynchronous mode, the pacemaker should produce pacing artifacts at the predetermined rate regardless of the child's underlying rhythm.

The clinician should document when and why transcutaneous pacing was implemented, periodic ECG rhythm strips documenting pacemaker status, any complications or adverse effects, and the following pacemaker parameters: pacing mode, pacing rate, stimulation threshold value, output setting, and percentage paced if in the demand mode.[56]

Transesophageal Pacing

Transesophageal atrial pacing was initially used with success in 1957[57] and is a semi-invasive method of temporarily pacing the atrium using an electrode catheter that is passed through the child's nares or mouth into the esophagus and placed behind the heart, specifically behind the left atrium. The proximal end of the catheter is attached to a stimulator or external pacemaker used to deliver energy. Because esophageal pacing of the ventricle is unreliable,[35] pacing of the atrium is the goal for this particular temporary pacing modality. The transesophageal electrode can also be used for recording electrical activity in the atrium for diagnostic purposes[58–60] (Fig. 4), as well as therapeutically to overdrive specific atrial reentrant tachyarrhyth-

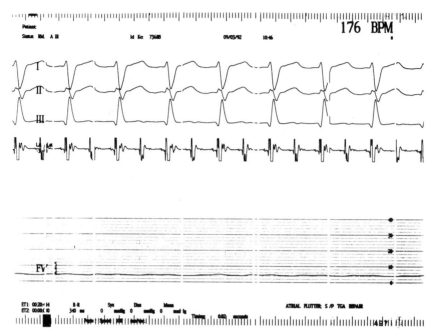

Figure 4. Surface ECG leads I, II, and III and a bipolar atrial electrogram recorded with a transesophageal pacing catheter. The temporary pacing catheter was used to help delineate the specific tachyarrhythmia mechanism in this postoperative Mustard patient. Atrial activity is difficult to discern from the surface ECG leads. Note the larger size of the atrial versus ventricular electrogram exhibited in this recording.

mias, including atrial flutter[58,61,62] (Fig. 5). It can also be used to assess the efficacy of antiarrhythmic drug therapy for SVT, to evaluate palpitations in children,[63] and to evaluate sinus and AV node function.[64]

The advantages of transesophageal pacing over other temporary pacing techniques include: 1) general anesthesia is not required for its use; 2) it can be used for bradycardia pacing in the presence of symptomatic bradycardia after successful SVT termination if AV node conduction is intact; and 3) it is useful in patients with limited venous access secondary to previous cardiac catheterizations and/or surgical procedures.[45] It can be used on an outpatient basis for overdriving paroxysmal SVTs that do not respond to other, less invasive maneuvers[65] and as a diagnostic tool to determine more definitive arrhythmia management, e.g., antiarrhythmic medications or radiofrequency ablation. The most common adverse effect of transesophageal pacing is esophageal discomfort.

Mechanism of Action

Transesophageal atrial pacing is achieved by placing an electrode catheter into the esophagus into a position directly behind the left atrium. The posterior left atrium is stimulated by the energy delivered through

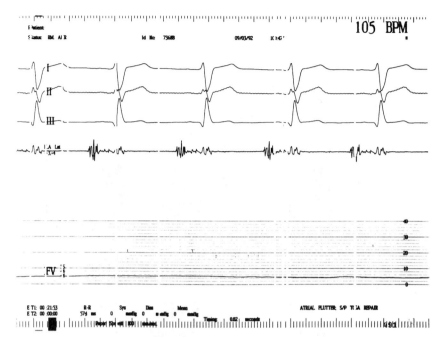

Figure 5. Surface ECG leads I, II, and III and a bipolar atrial electrogram recorded on the same patient in Figure 4. The tachycardia was overdriven with use of the temporary catheter, with resultant normal sinus rhythm as evidenced on this atrial electrogram. The P waves and the R waves are now similar in size.

the catheter's distal electrode through the esophagus *or* atrial activity is simply recorded in order to ascertain the atrium's role in a specific arrhythmia when it is not discernable on the surface ECG. Bipolar electrode catheters (Fig. 6) are used with a pacing current value of 10 to 20 mA (for consistent atrial capture) and a pulse width of 10 ms delivered by an external stimulator or temporary pacemaker.[35] Commercially available

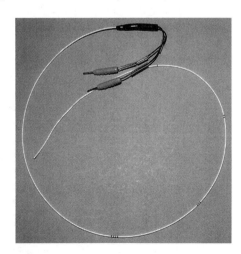

Figure 6. Bipolar transesophageal pacing catheter with tip electrodes. Distance markers for insertion can be seen in various areas on the catheter.

catheters used specifically for transesophageal pacing are generally available in the following French sizes: 4, 5, 7, and 10. The "pill" electrode, in which the tip of the electrode is covered by a gelatin capsule to ease swallowing, is an attractive option for children.[60] Alternatively, permanent pacing leads (Fig. 7) and electrophysiologic catheters made by a variety of manufacturers can also be used for this purpose; however, with the availability of a wide variety of transesophageal catheters, their use is on the decline.

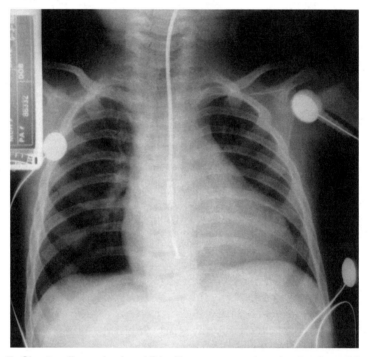

Figure 7. Chest radiograph of a child with a permanent pacing lead used for transesophageal pacing. The catheter is placed behind the left atrium, while surface ECG electrodes and leads are also evident.

For overdrive pacing of atrial tachyarrhythmias, a paced rate that is 10 to 30 bpm faster than the patient's measured atrial rate is delivered for approximately 30 seconds in order to "overdrive suppress" the arrhythmia with subsequent interruption of the reentry circuit (Fig. 8). Transesophageal electrophysiology testing is performed in a similar manner to intracardiac electrophysiology testing with the exception of ventricular stimulation. Once it has been determined that the transesophageal catheter is in proper position, atrial stimulation protocols are initiated. These protocols can include sinus node recovery times and sinoatrial conduction times, and are discussed in greater detail in the section on intracardiac electrophysiology testing in chapter 1.

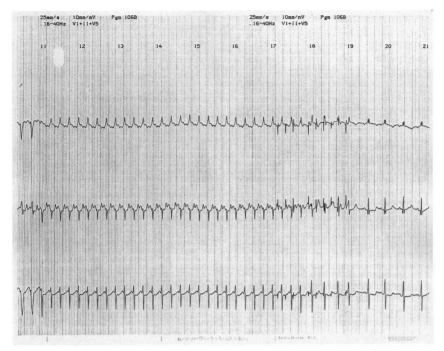

Figure 8. Surface ECG leads V$_1$, II, and V$_5$ recorded during an episode of supraventricular tachycardia. The tachycardia is overdriven by using 10 atrial paced beats at a rate slightly faster than the tachycardia rate, which results in tachycardia termination.

Amenable Arrhythmias

In most cases, transesophageal pacing is used to diagnose and terminate reentrant SVT. Specific arrhythmogenic substrates amenable to this type of temporary pacing include SVT associated with an accessory connection, including manifest and concealed WPW, AV node reentrant SVT, atrial flutter, and other IARTs. It may also be used to pace the atrium at high rates in order to produce second-degree AV block in patients with decreased cardiac output secondary to a rapid ventricular response to atrial tachycardia.

Implications for Clinicians

First and foremost, the patient and family must be educated about this particular method of temporary pacing before it is implemented. Since cooperation will be needed from the patient if the insertion is to be successful, the more information that can be provided, the better. For further discussion on patient and family education, please refer to the following section on patient and family considerations.

The transesophageal electrophysiology study itself may be carried out in a variety of settings. It can be performed in the ICU, the cardiac catheterization laboratory, or a designated procedure room. Regardless of where the procedure is performed, certain equipment must be readily available, including a surface ECG monitor capable of displaying a minimum of two channels, a noninvasive blood pressure monitor, a transcutaneous oxygen saturation monitor, external cardioverter/defibrillator pads and device, transesophageal catheters, and an external stimulator or pacemaker. Conventional temporary pacemakers are generally not used for transesophageal stimulation because of their short pulse durations (usually 2 ms or less) and their limited maximum outputs (only up to 20 mA). Because of the high output required for stimulation and the close proximity of the transesophageal catheter to the ventricle, ventricular stimulation is theoretically possible, necessitating the presence of an external defibrillator on standby.

Prior to the study, the patient should be NPO (nothing by mouth) for at least 3 hours. A consent form for the procedure, as well as IV access, should be obtained. IV fluids should be readily available although they are not always necessary. Care should be taken when determining which sedation agents will be used in order to avoid those that may affect conduction and/or inducibility. Pentobarbital or propofol may be less desirable for these reasons.

Prior to catheter insertion, the catheter should be measured against the patient to determine how much of it should be inserted. This is done by measuring the distance from the child's nares to the xiphoid process or using the child's height to estimate depth based on a previous study.[58] Once this has been accomplished, the catheter should be lubricated with an anesthetic ointment before it is inserted into the nares. Once the catheter is in position, the proximal end is attached to the recording device or stimulator depending on whether tachycardia determination or termination is desired, respectively. The two channels required for transesophageal electrophysiology testing include one that displays the left atrial electrogram (from the transesophageal catheter) and a surface ECG lead. Verification of transesophageal catheter placement can be determined by comparing the atrial electrogram with the P wave on the surface ECG if the patient is in normal sinus rhythm. The surface ECG is also used to determine the timing of ventricular activation in patients with ventricular preexcitation.

In general, when the procedure is performed in the ICU, a standard 12- to 15-lead ECG recorder can be used for recording both esophageal and surface ECGs. The electrode poles from the transesophageal catheter can be attached to the right and left arm lead inputs (lead I) or right arm and left leg (lead II), which go to the ECG machine. Surface ECG leads can then be displayed in two leads, while the transesophageal electrogram is displayed in either lead I or II. In the cardiac catheterization laboratory, a physiologic recording system and programmable stimulator are used to monitor, record, stimulate, and analyze data directly from the transesophageal catheter. A designated procedure room may use either one of these set-ups. Typical atrial stimulation protocols used for transesophageal electrophysiology testing can be found in chapter 1.

Once the procedure has been completed, the catheter is removed and the patient is returned to a recovery area, which may or may not be the same area where the procedure was performed. If no further testing or treatment is required, the sedated child can be discharged after meeting the discharge criteria for patients receiving IV sedation.[66]

Temporary Transvenous Pacing

Temporary transvenous pacing is an invasive technique in which a temporary pacing catheter is inserted into the heart, usually through a vein, and is commonly used as a temporary pacing modality.[67] This method is an attractive option for neonates with congenital complete AV block who require chronotropic support while awaiting permanent pacemaker placement or in patients with AV block inadvertently caused during a catheterization procedure. The catheter is generally placed/positioned through a vein into the right ventricle under fluoroscopic guidance; however, in the presence of a structurally normal heart, it can be done with echocardiographic guidance. Although rare in the pediatric population, temporary transvenous pacing catheters can be placed in the right atrium and/or coronary sinus. The one exception to the venous route is in the patient who has undergone a Fontan procedure (in which there is no venous access to the ventricle), where retrograde, arterial access to the left ventricle is required.

Common access routes in children include the internal jugular vein, the axillary vein, the subclavian vein, and the femoral vein. If the subclavian vein is used and endocardial permanent pacing is likely to follow, the temporary pacing catheter should be placed on the opposite side from where the permanent lead is to be placed. There are several types of catheters used for temporary transvenous pacing that are generally categorized into three basic types: balloon flotation, semiflotation, and traditional.[48] Additionally, electrode catheters used for intracardiac electrophysiology testing can be used for temporary transvenous pacing. In most pediatric centers, the most commonly used catheter is the balloon flotation catheter.

Temporary transvenous pacing is associated with a higher risk than are other temporary pacing modalities, primarily because of the invasive nature of this particular technique. Since the right ventricular myocardium is proportionally thinner in children versus adults, right ventricular perforation is a major concern, particularly in infants who require more than a few hours of pacing. Other potential complications include cellulitis, infection, catheter-induced arrhythmias, thrombus formation, bleeding, pneumothorax, arterial puncture/damage, lead dislodgment, pulmonary embolism, and venous obstruction. It is advisable to institute anticoagulation therapy in patients who are prone to thrombus formation, in patients with low cardiac output, and in patients with right-to-left or left-to-right intracardiac shunts.

Mechanism of Action

Temporary transvenous pacing leads work in the same way that placement of a permanent cardiac pacing lead works. In most cases, the temporary catheter is placed to the right ventricle and energy is delivered through the catheter into an electrode that is making direct contact with the ventricular myocardium. In most cases, a balloon-directed electrode catheter (as small as 3 Fr) is directed into the heart using a long accordionlike sterile cover that is secured to the sheath to permit later repositioning. The entrance of the catheter into the ventricle is often announced by the presence of catheter-induced PVCs.

Amenable Arrhythmias

The primary indication for temporary transvenous pacing in children is to provide temporary relief of bradycardia until a permanent pacing system can be safely implanted. Additionally, this method of temporary pacing can be used in patients with distal conduction disease requiring general anesthesia or in pacemaker-dependent patients undergoing pulse generator and/or lead replacement. Specific arrhythmias that are amenable to temporary transvenous pacing include sinus bradycardia, sick sinus syndrome, junctional bradycardia, and/or congenital or acquired second- or third-degree AV block.

Implications for Clinicians

The implications for clinicians caring for children with temporary transvenous pacing catheters are multifaceted and require that the clinician be aware of the potential complications of this particular technique as well as of specific signs that may alert one to these problems. Sterile technique should be maintained during insertion, regardless of where the procedure takes place. Additionally, securing the catheter and temporary pacemaker, verifying proper pacemaker function, sedation, and patient and family education are extremely important tasks that the clinician must undertake.

Once the catheter has been inserted and adequately positioned, the primary goal is to maintain that position and integrity until more permanent actions can be undertaken. Once the catheter is positioned and attached to the pulse generator, pacing should be verified by 12-lead ECG. Additionally, a portable chest roentgenogram should be performed to document lead placement as well as to evaluate for the presence of a pneumothorax. The catheter's exit/entry site should be covered with op-site and changed every 48 to 72 hours if the catheter is left in that long.[45] The excess catheter should be taped securely to the patient, with enough slack to prevent pulling with slight movements or patient repositioning. A stimulation threshold should be determined at this time, as should a sensing threshold. Once the stimulation threshold is determined, the external pacemaker output should be set two to three times higher than the threshold value. The sensitivity setting should be set two to three times less than the sensitivity threshold.

In most cases, the child will remain in the critical care setting for the duration of the catheter's placement, with continuous ECG, blood pressure, and oxygen saturation monitoring. In older children who are alert and cooperative, bed rest with no sedation may be adequate. In neonates, infants, and younger children, sedation is generally necessary to ensure catheter stability.

The clinician must be aware of the potential complications associated with temporary transvenous pacing. The two major serious complications are right ventricular perforation and lead dislodgment. Signs of perforation include loss of capture, a new-onset friction rub, or pericardial effusion/tamponade, the latter of which may be evidenced by unexplained sinus tachycardia and distant heart sounds upon auscultation. Lead dislodgment is estimated to occur in 25% of temporary transvenous lead systems[68] and is exhibited by loss of capture, loss of sensing, and atrial and ventricular ectopy. The signs and symptoms of site infection include fever, redness or swelling at the catheter site, and purulent drainage from the catheter site. Signs and symptoms of systemic infection or bacteremia include fever, loss of appetite, fatigue, elevated white blood cells/leukocytes, and increased blood sedimentation rate. Unfortunately, thrombus formation and/or venous obstruction may be difficult to ascertain and may only become apparent when further interventions are undertaken, such as dye injections used to delineate venous anatomy for permanent pacing leads or when trying to obtain venous access for cardiac catheterization procedures.

An evaluation of pacemaker function is critical after the catheter has been placed. In most cases, the mode of pacing used is ventricular demand (VVI), but occasionally it may be asynchronous (VOO). The physician's orders should include the following: the mode of pacing, the pacing rate, the output (usually in mA), and the sensitivity (in mV). The prescribed settings and the settings on the temporary pacemaker should be compared and any discrepancies clarified with the prescribing physician.

There are several things to consider when evaluating temporary pacemaker function. First and foremost, the clinician must determine if the pacemaker is capturing. In the VVI or VOO modes, this is evidenced by a pacemaker stimulus/spike that is followed by a QRS complex. This QRS complex is generally wider than the native QRS complex because of the abnormal depolarization caused by the temporary pacing lead. The pacemaker should only emit a stimulus if the patient's intrinsic ventricular rate is less than the prescribed/programmed pacing rate if in the demand mode. The pacemaker is sensing appropriately if the child's ventricular rate exceeds that of the prescribed pacing rate and no pacemaker spikes are emitted. For more information on pacemaker function, please refer to the section on epicardial pacing wires.

In most cases, the pacing and sensing thresholds are evaluated on a daily basis. The pacing threshold is the minimum amount of energy required to consistently result in depolarization, and is described as the numeric value that last captures 100% of the time. For example, the pacemaker is set at a numeric value of 10 mA and there is 100% capture of the ventricle. When the output value is decreased to 9 mA, it captures only every third beat. The pacing threshold in this case is 10 mA. The sensing threshold is the minimum intracardiac signal required to trigger or to inhibit a cardiac pacing stimulus, and it must be obtained when a spontaneous rhythm (versus a paced rhythm) is present. If the sensitivity setting is 5 mV and the patient's ventricular rate is faster than the prescribed pacing rate, the pacemaker is said to be sensing appropriately. If the sensitivity is set to 6 mV and random pacing spikes start appearing on the surface ECG without regard to the intrinsic QRS, the pacemaker is no longer sensing. This is due to the fact that the intrinsic signal (or QRS) is now too small for the pacemaker to recognize and it thinks there is no spontaneous depolarization, so it delivers a stimulus. In this particular example, the signal height of the intrinsic deflection is somewhere between 5 and 6 mV and the sensing threshold is 5 mV.

The pacemaker output and sensitivity settings should never be left at the threshold values as there are many things that can alter the thresholds, such as electrolyte imbalances, CHF, and medications. In general, the pacing output is set three times higher than the pacing threshold in order to provide an adequate safety margin, and the sensitivity is set to a value two times more sensitive (more sensitive meaning a lower numeric value) than the value just prior to loss of sensing. The patient's underlying rhythm should be ascertained by slowly decreasing the pacing rate until a ventricular escape beat occurs, NOT by suddenly turning off the temporary pacemaker.

Documentation for the patient undergoing temporary transvenous pacing should include the pacing indication, a periodic ECG rhythm strip documenting pacemaker function/status, hemodynamic assessment, stimulation and sensitivity thresholds, percentage paced (versus sensed) beats, type of catheter used and insertion site, and the following pacemaker parameters: pacing mode, pacing rate, output, and sensitivity.

Epicardial Pacing Wires

Temporary epicardial pacing wires are routinely placed at the time of open heart surgery and may or may not be used in the immediate postoperative period. The safety and efficacy of temporary epicardial pacing wires in the pediatric population has been validated by Yabek et al.[69] in more than 100 patients. This method of temporary pacing can be used to: 1) improve overall hemodynamics by improving cardiac output through increased rate and AV synchrony; 2) suppress ectopy; 3) terminate reentrant arrhythmias; and 4) record intrinsic electrical activity when rhythm abnormalities are difficult to ascertain from the surface ECG.

At the time of open heart surgery, the polyethylene- or Teflon-coated steel wires are sewn directly onto the epicardial surface of the right atrium and right ventricle in most cases because of their anterior anatomic location when the chest is open. Obviously in children with complex congenital heart defects, the wires may be placed in alternate anatomic locations. Prior to chest closure, the wires are pulled through the chest wall. It is not common practice to evaluate their function at the time of surgery and, in fact, it is better to evaluate pacing and sensing functions when the patient is normothermic.

As is standard in most institutions, the atrial wires are located to the right of the sternum at the subcostal region and the ventricular wires to the left of the sternum in the same location. The wires are generally removed within 48 to 72 hours after surgery, but may be used longer (up to 10 days) in patients with surgically acquired AV block or symptomatic bradycardia. A major advantage of using epicardial pacing wires over other temporary pacing modalities is the ability to use a variety of pacing modes, specifically the dual chamber modes. Additionally, there is less pain and discomfort with this technique compared with others, and use of this technique rarely requires sedation. Disadvantages include infection (rare), exit block, and cardiac tamponade (after wire removal). The biggest problem is that of exit block, in which the energy requirements exceed that which the pacemaker is able to provide. Not only are pacing thresholds affected by scar tissue formation at the suture site, but also by high catecholamine states, hypothermia, alkalosis, hypoxia, and hypokalemia.

Mechanism of Action

Postoperative epicardial pacing wires provide direct stimulation of the myocardium through energy delivered by an external pulse generator. The terminal end of the wire has a pin that can be attached directly to the pulse generator or to a cable that then attaches to the pulse generator. In most cases, the bipolar configuration is used, in which the electrical circuit is between the two sets of lead wires that are attached directly to the heart. The unipolar configuration requires that a skin electrode be placed and the electrical circuit is then between a single lead wire and the skin electrode. The terminal pins are then connected to the external pulse generator (Figs. 9 and 10). The atrial wires can also be used to record intrinsic atrial activity (i.e., an atrial electrogram) when it is difficult to discern the patient's rhythm from the surface ECG. Instructions for obtaining an atrial electrogram using postoperative epicardial pacing wires can be found in Table 2.

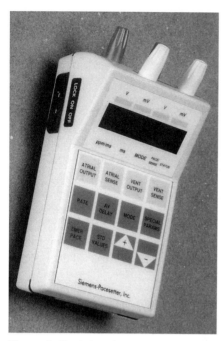 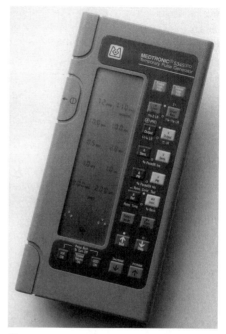

Figure 9. Dual chamber temporary pacemaker.

Figure 10. Dual chamber temporary pacemaker with liquid crystal display.

Amenable Arrhythmias

Arrhythmias that are amenable to temporary epicardial pacing include bradyarrhythmias and tachyarrhythmias. Bradyarrhythmias include sinus bradycardia, junctional bradycardia, and second- or third-degree AV block. Tachyarrhythmias include reentrant SVTs such as reentrant tachycardia using a bypass tract, AVNRT, atrial flutter, and other IARTs. An additional tachyarrhythmia that is amenable to this type of temporary pacing is JET. This arrhythmia is generally temporary, but can be deadly if not controlled. In patients with postoperative JET, the temporary pacing wires are

Table 2
Obtaining an Atrial Electrogram Using
Temporary Epicardial Pacing Wires

1. Always wear gloves when manipulating the temporary wires.
2. Use the wires located on the patient's RIGHT, which are the atrial wires.
3. Apply ECG electrodes to: left arm (LA), right leg (RL), V_1, and V_5, and attach to corresponding leads.
4. Attach atrial wires to ECG leads right arm (RA) and left leg (LL).
5. Program rhythm strip to: $V_1 + II + V_5$.
6. Press record rhythm at 25 mm/s, 10 mm/mV, and 100 Hz.
7. Lead II will exhibit atrial electrogram and leads V_1 and V_5 will exhibit surface ECG.

not used to terminate the tachycardia, but rather to improve cardiac output and provide AV synchrony by pacing the atrium at a rate slightly faster than the junctional rate. Additionally, these patients may benefit from pacing the atrium at rapid enough rates to produce 2:1 AV block. This results in a slower ventricular rate, which is intended to improve overall hemodynamics by improving cardiac output.

Implications for Clinicians

The implications for clinicians caring for children who require use of their temporary epicardial pacing wires are multifaceted. An IV line should be in place in addition to continuous ECG monitoring in patients undergoing temporary pacing. If the wires are not in use, they should be secured to the patient's chest until their removal. The wires can be wrapped around a 2 × 2 gauze, placed in a finger cot, and taped to the child's chest. Although site infection is rare, a betadine or similar solution should be applied to the exit site every 24 hours and as needed. The following discussion includes the implications for clinicians as they relate to attaching the temporary wires to an external pulse generator, securing the pacing system, batteries, evaluation of pacemaker function, and troubleshooting.

Attaching the Wires

The clinician should use extreme caution when handling the external pins of the temporary pacing wires. The wires are in direct contact with the myocardium, providing a low-resistance path for electrical current allowing even static electricity to result in an arrhythmia.[70] Although rare, VF can result from current leakage, making contact with unprotected terminals. First and foremost, any individual handling the terminal pins or exposed wires must wear rubber gloves[71] and avoid contact with any electrically operated device, including lights, monitors, x-ray equipment, radios, television, and respiratory therapy equipment, until the wires are securely attached to the external pulse generator. Once the terminal pins are exposed, they can be inserted directly into the receptacles of the pulse generator or to a connector cable, which may use alligator clips or a more secure thumbwheel set screw connection. These connections should be assessed by the clinician every 8 hours for intactness.[72] In unstable or hemodynamically compromised patients, the ventricular wires should be attached first. Once attached to the pulse generator, the pacemaker settings should be set according to the physician's orders. For further information regarding pacemaker function, please refer to the separate section on evaluation of pacemaker function.

Securing the Pacing System

Once everything is connected, it must be secured to the patient. There should be enough slack in the wires and/or cable to allow patient movement, and the pacemaker should be attached to the patient or placed in a carrying pouch such as those used for ambulatory telemetry monitors. It may be attached to the patient's leg or chest (for infants) with proper measures taken to prevent disconnection and/or wire dislodgment. Older style temporary pacemakers with analog controls have a plastic cover that slides over the dials to prevent the child from inadvertently changing any of the settings (Fig. 11). When the device is secured, it is important that this plastic cover be easily removable by the clinician in the event that quick changes are necessary. Newer devices with digital controls have a "lock" button that requires more ingenuity to change the settings, thus preventing inadvertent patient readjustments.

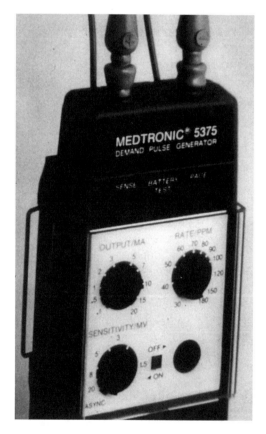

Figure 11. Older style single chamber temporary pacemaker with slideable plastic cover over the pacemaker setting dials.

Batteries

Extra batteries should be placed at the patient's bedside when a temporary pacemaker is in use. Optimally, the batteries should be changed prior to attaching the pulse generator to the pacing wires, since it is best to change them when the device is not in use; however, most devices will continue to operate for 10 to 15 seconds once the battery is removed. When the batteries are changed, the clinician should place a piece of tape on the pacemaker with the date, time, and initials to denote this change. Although hospital policy varies, the authors recommend changing the pacemaker batteries every 3 weeks when the device is not in use and every 24 hours when it is in use. Although rare, a second pacemaker should be available in case of device malfunction.

Evaluation of Pacemaker Function

In order to ascertain if the temporary pacemaker is functioning properly, the two most basic things (and minimal things) that the clinician must know are the pacemaker's prescribed mode of operation and the pacing rate. The generic mode code for cardiac pacemakers can be found in chapter 7. There are four basic factors to consider when evaluating pacemaker function: pacing, capture, sensing, and the pacing interval. Specific questions to ask oneself in order to evaluate these four factors, respectively, are: 1) Is the pacemaker pacing/firing at all and if so, is it at the preset rate? 2) Is a cardiac response elicited when the pacemaker fires? 3) Is the patient's intrinsic rhythm recognized? 4) What is the interval between paced beats and does it correlate with the prescribed pacing rate? By answering these basic questions, the clinician should be able to determine if the pacemaker is functioning properly and, if not, easily identify the area where the problem is originating (i.e., sensing or pacing). Evaluation of the pacing rate should be made by manual calculation using a printed rhythm strip, not by using the heart rate displayed on the cardiac monitor, which can be distorted by artifact or electrode movement.

When using epicardial pacing wires as a method for temporary pacing, the clinician now has more choices available for pacing modes. When using the single chamber modes, the determination of appropriate pacemaker function is relatively simple. First, the clinician must determine if the pacemaker is capturing. In the VVI or VOO modes, this is evidenced by a pacemaker stimulus/spike followed by a QRS complex that is generally wider than the patient's native QRS complex. In the AAI or AOO modes, capture is evidenced by a P wave following each pacemaker spike. Depending on where the atrial electrode is making contact with the atrium, the P wave may be positive or negative and may or may not have a similar appearance to the child's native P wave.

During use of a dual chamber pacing mode, evaluation of pacemaker function becomes slightly more complicated. The device can pace DOO (asynchronous pacing), DVI (AV sequential pacing), or DDD (atrial synchronous pacing). The most commonly used mode is the DDD mode, because this mode most closely mimics normal cardiac conduction. The asynchronous mode (DOO) is rarely used and the DDI mode can be used in patients who need AV synchrony but who have concomitant, intermittent atrial tachyarrhythmias in which atrial tracking is not desired. The advent of newer temporary pacemakers with the DDD mode has virtually eliminated the use of the DVI mode, which for a long time was the only dual chamber mode available in temporary pacemakers.

Since the DDD mode is the preferred pacing mode for children after CHD surgery, several issues warrant discussion. The DDD mode incorporates virtually every other pacing mode and can thus function in a variety of ways. In most cases, the pacing indication in patients with temporary epicardial pacing wires is AV block. Additional parameters that the clinician must be knowledgeable about in a dual chamber pacemaker include lower rate, upper rate, AV delay, and upper rate limit behavior. The lower rate in a DDD pacemaker is the lowest possible atrial rate. The upper rate is the highest rate that the ventricle is allowed to "track" the atrium in a 1:1 manner. The AV delay (synonymous with the PR interval) is the time from an atrial event (either sensed or paced) to a ventricular event (either sensed or paced). The upper rate limit behavior is a built-in mechanism to control the ventricular rate in the presence of rapid atrial rates, such as those seen in patients with atrial flutter.

When DDD pacemakers are used for temporary pacing in children after cardiac surgery, the clinician must be knowledgeable enough regarding the aforementioned parameters in order to determine if the device is working properly. A common assumption by clinicians is that the pacemaker is not working properly when it is exhibiting upper rate limit behavior. Since many of these children will exhibit sinus tachycardia in the ICU when emerging from anesthesia, this is a common occurrence. In general, the child's sinus node function is normal and the pacemaker is being used for some degree of AV block. As the sinus rate increases, the pacemaker "tracks" the atrium, waits for the programmed AV delay criteria to be met, and then paces the ventricle at the same rate as the sensed atrial rate. If the upper rate of the DDD pacemaker is exceeded, upper rate limit behavior is automatically implemented by the device. This behavior, in most cases, is Wenckebach in which every third or fourth P wave is not followed by a paced QRS complex. The pacemaker is in fact not malfunctioning but only doing the job it was told to do. In many cases, the P wave that was not followed by a paced QRS is then followed by an atrial pacing spike because the lower rate criteria have now been met. For more in-depth information regarding pacemaker function, please refer to chapter 7.

Documentation for the patient using epicardial pacing wires for temporary pacing should include an ECG rhythm strip before and after initiation of pacing, every 8 hours, and when their are changes in the patient's rhythm or hemodynamic status.[72] The clinician should document the child's clinical assessment including LOC, color, peripheral pulses, blood pressure, and respiratory status. Additional documentation should include the stimulation and sensitivity thresholds, percentage of paced (versus sensed) beats, pacing system polarity, the child's underlying rhythm, and the following pacemaker parameters: pacing mode, pacing rate, output, AV interval (in dual chamber devices), and upper rate limit (in dual chamber devices in DDD mode).

Troubleshooting

Many unexpected things can happen during the use of temporary epicardial pacing wires. As previously mentioned, the wires tend to form scar tissue at the suture site, which can cause an elevation in the pacing thresholds. In the case of a significant rise in the pacing threshold, IV or oral steroid therapy may be warranted. If the patient is able to tolerate oral administration, prednisone is used at a starting dosage of 60 mg/m^2/day or, if the IV route is preferred, Decadron 1 to 2 mg is used.

In the case of wire breakage or loss of the terminal connection pin, a bipolar system can be converted to a unipolar system by using a skin electrode. If this is not successful or if there is only one wire to begin with, the wire can still be used if the protective coating is shaved off and the exposed wire inserted directly into the pulse generator or to the pacing cable. This latter technique should only be used in emergent situations and if the patient is hemodynamically compromised.

Due to the proximity of the phrenic nerve to the epicardial wire placement site, the tip of the wire occasionally paces the diaphragm. This is also known as extracardiac or diaphragmatic pacing and is more likely to occur when the unipolar configuration is used. The patient will exhibit chest wall stimulation or complain of hiccoughs while the pacemaker is pacing. If the temporary pacemaker allows manipulation of pulse width/duration, it should be increased while the output or pulse amplitude is decreased. The pacing threshold must be reevaluated at these settings and an adequate safety margin provided. If the pulse width is not changeable, the polarity of the two wires can be reversed, simply by reversing the connector pins. In some cases, phrenic nerve stimulation can occur when the patient assumes various positions. The patients should be encouraged to avoid these positions until a more permanent solution can be obtained.

Patient and Family Considerations

Patient and family education is extremely important when caring for children who undergo temporary pacing therapy for transient or permanent cardiac rhythm disturbances. The clinician must first assess the patient and family's basic level of understanding in order to develop a specific educational plan that will best meet the individual needs of each specific family. Information should be provided in a brief and simple format and repeated often. These families are often under stress and have difficulty retaining information that the clinician provides. Any written material that can be provided is a useful adjunct. The following discussion is divided into sections specific to the particular pacing modality being used.

Noninvasive Transcutaneous Pacing

In many instances, this temporary pacing modality is used in emergent or urgent situations and very little time is available for patient and family education. Due to the somewhat violent appearance that this treatment modality provokes, it is important to reassure the family that as soon as the child is stabilized, sedation will be given in order to make their child more comfortable. Additionally, it should be reiterated that this treatment modality will only be used temporarily until other measures can be undertaken.

Transesophageal Pacing

In older children, transesophageal pacing can be performed without sedation. Education and preparation prior to the implementation of transesophageal pacing is critical if the patient is to be even slightly cooperative. In the older child who can understand instructions, gaining his or her trust is paramount. The child should be prepared for anything and everything that he or she will experience during the procedure, such as esophageal discomfort, the sensation of heart burn, coughing, hiccoughing, and the sensation of irregular and rapid heartbeats. It may also be helpful to use lower current levels with gradual increases until the patient experiences what it feels like for the catheter to stimulate and capture the heart. Stopping the stimulation immediately will reassure the child that the sensations are only temporary and that they will go away once the stimulation has ceased.

Depending on the specific clinical situation, parents may or may not be allowed to stay with the child during this procedure. If they are allowed to stay, certain limits must be imposed on their behavior for the duration of the study prior to treatment initiation. If they are not allowed to stay, they should be informed of the expected duration of the procedure and where to wait until the procedure has been completed.

Temporary Transvenous Pacing

The need for a temporary transvenous pacemaker can be urgent or emergent, depending on the child's presenting symptomatology or planned intervention. In some cases, a temporary transvenous pacemaker is placed prior to pulse generator replacement in pacemaker-dependent patients or in patients with permanent pacemakers who must undergo other surgeries in which electrocautery is necessary. Depending on the specific clinical situation, the clinician may or may not have the time to fully educate the patient and family. In an emergency situation, patient and family education may consist of a brief explanation of what is expected to happen, with assurance that additional information will be given once the child has been stabilized. For patients who undergo temporary transvenous pacing on a nonemergent basis, the clinician should explain the specifics of the procedure, the anticipated duration of the procedure, and what to expect after the procedure. It should be explained to both the patient and family that the temporary catheter will remain in use until the situation resolves or until more permanent measures can be implemented. The clinician should reiterate that activity will be restricted, bed rest will be required, and sedation will be used in order to prevent catheter dislodgment in younger children who are unable to cooperate.

Postoperative Epicardial Pacing Wires

Patients may or may not return from open heart surgery with their epicardial pacing wires in use. If they are being used, the nurse caring for the patient should explain to the family why they are needed and that, in most cases, they are only required on temporary basis. The provision of information and support is critical at this time because of the high anxiety level associated with any open heart procedure. If the child is awaiting placement of a permanent cardiac pacemaker, it is important for the clinician to explain to the patient and family that permanent and temporary devices are very different, particularly in regard to the size of the pulse generator.

Since many children experience temporary AV block following CHD surgery, it is often necessary to use the epicardial pacing wires for an extended period, e.g., 10 to 14 days. Parents often become frustrated and misunderstand why the wait is necessary. It is important that the clinician explain to the patient and family in terms that they can understand that waiting is much better than prematurely implanting a permanent device. It should be stressed that once a permanent device is implanted, it must be continuously evaluated and replaced. By emphasizing why the wait is necessary, the clinician can assist parents in their own understanding so that they in turn can assist in explaining things to their child.

Synchronized Cardioversion

Synchronized, direct current cardioversion is generally used in children to convert hemodynamically unstable SVTs or VT, or in cases where other treatment modalities have failed. It may also be used to electively convert asymptomatic atrial flutter or fibrillation in patients who have undergone previous surgery for CHD. It is the only nonpharmacologic method for converting atrial fibrillation to normal sinus rhythm.

Mechanism of Action

It is hypothesized that the mechanism of arrhythmia termination by use of transthoracic electric shocks is that some proportion of the myocardium must be depolarized so that the remainder of the muscle is inadequate to maintain the arrhythmia.[73] This and other hypotheses for the mechanism of action for electrical countershock of ventricular defibrillation[74,75] may or may not apply to atrial arrhythmias requiring synchronized cardioversion.[76]

In contrast to conventional external defibrillation, synchronized cardioversion delivers a shock that is synchronized with the heart's ventricular activity. The external defibrillator is set to "Sync" mode, the R wave is detected, and the shock is delivered through the chest wall during ventricular depolarization. The synchronization is to prevent the shock from being delivered during ventricular repolarization (i.e., the T wave), resulting in VF.

Amenable Arrhythmias

Arrhythmias that are amenable to synchronized, direct current cardioversion include atrial flutter, atrial fibrillation, other IARTs, SVTs due to an accessory pathway, AVNRT, and reentrant VT. Synchronized cardioversion is not generally useful for arrhythmias secondary to an automatic or ectopic focus, specifically AETs and JETs. Additionally, it is rarely if ever useful for children with chaotic or multifocal atrial tachycardias; however, failure to terminate a rhythm with synchronized cardioversion is occasionally part of the diagnostic cascade used to identify an automatic mechanism underlying atrial, junctional, or ventricular tachycardias.

Implications for Clinicians

Clinicians caring for children undergoing synchronized cardioversion have various responsibilities.[77] First and foremost is the ongoing assessment of the child's hemodynamic status. Since this particular treatment modality can be used in one of two basic scenarios, the implications for caregivers can be slightly different. This particular treatment modality is either used as an emergent treatment for hemodynamically unstable SVT (and in some cases, VT) or electively in select patients with atrial flutter or fibrillation. The commonalities between the two are discussed first, followed by the planned interventions associated with the latter scenario.

Synchronized cardioversion can be carried out in the emergency room, the ICU, or the cardiac catheterization laboratory. Optimally, the patient should be without food and fluids for approximately 4 hours prior to the procedure, but this is not always possible if emergency cardioversion is required. The patient should be attached to a continuous ECG monitor, noninvasive blood pressure monitor, and transcutaneous oxygen monitor. IV access should be obtained prior to cardioversion, and sedation agents administered if possible. Additional necessary equipment includes airway management equipment, appropriately sized pad or paddles, and an external defibrillator that is also capable of bradycardia pacing.

The electrode paddle size is recommended as follows by the American Heart Association manual on Pediatric Advanced Life Support[16]: 4.5 cm for infants and 8 or 13 cm for children. Since electrode size has been determined to be the major determinant of transthoracic impedance in children, Atkins and colleagues[78] recommend the use of larger electrodes when the child's thorax is large enough to permit electrode-to-chest contact over the entire surface; this occurs when the child reaches a weight of approximately 10 kg. This applies to preapplied self-adhesive electrode pads as well. Samson and colleagues[79] evaluated various sizes of electrode pads in 25 children, and offer the following final recommendations: a pad diameter of 5.8 cm should be used for infants less than 1 year of age and a pad diameter of 7 cm should be used for older children.

The most commonly used position for paddles or self-adhesive electrode pads is the anterolateral position. One electrode is placed on the anterior chest over the heart and the other on the back over the apex. The standard position requires that the electrode be placed on the upper right chest below the clavicle and the other to the left of the nipple in the anterior axillary line. In patients with permanent cardiac devices, the electrode paddles/pads should be placed as far away from the pulse generator as possible (see chapter 7 for additional information). When paddles are used, an electrode cream or gel is required to act as a low-impedance interface. Unacceptable substitutes for electrode gel include sonographic gels, which are poor electrical conductors, saline-soaked pads, which have variable conductivity and tend to drip, and alcohol pads, which produce a fire hazard and can produce serious chest burns.[16]

Toto[80] recommends plugging the defibrillator in, even if it is battery operated, prior to using it for cardioversion or defibrillation. The ECG monitor on the defibrillator should be assessed for monitor artifact and, if noted, the electrodes should be repositioned. Prior to any synchronized cardioversion, the clinician must ensure that the external defibrillator is in the "Sync" position (Fig. 12). This is generally verified by markers (i.e., lines or dots) on the QRS complex on the surface ECG. If the lines or dots are not present, the shock may not be synchronized to the R wave and may inadvertently result in VF.

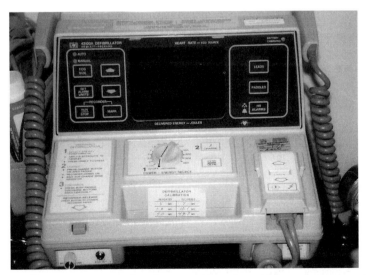

Figure 12. External defibrillator/cardioverter. Note the middle square where the energy is selected. The unnumbered square to the right denoted "SYNC/DEFIB" is critical when determining whether R wave synchronization is to be used.

The energy dose for a standard synchronized cardioversion in the pediatric patient is 0.5 to 1.0 J/kg of body weight. The energy level is selected, but prior to energy delivery the defibrillator's capacitors must be charged. Once the capacitors are charged, the rhythm is reevaluated. If the arrhythmia is still present, the clinician should ensure that everyone is "clear" from the patient. The discharge buttons are depressed simultaneously and are held until the energy is released. If the initial energy dose is not successful in converting the arrhythmia, a repeat dose of 2 J/kg may be given. If multiple attempts are necessary for arrhythmia conversion, each shock should be separated by at least 2 minutes to reduce myocardial injury, especially in infants and small children.

After successful cardioversion, the patient should undergo continuous ECG and vital sign monitoring, with a specific emphasis on airway patency and respiratory status. Documentation should include the patient's initial rhythm with ECG strip, the amount of energy delivered, if multiple attempts were necessary and if so how many, and the rhythm with ECG strip following the cardioversion. The clinician should also assess the child's skin where the pads or paddles were placed and note any irregularities.

Patients who undergo elective cardioversion are generally patients with postoperative atrial arrhythmias. In such cases, the patient should be NPO for at least 4 hours prior to cardioversion and the clinician should ensure that consent for the cardioversion has been obtained. An assessment of any medications that the patient is currently taking should be included in the preprocedural assessment. Most elective cardioversions are performed in the ICU or cardiac catheterization laboratory, but they can be performed in the operating room as well. Most patients receive conscious or deep sedation for the procedure.

Two issues that are specific to cardioversion of tachyarrhythmias in patients after surgery for CHD warrant further discussion. First, many of these patients have undergone Fontan, Mustard, or Senning repairs and are at risk for bradycardia post cardioversion. Temporary bradycardia pacing must be available for these patients undergoing synchronized cardioversion, and special attention must be paid to those who also receive antiarrhythmic medications and those undergoing initial cardioversion in whom the response to tachycardia termination is unknown.[81] Second, since these patients are also prone to clot formation, a transesophageal echocardiogram should be performed prior to cardioversion to assess for the presence of atrial thrombi. Feltes and Friedman[82] have reported that transesophageal echocardiography is far superior in detecting atrial thrombi (8 of 19 patients) compared to transthoracic (1 in 19 patients) echocardiography. Controversy remains over whether these patients should receive anticoagulation therapy prior to undergoing elective cardioversion.

Patient and Family Considerations

In order to provide expert patient and family education for patients undergoing emergent or elective cardioversion, the clinician should first assess the patient and family's basic level of understanding and then develop a specific educational plan to best meet their specific educational needs. It is important at this time to dispel any myths regarding the procedure that may be propagated by the media so that parents will have an accurate understanding of what is to take place with their child. It is best if information is provided in a brief and simple format and repeated often.

Depending on the specific clinical situation, the clinician may or may not have the time to fully educate the patient and family. In an emergency situation, patient and family education may consist of a brief explanation of what is expected to happen, with assurance that additional information will be provided once the child has been stabilized. In elective procedures in which the clinician has more time to prepare the patient and family, an explanation should be given, including the following: the specifics of the procedure, the anticipated duration of the procedure, and what to expect after the procedure. The clinician should reiterate to the family that a designated individual will keep them informed of their child's condition throughout the procedure.

External Defibrillation

External defibrillation or electrical countershock is generally used in children for VF or for pulseless VT or torsades de pointes in which synchronization to the R wave is not possible (Fig. 13).

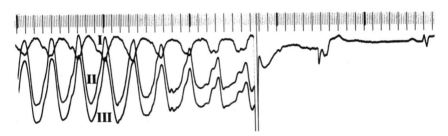

Figure 13. Surface ECG leads I, II, and III on a patient exhibiting torsades de pointes. External defibrillation was successful in restoring normal sinus rhythm.

Mechanism of Action

Unlike synchronous cardioversion, which is timed, external defibrillation is the untimed depolarization of a critical mass of myocardial cells that allows the initiation of an organized spontaneous beat. As previously stated, one hypothesis for the termination of VF using electrical countershock is that some proportion of the myocardium is depolarized in order to make the remainder of the muscle unable to sustain the arrhythmia.[73] For fibrillation, there is evidence that virtually all cells in the affected chamber must be depolarized to prevent immediate recurrence of the fibrillation.

Amenable Arrhythmias

The primary arrhythmia that is amenable to external defibrillation is VF. In cases in which synchronization to the QRS is not possible, pulseless VT or torsades de pointes may respond to defibrillation.

Implications for Clinicians

The clinician caring for children requiring external defibrillation is presented with many challenges. It is important when evaluating the monitored patient with suspected VF that the clinician assess the patient and not the monitor, since ECG electrode displacement is very similar in appearance to VF on surface ECG.[83] Obviously, the clinician should first assess the child's airway, breathing, and circulation as delineated by the American Heart Association's basic life support. The pulse assessment includes palpation of the brachial artery in the infant and the carotid artery in the child and young adult. The femoral artery can also be used in infants. It is important with VF or pulseless VT that the clinician continue cardiopulmonary resuscitation with as little interruption as possible.[16]

The electrode paddle size is the same as that recommended for synchronized cardioversion: 4.5 cm for infants and 8 or 13 cm for children.[16] Again, Atkins and colleagues[78] recommend the use of larger electrodes when the child's thorax is large enough to permit them. The paddles or pads may be placed in one of two positions: 1) the upper right chest below the clavicle and the other to the left of the nipple in the anterior axillary line (standard), or 2) the anterior chest over the heart and the other on the back over the apex (anterolateral). In patients with permanent cardiac devices, the paddles or pads should be placed as far away from the device as possible (see chapter 7 for additional information). When the paddles are used, an electrode cream or gel that acts as a low-impedance interface is applied prior to paddle placement.

The defibrillator should be plugged in prior to defibrillation, regardless of whether it is battery operated. Prior to defibrillation, the clinician should ensure that the device is NOT in the "Sync" position and the device should be powered on. The energy dose for a standardized external defibrillation is 2.0 J/kg of body weight.[16] The calculated energy dose should be set, followed by the charging of the defibrillator's capacitors. If self-adhesive electrodes are not being used, the paddles should be applied to the chest after gel has been applied, with temporary cessation of chest compressions. Once the capacitors are charged, the rhythm is reevaluated. The clinician should ensure that everyone is "clear" and, with firm pressure to the paddles, press the discharge buttons and hold them until the energy is delivered. If the initial energy dose is not successful in terminating the tachyarrhythmia, a repeat dose of 4 J/kg of body weight should be used.[16]

After successful defibrillation, the clinician should assess the child for any adverse effects, such as skin abrasions or burns.[77] Skin burns or abrasions can result from an inadequate amount or an excessive amount of gel between the skin and electrode pads or paddles in addition to inadequate skin contact.[77] Minor abrasions or burns can be treated with topical hydrocortisone cream. The child should undergo continuous ECG monitoring to assess for rhythm recurrence while efforts are undertaken to determine the etiology of the episode and plan further treatment modalities.

Patient and Family Considerations

Patients who require external defibrillation require cardiopulmonary resuscitation. This is an incredibly difficult time for parents, and communication from the health care team is critical. A designee should ensure that the parents receive information at frequent intervals during their child's resuscitation. This information should be provided in a quiet, private area, away from other patients and family members. The family should be given the opportunity to contact relatives for support and ancillary services should be notified by the clinician of the child's critical condition. These services include clergy, social services, and/or psychiatry services.

The parents of a child with VF or pulseless VT requiring defibrillation will be in a state of shock, disbelief, denial, and often guilt. Any information regarding the families' previous coping strategies should be incorporated into the overall plan of care. Parents may respond to their child's situation with anticipatory grief, denial, withdrawal, and avoidance, or all of these reactions.[84] If the child dies, the clinician should give the parents an opportunity to see their child at his or her bedside. The parents will need much support from the nurse at this time. This support consists of answering questions that the parents may have, or simply a nonverbal presence. The clinician can also assist parents by providing a quiet place to telephone relatives as well as helping them to coordinate funeral arrangements.

Automated External Defibrillation

Since their initial description more than 20 years ago,[85] automatic external defibrillators (AEDs) have become widespread in their usage in the adult who experiences an out-of-hospital cardiac arrest. Their accuracy and success in rescuing adults with VT and VF have been well documented.[86–88] AED use is becoming more widespread, as evidenced by its use on airplanes[89,90] and by police officers.[91] One study has even evaluated its use by sixth graders,[92] while others are using AEDs to train nurses[93,94] and other first responders.[95] Although their use has been limited primarily to adults, they are gaining popularity in the pediatric population, since several studies reveal that children experience more frequent out-of-hospital VF than originally thought.[96,97] Additionally, children also have improved survival when treated rapidly by emergency response systems.[96–98] Currently, the

American Heart Association recommends AEDs for use in children older than 8 years of age.[99]

The only published study of AED use in the pediatric population was published in 1998 by Atkins and colleagues.[100] This study evaluated the accuracy and effective treatment of AEDs in adolescents with VF. While the study validated the use of AEDs in adolescents, the authors recommend certain modifications in AED design for pediatric use, specifically the rhythm detection algorithm, the energy dose, and the electrode paddle size. Currently, AEDs deliver a set energy dose with no way to alter that dose. Smaller children require smaller doses and the currently available dose of 200 J is inappropriate for them. The authors also suggest that the use of separate pediatric paddles for children greater than 8 years of age is not necessary.[100] Issues regarding detection rates require further assessment in children, since sinus tachycardia rates are generally higher in children versus adults.

Mechanism of Action

The mechanism of action of the AED is similar to that of a conventional external defibrillator with the exception that the AED uses a detection algorithm to determine the patient's arrhythmia. A microprocessor inside the device interprets/analyzes the rhythm through the adhesive electrodes that are placed on the patient's chest. In the event that the arrhythmia meets the detection criteria, most devices provide voice prompts to assist the rescuer in charging and delivering the shock. If the rhythm does not meet the criteria for a "shockable" arrhythmia, the AED will not advise a shock and will continue to monitor the rhythm.

Amenable Arrhythmias

The only arrhythmias at this time that will benefit from the use of an AED are VF or fast VT. Specific pediatric patient populations that may potentially benefit from AED use are those in which there is a life-threatening arrhythmia. Specific patient populations include patients with long QT syndrome, idiopathic VF, and VT/VF after surgery for CHD.

Implications for Clinicians

Currently, the American Heart Association includes training for health care providers in the use of AEDs in their basic lifesaving courses designed for the health care provider. Since the safety and efficacy of the use of AEDs in hospitals has been evaluated,[93,94] it is anticipated that this type of immediate arrhythmia management technique will become commonplace in the hospital setting to be used by registered nurses to decrease the time to first shock, thereby improving resuscitation outcome in some cases.

Patient and Family Considerations

Families are now able to obtain more information regarding their child's medical condition and potential treatment modalities through the Internet. Many will research these treatment options and have valid and educated questions for their health care providers. In specific clinical situations, at-home availability of AEDs is a viable treatment option. Patient and family education regarding AEDs should include the advantages and disadvantages of home AED use as well as the potential cost. Some third party payers will pay for the device if the physician deems it medically necessary and will provide a prescription for it.

In summary, the initial or immediate management of a child's arrhythmia is multifaceted and depends on the child's overall hemodynamic status as well as the arrhythmia mechanism. In most cases, the arrhythmia mechanism is easily identified, but in some cases, immediate arrhythmia management techniques can assist the clinician in making this determination. Whether or not a simple vagal maneuver, antiarrhythmic drug, temporary pacing, or cardioversion/defibrillation is used to terminate a cardiac arrhythmia, the clinician has the responsibility both to himself and the patient to be as knowledgeable as possible regarding the how, the whys, and the when of each of the treatment modalities used for immediate arrhythmia management in children.

References

1. Ludomirsky A, Garson A Jr.: Supraventricular tachycardia. In Gillette PC, Garson A Jr. (eds.): Pediatric Arrhythmias: Electrophysiology and Pacing. Philadelphia: WB Saunders Company; 1990:380–426.
2. Hayes DL, Maue-Dickson W, Stanton MS: Dictionary of Cardiac Pacing Electrophysiology and Arrhythmias. Miami Lakes: Peritus Corporation; 1993.
3. Wilbur SL, Marchilinski FE: Adenosine as an antiarrhythmic agent. Am J Cardiol 1997; 79:30–37.
4. Till J, Shinebourne EA, Rigby ML, et al: Efficacy and safety of adenosine in the treatment of supraventricular tachycardia in infants and children. Br Heart J 1989; 62:204–211.
5. Epstein ML, Kiel EA, Victorica BE: Cardiac decompensation following verapamil therapy in infants with supraventricular tachycardia. Pediatrics 1985; 75:737–740.
6. Zeigler VL: Adenosine in the pediatric population: Nursing implications. Pediatr Nurs 1991; 17:600–602.
7. Shryock JC, Boykin MT, Hill JA, et al: A new method of sampling blood for measurement of plasma adenosine. Am J Physiol 1990; 258:H1232-H1239.
8. Moser GH, Schrader J, Deussen A: Turnover of adenosine in plasma of human and dog blood. Am J Physiol 1989; 256:C799-C806.
9. Opie LH, Chatterjee K, Frishman W, et al (eds.): Drugs for the Heart. 4th ed. Philadelphia: WB Saunders Company; 1995:207–246.
10. Camm AJ, Garratt CJ: Adenosine and supraventricular tachycardia. N Engl J Med 1991; 325:1621–1629.
11. Malcolm AD, Garratt CJ, Camm AJ: The therapeutic and diagnostic cardiac electrophysiologic uses of adenosine. Cardiovasc Drugs Ther 1993; 7:139–147.
12. Perry JC, Knilans TK, Marlow D, et al: Intravenous amiodarone for life-

threatening tachyarrhythmias in children: 135 cases. J Am Coll Cardiol 1993; 22:95–99.

13. Figa FH, Gow RM, Hamilton RM, et al: Clinical efficacy and safety of intravenous amiodarone in infants and children. Am J Cardiol 1994; 74:573–577.

14. Perry JC, Fenrich AL, Hulse JE, et al: Pediatric use of intravenous amiodarone: Efficacy and safety in critically ill patients from a multicenter protocol. J Am Coll Cardiol 1996; 27:1246–1250.

15. Perry JC: Medical antiarrhythmic therapy. In Gillette PC, Garson A Jr. (eds.): Clinical Pediatric Arrhythmias. 2nd ed. Philadelphia: WB Saunders Company; 1999:231–248.

16. American Heart Association/American Academy of Pediatrics. Textbook of Pediatric Advanced Life Support. Dallas: American Heart Association; 1997.

17. Holder DA, Sniderman AD, Fraser G, et al: Experience with bretylium tosylate by a hospital cardiac arrest team. Circulation 1977; 55:541–544.

18. Stang JM, Washington SE, Barnes SA, et al: Treatment of prehospital refractory ventricular fibrillation with bretylium tosylate. Ann Emerg Med 1984; 13:234–236.

19. Rainey P: Digibind and free digoxin. Clin Chem 1999; 45:719–721.

20. Marcus FI: Digitalis. In Schlant RC, Alexander RW, O'Rourke RA (eds.): The Heart. 8th ed. New York: McGraw-Hill; 1994:573–588.

21. Wellens HJJ, Durrer D: Effect of digitalis on atrioventricular conduction and circus-movement tachycardias in patients with Wolff-Parkinson-White syndrome. Circulation 1973; 47:1229–1233.

22. Byrum C, Wahl RA, Behrendt DM, et al: Ventricular fibrillation associated with the use of digitalis in a newborn infant with Wolff-Parkinson-White syndrome. J Pediatr 1982; 101:400–403.

23. Esmolol Research Group: Intravenous esmolol for the treatment of supraventricular tachyarrhythmia: Results of a multicenter, baseline controlled safety and efficacy study in 160 patients. Am Heart J 1986; 112:498–505.

24. Trippel DL, Wiest DB, Gillette PC: Cardiovascular and antiarrhythmic effects of esmolol in children. J Pediatr 1991; 119:142–147.

25. Miller S, Fiorvanti J (eds.): Pediatric Medications: A Handbook for Nurses. St. Louis: Mosby-Year Book, Inc.; 1997:1–844.

26. Felps SJ, Hak EB (eds.): Guidelines for Administration of Intravenous Medications to Pediatric Patients. 5th ed. Bethesda: American Society of Health-System Pharmacists; 1996:1–188.

27. Gallick D, Altamirano J, Singh BN: Restoring sinus rhythm in patients with atrial flutter and fibrillation: Pharmacologic or electrical cardioversion? J Cardiovasc Pharmacol Ther 1997; 2:135–144.

28. Li H, Natale A, Tomassoni G, et al: Usefulness of ibutilide in facilitating successful external cardioversion of refractory atrial fibrillation. Am J Cardiol 1999; 84:1096–1098.

29. Stambler BS, Wood MA, Ellenbogen KA, et al: Efficacy and safety of repeated intravenous doses of ibutilide for rapid conversion of atrial flutter or fibrillation. The Ibutilide Repeat Dose Study Investigators. Circulation 1996; 94:1613–1621.

30. Roden DM: Ibutilide and the treatment of atrial arrhythmias. A new drug "almost unheralded" is now available to US physicians. Circulation 1996; 94:1499–1502.

31. Sager PT: New advances in class III antiarrhythmic drug therapy. Curr Opin Cardiol 2000; 15:41–53.

32. Kowey PR, VanderLugt JT, Luderer JR: Safety and risk/benefit analysis of ibutilide for acute conversion of atrial fibrillation/flutter. Am J Cardiol 1996; 78(suppl 8A):46–52.

33. Pill MV: Ibutilide: A new antiarrhythmic agent for the critical care environment. Crit Care Nurs 1997; 17:19–22.

34. Reder RF, Rosen MR: Basic electrophysiologic principles: Application to treatment of dysrhythmias. In Gillette PC, Garson A Jr. (eds.): Pediatric Cardiac Dysrhythmias. NY: Grune & Stratton; 1981:121–143.
35. Silka MJ: Emergency management of arrhythmias. In Deal BJ, Wolff GS, Gelband H (eds.): Current Concepts in Diagnosis and Management of Arrhythmias in Infants and Children. Armonk, NY: Futura Publishing Company, Inc.; 1998:309–328.
36. Gorgels APM, van den Dool A, Hofs A, et al: Comparison of procainamide and lidocaine in terminating sustained monomorphic ventricular tachycardia. Am J Cardiol 1996; 78:43–46.
37. Garson A Jr., Kugler JD, Gillette PC, et al: Control of late postoperative ventricular arrhythmias with phenytoin in young patients. Am J Cardiol 1980; 46:290–294.
38. Vaughn Williams EM: A classification of antiarrhythmic actions reassessed after a decade of new drugs. J Clin Pharmacol 1984; 24:129–147.
39. Garson A Jr.: Ventricular dysrhythmias. In Gillette PC, Garson A Jr. (eds.): Pediatric Cardiac Dysrhythmias. NY: Grune & Stratton; 1981:295–360.
40. Zoll PM: Resuscitation of the heart in ventricular standstill by external electric stimulation. N Engl J Med 1952; 248:768–771.
41. Beland MJ, Hesslein PS, Findlay CD, et al: Noninvasive transcutaneous cardiac pacing in children. Pacing Clin Electrophysiol 1987; 10:1262–1270.
42. Gamrath B, Del Monte L, Richards K: Noninvasive pacing: What you should know. J Emerg Nurse 1998; 24:223–230.
43. Zoll PM, Zoll RH, Falk RH, et al: External noninvasive temporary pacing: Clinical trials. Circulation 1985; 71:937–944.
44. Falk RH, Zoll PM, Zoll RH: Safety and efficacy of noninvasive cardiac pacing. N Engl J Med 1983; 309:1166–1168.
45. Taylor S: Temporary pacing in children. In Gillette PC, Zeigler VL (eds.): Pediatric Cardiac Pacing. Armonk, NY: Futura Publishing Company; 1995:115–148.
46. Moak JP: Electrical treatment of arrhythmias. In Garson A Jr., Bricker JT, McNamara DG (eds.): The Science and Practice of Pediatric Cardiology. Philadelphia: Lea & Febiger; 1990:2162–2172.
47. Moses HW, Moulton KP, Miller BD, Schneider JA: A Practical Guide to Cardiac Pacing. 4th ed. Boston: Little, Brown and Company; 1995:89–112.
48. Wharton JM, Goldschlager N: Temporary cardiac pacing. In Saksena S, Goldschlager N (eds.): Electrical Therapy for Cardiac Arrhythmias: Pacing, Antitachycardia Devices, Catheter Ablation. Philadelphia: WB Saunders Company; 1990:107–138.
49. Sharkey SW, Chaffee V, Kaspner S: Prophylactic external pacing during cardioversion of atrial tachyarrhythmias. Am J Cardiol 1985; 55:1632–1634.
50. Rein AJ, Cohen E, Weiss A, et al: Noninvasive external pacing in the newborn. Pediatr Cardiol 1999; 20:290–292.
51. Beland MJ: Noninvasive transcutaneous cardiac pacing in children. In Birkui PJ, Trigano JA, Zoll PM (eds.): Noninvasive Transcutaneous Cardiac Pacing. Mount Kisco, NY: Futura Publishing Company, Inc.; 1993:91–98.
52. Zoll PM: Noninvasive temporary pacing. In Bartecchi CE, Mann DE (eds.): Temporary Cardiac Pacing. Chicago: Precept Press Inc.; 1990:124–136.
53. Appel-Hardin S, Dente-Cassidy AM: How to use a noninvasive temporary pacemaker. Nursing 91 1991; 21:58–64.
54. Coté CJ: Sedation for the pediatric patient: A review. Pediatr Clin North Am 1994; 41:31–58.
55. Zeigler VL, Brown LE. Conscious sedation in the pediatric population: Special considerations. Crit Care Clin North Am 1997; 9:381–394.
56. Kincade SL: Transcutaneous pacing. In Kincade SL, Lohrman J (eds.): Criti-

cal Care Nursing Procedures: A Team Approach. Philadephia: BC Decker, Inc.; 1990:72–75.

57. Shafiroff BGP, Linder J: Effects of external electrical pacemaker stimuli on the human heart. J Thorac Surg 1957; 33:544–550.

58. Benson DW Jr., Dunnigan A, Benditt DG, et al: Transesophageal cardiac pacing: History, application, technique. Clin Prog Pacing Electrophysiol 1984; 2:360–372.

59. Gallagher JJ, Smith WM, Kasall J, et al: Use of the esophageal lead in the diagnosis of mechanisms of reciprocating tachycardia. Pacing Clin Electrophysiol 1980; 3:440–451.

60. Schittger I, Rodriguez IM, Winkle RA: Esophageal electrocardiography: A new technology revives an old technique. Am J Cardiol 1986; 57:604–607.

61. Benson DW Jr., Dunnigan A, Benditt DG, et al: Transesophageal study of infant supraventricular tachycardia: Electrophysiologic characteristics. Am J Cardiol 1983; 52:1002–1006.

62. Dick M II, Scott WA, Serwer GS, et al: Acute termination of supraventricular tachyarrhythmias in children by transesophageal pacing. Am J Cardiol 1988; 61:925–927.

63. Benson DW Jr., Dunnigan A, Sterba R, et al: Atrial pacing from the esophagus in the diagnosis and management of tachycardia and palpitations. J Pediatr 1983; 102:40–46.

64. Blomström-Lundquist C, Edvardsson N: Transesophageal versus intracardiac atrial stimulation in assessing electrophysiologic parameters of the sinus and AV nodes and of atrial myocardium. Pacing Clin Electrophysiol 1987; 10:1081–1095.

65. Campbell RM, Dick M II, Jenkins JM, et al: Atrial overdrive pacing for conversion of atrial flutter in children. Pediatrics 1985; 75:730–736.

66. American Academy of Pediatrics, Committee on Drugs: Guidelines for monitoring and management of pediatric patients during and after sedation for diagnostic and therapeutic procedures. Pediatrics 1992; 89:1110–1115.

67. Cottle S: Temporary transvenous cardiac pacing. Nurs Times 1999; 93:48–51.

68. Silver MD, Goldschlager N: Temporary transvenous cardiac pacing in the critical care setting. Chest 1988; 93:607–613.

69. Yabek SM, Bechara FA, Berman W, et al: Use of atrial epicardial electrodes to diagnose and treat postoperative arrhythmias in children. Am J Cardiol 1980; 46:285–289.

70. Hickey CS, Baas LS: Temporary cardiac pacing. AACN Clin Issues Crit Care Nurs 1991; 2:107–117.

71. Baas LS: Care of the cardiac patient. In Kinney M, Packa D (eds.): Andreoli's Comprehensive Cardiac Care. 8th ed. St Louis: Mosby-Year Book, Inc.; 1996:276–341.

72. Kincade SL: Initiation of epicardial pacing. In Kincade SL, Lohrman J (eds.): Critical Care Nursing Procedures: A Team Approach. Philadephia: BC Decker, Inc.; 1990:87–95.

73. Zipes DP, Fischer J, King RM, et al: Termination of ventricular fibrillation in dogs by depolarizing a critical amount of myocardium. Am J Cardiol 1975; 36:37–44.

74. Shibata N, Chen PS, Dixon EG, et al: Epicardial activation after unsuccessful defibrillation shocks in dogs. Am J Physiol 1988; 255:H902-H909.

75. Jones DL: Waveforms for implantable cardioverter defibrillators and transchest defibrillation. In Tacker WA (ed.): Defibrillation of the Heart. St. Louis: Mosby-Year Book, Inc.; 1994:46–81.

76. Kerber RE: External direct current cardioversion-defibrillation. In Zipes DP, Jalife J (eds.): Cardiac Electrophysiology: From Cell to Bedside. 2nd ed. Philadelphia: WB Saunders Company; 1995:1360–1365.

77. Suddaby EC, Riker SL: Defibrillation and cardioversion in children. Pediatr Nurs 1991; 5:477–481.

78. Atkins DL, Sirna S, Kieso R, et al: Pediatric defibrillation: Importance of paddle size in determining transthoracic impedance. Pediatrics 1988; 82:914–918.
79. Samson RA, Atkins DL, Kerber RE: Optimal size of self-adhesive preapplied electrode pads in pediatric defibrillation. Am J Cardiol 1995; 75:544–545.
80. Toto KH: Cardioversion. In Kincade SL, Lohrman J (eds.): Critical Care Nursing Procedures: A Team Approach. Philadephia: BC Decker, Inc.; 1990:117–121.
81. Sokoloski MC: Tachyarrhythmias confined to the atrium. In Gillette PC, Garson A Jr. (eds.): Clinical Pediatric Arrhythmias. 2nd ed. Philadelphia: WB Saunders Company; 1999:78–96.
82. Feltes TF, Friedman RA: Transesophageal echocardiographic detection of atrial thrombi in patients with non-fibrillation atrial tachyarrhythmias and congenital heart disease. J Am Coll Cardiol 1994; 24:1365–1370.
83. Silka MJ, Garson A Jr.: Ventricular arrhythmias. In Gillette PC, Garson A Jr. (eds.): Clinical Pediatric Arrhythmias. 2nd ed. Philadelphia: WB Saunders Company; 1999:121–145.
84. Miles MS, Warner JB: The dying child in the intensive care unit. In Hazinski MF (ed.): Nursing Care of the Critically Ill Child. 2nd ed. St. Louis: Mosby-Yearbook, Inc.; 1992:101–116.
85. Diack AW, Welborn WS, Rullman RG, et al: An automatic cardiac resuscitator for emergency treatment of cardiac arrest. Med Instrum 1979; 13:78–83.
86. Stults KR, Brown DD, Kerber RE: Efficacy of an automated external defibrillator in the management of out-of-hospital cardiac arrest: Validation of the diagnostic algorithm and initial clinical experience in a rural environment. Circulation 1986; 73:701–709.
87. Weaver WD, Hill D, Fahrenbruch CE, et al: Use of the automatic external defibrillator in the management of out-of-hospital cardiac arrest. N Engl J Med 1988; 319:661–666.
88. Cummins RO, Eisenberg MS, Litwin PE, et al: Automatic external defibrillators used by emergency medical technicians: A controlled clinical trial. JAMA 1987; 257:1605–1610.
89. Zimmermann PG: Something special in the air: Automatic external defibrillators on American Airlines planes. J Emerg Nurs 1997; 23:340–342.
90. Zimmermann PC, Campbell L: Automatic external defibrillators on commercial airlines. J Emerg Nurs 1999; 25:166.
91. Mosesso VN Jr., Davis EA, Auble TE, et al: Use of automated external defibrillators by police officers for treatment of out-of-hospital cardiac arrest. Ann Emerg Med 1998; 32:200–207.
92. Gundry JW, Comess KA, Derook FA, et al: Comparison of naive sixth-grade children with trained professionals in the use of an automated external defibrillator. Circulation 1999; 100:1703–1707.
93. Klein A: Towards early defibrillation—a nurse training programme in the use of automated external defibrillators. Resuscitation 1996; 31:173–174.
94. Warwick JP, Mackie K, Spencer I: Towards early defibrillation—a nurse training programme in the use of automated external defibrillators. Resuscitation 1995; 30:231–235.
95. Kaye W, Mancini ME, Giuliano KK, et al: Strengthening the in-hospital chain of survival with rapid defibrillation by first responders using automated external defibrillators: Training and retention issues. Ann Emerg Med 1995; 25:163–168.
96. Mogayzel C, Quan L, Graves JR, et al: Out-of-hospital ventricular fibrillation in children and adolescents: Causes and outcome. Ann Emerg Med 1995; 25:484–491.
97. Safranek DJ, Eisenberg MS, Larsen MP: The epidemiology of cardiac arrest in young adults. Ann Emerg Med 1992; 21:1102–1106.
98. Ronco R, King W, Donley DK, et al: Outcome and cost at a children's hospital

following resuscitation for out-of-hospital cardiopulmonary arrest. Arch Pediatr Adolesc Med 1995; 149:210–214.

99. Emergency Cardiac Care Committee and Subcommittees AHA. Guidelines for cardiopulmonary resuscitation and emergency cardiac care. IV. Pediatric advanced life support. JAMA 1992; 268:2262–2275.

100. Atkins DL, Hartley LL, York DK: Accurate recognition and effective treatment of ventricular fibrillation by automated external defibrillators in adolescents. Pediatrics 1998; 101:393–397.

Appendix 4–1
Intravenous Agents Used for Immediate Arrhythmia Management in Children

Drug	Dosage	Onset of Action	Potential Adverse Effects	Drug Interactions	Cardiovascular Contraindications	Comments
Adenosine (Adenocard)	100–150 µg/kg given rapid IV push followed quickly with saline flush; double dose sequentially to maximum of 300 µg/kg or the adult dose of 6–12 mg	<5 seconds	Dyspnea, shortness of breath, bronchospasm, headache, facial flushing, chest pressure/pain, sinus brady-cardia, AV block/asystole, ventric-ular ectopy, atrial fibrillation, tor-sades de pointes, sweating, palpitations, hypotension	• Theophylline (makes adeno-sine less effective) • Carbamazepine (may result in increased degree of AV block) • Dipyridamole (requires using a lower dose of adenosine) • Digoxin (may be associated with increased risk of VF) • Diazepam (potentiates effects of adenosine)	• Prolonged QT interval • Second- or third-degree AV block, except in presence of temporary/ permanent pacemaker • Sick sinus syndrome	• Have defibrillator available when administering, in the event of ventricular rate acceleration, torsades de pointes, or VF • Caffeine makes adenosine less effective • Avoid or use with caution in patients with asthma secondary to bronchoconstriction • Use with caution in patients receiving digoxin and verapamil • Incompatible with any drug in solution or syringe

Appendix 4–1

Intravenous Agents Used for Immediate Arrhythmia Management in Children (*cont.*)

Drug	Dosage	Onset of Action	Potential Adverse Effects	Drug Interactions	Cardiovascular Contraindications	Comments
Amiodarone (Cordarone)	Bolus: 5mg/kg (1 mg/kg over 5 minutes) OR 2.5 mg/kg given twice Infusion: 10–15 mg/kg/day	Within 5 minutes of initial bolus	Hypotension, sinus bradycardia or sinus arrest, AV block	• Digoxin (causes ↑ level of digoxin) • Procainamide (causes ↑ level of procainamide) • Quinidine (causes ↑ level of quinidine) • Flecainide (causes ↑ level of flecainide) • Phenytoin (causes ↑ levels of phenytoin and amiodarone) • Warfarin (causes ↑ PT and INR values)	• Sick sinus syndrome except in presence of temporary/permanent pacemaker • AV block except in presence of temporary/permanent pacemaker • Cardiogenic shock	• Monitor blood pressure, heart rate, and rhythm continuously • Transient hypotension can be treated with volume or calcium chloride infusion • Due to vasodilatory effect, may potentiate effects of certain antihypertensives
Atropine Sulfate (Atropine)	0.02–0.04 mg/kg with a minimum dose of 0.1 mg; can be repeated after 5 minutes to a maximum	2–4 minutes	Tachycardia, dry mouth, blurred vision, constipation, urinary retention, CNS symptoms, hyperthermia,	• Phenothiazines (increased anticholinergic effect) • Quinidine (increased anticholinergic	• Tachyarrhythmias • Asthma • Myocardial ischemia • Acute hemorrhage	• May be given endotracheally and intraosseously • May cause paradoxical bradycardia in infants, especially with slow IV

Drug	Dose	Onset	Side effects	Drug interactions	Contraindications/cautions	Comments
	cumulative dose of 1.0 mg for a child and 2.0 mg for an adolescent		dilated pupils, flushed/dry skin, worsening of AV block, PVCs, ventricular tachycardia, hypertension, hypotension	effect) • Procainamide (increased anticholinergic effect)		administration • Not stable in alkaline solutions • Helpful in patients with vagally mediated bradycardia • Helpful for bradycardia/AV block in patients with neurologic injuries • Monitor ECG for heart rate and rhythm continuously
Bretylium tosylate (Bretylol)	Bolus: 5mg/kg/dose every 15–30 min up to 30 mg/kg; Infusion: 15–30 µg/kg/min	Within 5 minutes	Hypotension, nausea, vomiting, transient hypertension, bradycardia, anginal pain, transient arrhythmias	Digoxin (may worsen the arrhythmia—aggravates digoxin toxicity; this is controversial) • Quinidine (reverses local anesthetic effects) • Tricyclic antidepressants (causes a ↓ in Bretylium's synaptic effects) • Sympathomimetics (enhances sympathomimetic effects)	Digoxin toxicity • Patients with aortic stenosis • Patients with pulmonary hypertension	Give 5 mg/kg then defibrillate • If VF persists, give 10 mg/kg and defibrillate again • For ventricular tachycardia in the conscious patient, give 5 mg/kg over 8–10 minutes to alleviate nausea and vomiting • Monitor blood pressure, heart rate, and rhythm continuously • Use with extreme caution in patients with aortic or subaortic stenosis

Appendix 4–1
Intravenous Agents Used for Immediate Arrhythmia Management in Children (*cont.*)

Drug	Dosage	Onset of Action	Potential Adverse Effects	Drug Interactions	Cardiovascular Contraindications	Comments
Digoxin Immune Fab (Digibind)	SEE TEXT	5–10 minutes	Congestive heart failure and rapid ventricular rates (both caused by reversal of digoxin effects), hypokalemia, hypersensitivity reactions, increased respiratory rate, and decreased respiratory function.	None known	• Absence of life-threatening symptomatology	• Continuous ECG monitoring • Response is nearly immediate • Give IV over 15–30 minutes through 0.22-micron filter • Dilute with 0.9% NaCl • Digoxin serum concentrations are inaccurate until Digibind clears from body (usually 2 days) • Monitor potassium levels (digoxin intoxication causes elevations, but Digibind administration can cause decreased levels)

| Digoxin (Lanoxin) | Total digitizing dose:* **Preemie infant:** 20 μg/kg; **Full-term newborn:** 30 μg/kg; **Infant** <2 yrs.: 40–50 μg/kg; **Children** >2 yrs.: 30–40 μg/kg. *Total loading dose is divided into three doses: dose #1 is 50% of total, doses #2 and #3 are 25% of total; doses are given every 8 hours over 24 hours. Maintenance dose: 25% of total digitizing does q 12 hours | 5–30 minutes | Nausea, vomiting, anorexia, headache, fatigue, visual changes, drowsiness (all of the former in smaller sized patients), sinus bradycardia, AV block, atrial tachycardia, accelerated junctional rhythm, PACs, PVCs, lethargy | • Quinidine (results in ↑ digoxin level – approximately double)
• Amiodarone (results in ↑ digoxin level)
• Propafenone (results in ↑ digoxin level and ↓ inotropic effect)
• Diuretics (may make patient more prone to hypokalemia)
• ACE inhibitors (may precipitate renal failure)
• Sympathomimetics (↑ arrhythmias)
• Verapamil (results in ↑ digoxin level)
• β-blockers (↑ digoxin toxicity, ↓ inotropic effect)
• Rifampin (↓ digoxin effect) | • Hypertrophic obstructive cardiomyopathy (may worsen outflow obstruction)
• WPW (may enhance accessory pathway conduction; in presence of atrial flutter, rapid conduction may result in VF)
• AV block (without pacemaker)
• Unrepaired tetralogy of Fallot | • Renal dysfunction can prolong digoxin half-life for as long as 1 week
• Digoxin toxicity more likely if hypokalemic or hypercalcemic
• Monitor heart rate, rhythm, and PR interval continuously
• Monitor serum potassium, magnesium, and calcium in select patients |

Appendix 4–1
Intravenous Agents Used for Immediate Arrhythmia Management in Children (cont.)

Drug	Dosage	Onset of Action	Potential Adverse Effects	Drug Interactions	Cardiovascular Contraindications	Comments
Esmolol (Brevibloc)	Load: 500 μg/kg over 1–2 minutes Maintenance: 50–200 μg/kg/minute	Within 1–2 minutes	Hypotension, dizziness, somnolence, headache, agitation, fatigue, nausea and vomiting, bronchospasm, irritation at IV site, bradycardia, AV block, ↓ CO, pallor, flushing	• Digoxin (causes ↑ in serum concentration of digoxin 10%–20%) • Morphine sulfate (may cause ↑ in esmolol serum concentration) • Succinylcholine (esmolol may cause prolonged neuromuscular blockade) • Lidocaine (esmolol may cause ↑ effects) • Disopyramide (esmolol may cause ↑ effects)	Sinus bradycardia, second- or third-degree AV block without pacemaker, cardiogenic shock, overt heart failure.	• Use with caution in patients with ↓ renal function, diabetes, or bronchospasm • Effects subside within 1–2 minutes, complete reversal within 30 minutes • Solution is incompatible with diazepam, furosemide, sodium bicarbonate, and thiopental sodium • Best administered using an infusion control device • Recommended only for short-term use (<48 hours) • Avoid extravasation (very acidic solutions can lead to skin necrosis)

Drug	Dose	Onset	Side Effects	Interactions	Contraindications	Nursing Considerations
Ibutilide (Corvert)	Adults: 10–25 µg/kg bolus over 10 minutes; may repeat in 10 minutes	10–30 minutes	AV block, QT prolongation, bradycardia, constipation, serious proarrhythmia including the development of polymorphic ventricular tachycardia and torsades de pointes	• Class Ia and III drugs (potentiates effects of all drugs) • Phenothiazines, tricyclic antidepressants, tetracyclines (prolongs QT interval)	• Hypersensitivity to ibutilide	• Continuous ECG monitoring during administration and at least 4 hours after infusion OR until QTc has returned to baseline • Do not give Class Ia or Class III drugs within 4 hours of ibutilide administration
Isoproterenol (Isuprel)	0.05 to 1.0 µg/kg/min (increase infusion rate every 5 minutes until desired effect seen) Continuous infusion: 20–50 µg/kg/minute	Within 1½ to 2 minutes	Tachycardia, palpitations, nausea, vomiting, facial flushing, dizziness, nervousness, hyperglycemia, headache, tremor, sweating, irritability, chest pain, bronchial irritation	• Sympathomimetics (↑ risk of arrhythmia) • Propranolol and other β-blockers (decreased effects of isoproterenol)	• Patients with myocardial ischemia • Arrhythmias secondary to digoxin toxicity	• Causes ↑ in pulse pressure characterized by ↓ in diastolic and ↑ in systolic pressure • Continuous ECG monitoring • Increases myocardial oxygen consumption • Administer using infusion pump • Drug decomposes rapidly in alkaline solutions

Appendix 4–1
Intravenous Agents Used for Immediate Arrhythmia Management in Children (cont.)

Drug	Dosage	Onset of Action	Potential Adverse Effects	Drug Interactions	Cardiovascular Contraindications	Comments
Lidocaine (Xylocaine)	Load: 1 mg/kg every 5 minutes × 3 doses Infusion: 20–50 µg/kg/min	45–90 seconds	Tinnitus, perioral paresthesias, altered sensorium, seizures, confusion, tremor, lethargy, somnolence, stupor, restlessness, slurred speech, muscle twitching, blurred vision, apnea, altered mental status, anxiety, agitation, bradycardia, hypotension, and respiratory depression	• Cimetidine (reduces hepatic clearance of lidocaine) • β-blockers (reduce hepatic clearance of lidocaine) • Phenytoin (additive cardiac depressive effects) • Procainamide (additive cardiac depressive effects) • Quinidine (additive cardiac depressive effects)	• Severe sinus and AV node dysfunction without pacemaker	• Can be given endotracheally or intraosseously • Continuous ECG monitoring • Use decreased dose in patients with congestive heart failure or liver failure • Serum concentrations range from 2 to 5 µg/mL. • Monitor potassium levels—more effective with higher potassium levels • Reduce dose when using with halothane

Drug	Dose	Onset	Side Effects	Drug Interactions		Nursing Considerations
Phenytoin (Dilantin)	15 mg/kg over 1 hour: give 1/12 of total dose every 5 minutes	1–2 hours	Bradycardia, ↓ myocardial contractility, hypotension, vertigo, lethargy, confusion, slurred speech, dizziness, and burning at injection site, ataxia, nervousness, twitching, headache, bradycardia, rash, nausea and vomiting, nystagmus.	• Verapamil (potentiates verapamil effect) • Wafarin (may result in ↓ PT and INR values) • Isoniazid (↓ phenytoin metabolism) • Diazepam (↓ phenytoin metabolism) • Phenobarbital (enhances phenytoin metabolism) • Carbamazepine (enhances phenytoin metabolism) • Amiodarone (↑ phenytoin metabolism)	• Pregnancy	• Dairy products may ↓ absorption • Continuous ECG monitoring • Serum concentration 10–20 µg/mL • May cause urine discoloration • Prolonged elimination half-life in infants (up to 24 hours) • Inject undiluted and flush with normal saline immediately following administration • Begin oral administration simultaneously • May cause local vein irritation, inflammation, necrosis, and sloughing *with or without* signs of infiltration

Appendix 4–1

Intravenous Agents Used for Immediate Arrhythmia Management in Children (cont.)

Drug	Dosage	Onset of Action	Potential Adverse Effects	Drug Interactions	Cardiovascular Contraindications	Comments
Procainamide (Pronestyl)	Load: Infants: 7–10 mg/kg over 30–45 minutes; Older children: Bolus of 15 mg/kg Infusion: 40–50 µg/kg/min (infants occasionally need up to 100 µg/kg/min to maintain therapeutic serum concentration)	Within 30 minutes	• Hypotension, ↑ ventricular response with atrial flutter, bradycardia, asystole, depressed ventricular function, AV block, fever, myalgia, confusion, dizziness, and headache	• Amiodarone (causes ↑ in serum concentration) • Cimetidine (prolongs procainamide elimination half-life) • Anticholinergics (additive anticholinergic effects) • Digoxin (↑ digoxin serum concentration)	• Second- or third-degree AV block without pacemaker • Torsades de pointes • Congestive heart failure • Prolonged QT interval	• Decrease dose when patient also receiving cimetidine • Continuous ECG monitoring • Monitor serum concentration of procainamide (4–8 µg/mL) and NAPA (10–30 µg/mL) • NAPA is active metabolite of procainamide • Continuous ECG and blood pressure monitoring • Monitor potassium levels (↓ level may lead to ↑ arrhythmias)

ACE = angiotensin-converting enzyme; AV = atrioventricular; CNS = central nervous system; INR = international normalized ratio; IV = intravenous; NAPA = N-acetyl procainamide; PAC = premature atrial contraction; PVC = premature ventricular contraction; PT = prothrombin time; VF = ventricular fibrillation; WPW = Wolff-Parkinson-White.

Chapter 5

Long-Term Antiarrhythmic Drug Therapy

Debra G. Hanisch, RN, MSN, CPNP and George F. Van Hare, MD

The management of arrhythmias in children is evolving rapidly. Even with the introduction of radiofrequency ablation in the late 1980s, many situations remain in which antiarrhythmic medications play an important role in the treatment of pediatric arrhythmias. Antiarrhythmic agents, namely digoxin, quinidine, procainamide, mexiletine, phenytoin, flecainide, propafenone, propranolol, atenolol, sotalol, amiodarone, and verapamil, may be used for suppression of atrial and ventricular tachyarrhythmias in infants and young children until they reach a favorable size for elective radiofrequency ablation or while awaiting potential spontaneous resolution of their arrhythmia. These agents may be prescribed for the long term in others for whom radiofrequency ablation is not indicated or has been unsuccessful. β-Blockers such as propranolol, atenolol, or metoprolol are often combined with device therapy for management of patients with long QT syndrome (LQTS).

Of all the antiarrhythmic drugs that have Food and Drug Administration (FDA) approval for use in adults, only five have specific approval for pediatric use. These agents are digoxin, propranolol, phenytoin, lidocaine, and disopyramide. This is not due to any specific information indicating any untoward risks for most drugs, but rather is due to a lack of pharmacokinetic, efficacy, and safety data gathered in children as part of the regulatory approval process. Despite the lack of well-established pediatric guidelines, it is important for nurses and other clinicians who administer these drugs to children in the hospital setting and educate families about administering them in the home to be knowledgeable about the

From Zeigler VL, Gillette PC: *Practical Management of Pediatric Cardiac Arrhythmias.* Armonk, NY: Futura Publishing Co., Inc.; ©2001.

pharmacologic issues related to their use. This chapter focuses on long-term antiarrhythmic drug therapy in infants and children, with a brief overview of pediatric pharmacokinetics, pharmacodynamics, and classification of drugs followed by an emphasis on actions and uses, dosing and administration, implications for clinicians, and patient and family considerations for specific agents. Finally, special considerations as they apply to children receiving antiarrhythmic drugs are also reviewed.

Pediatric Pharmacokinetics/Pharmacodynamics

Pharmacokinetics refers to the relationship between the dose of a medication and the blood concentration. It is influenced by absorption, distribution, metabolism, and excretion.[1,2] In infants, gastric secretion is decreased for the first 3 months and gastric emptying is delayed for the first 6 months.[3] This slows absorption of most drugs and may affect peak serum concentrations. In the first 2 years of life, infants have a larger volume of distribution and decreased protein binding, both of which result in a lower serum concentration for a given dose.[4] Absorption and distribution may also be influenced by certain clinical conditions, e.g., congestive heart failure (CHF). Due to immaturity of enzyme systems and renal function, metabolism and excretion are diminished for the first 6 months of life, but between 6 months and adolescence, they are slightly better than adult metabolism and excretion.[1] Clinical conditions associated with hepatic or renal dysfunction result in impairment of metabolism or excretion of most drugs. Pharmacodynamics refers to the relationship between the serum concentration of a drug and the drug's clinical effect. Differences between children and adults will exist because of differences in the underlying mechanisms responsible for the arrhythmias. Furthermore, basic developmental differences between children and adults may account for altered pharmacodynamics. Common terminology used when discussing pharmacologic agents can be found in Table 1.

Given these differences between children and adults, some factors would lead one to administer a relatively higher dose of a drug to children while other factors suggest the opposite. Garson[1] recommends, in general, choosing a relatively smaller dose for infants and a relatively larger dose for children. Ideally, doses should be calculated based on body surface area rather than weight alone whenever possible. Body surface area is directly proportional to intestinal surface area, total body water and cardiac output, hepatic blood flow, and glomerular filtration, which are principle determinants of absorption, distribution, metabolism, and excretion, respectively.

Classification of Drugs

In 1981, Vaughan Williams[5] developed a classification system to describe the antiarrhythmic action of certain drugs. This classification system, which was revised in 1984,[6] has since been the most widely accepted

Table 1
Commonly Used Pharmacologic Terms

Bioavailability	The extent to which a drug reaches its site of action (different from potency) or the fraction of a drug absorbed into the systemic circulation
Clearance	A measure of the body's ability to eliminate a drug
Half-life	The time it takes for the plasma concentration (or amount of drug in the body) to be reduced by 50%
Loading dose	One or a series of doses that may be given at the onset of therapy aimed at achieving the target concentration rapidly
Peak level	The highest concentration a drug reaches after a number of doses have been administered
Toxicity	A state of harmful adverse effects caused by a specific agent
Trough level	The lowest concentration a drug reaches between doses
Volume of distribution	A measure of the apparent space in the body available to contain a drug

Sources: Benet LZ, Kroetz DL, Sheiner LB: Pharmocokinetics: The dynamics of drug absorption, distribution, and elimination. In Hardman JG, Limbird LE, Molinoff PB, et al. (eds.): Goodman and Gilman's The Pharmacological Basis of Therapeutics. 9th ed. New York: McGraw Hill; 1996:3–27.
Miller S, Fioravanti J (eds.): Pediatric Medications: A Handbook for Nurses. St. Louis: Mosby-Year Book Inc.; 1997:1–10.

means to classify antiarrhythmic agents To summarize briefly, Class I agents, sometimes referred to as local anesthetics, are sodium channel blockers, in which membrane-active agents work on the fast sodium channels by inhibiting depolarization. These agents primarily slow conduction within the heart and depress automaticity and are subdivided into three different subsets according to their specific effects on refractoriness of the cardiac action potential. Class Ia agents prolong refractoriness, Class Ib agents shorten refractoriness, and Class Ic agents produce only minor changes in refractoriness. Class II agents are β-adrenergic blockers, which decrease sympathetic activity by competitively blocking β-adrenergic receptors. This results in slowed conduction, depressed automaticity, and an increase in the effective refractory period of the atrioventricular (AV) node. Class III agents prolong repolarization and refractoriness by delaying the inward flux of potassium that drives repolarization. Class III agents also have important antifibrillatory effects. Class IV agents are calcium channel blockers, which primarily inhibit the slow inward flux of calcium. These agents act to primarily depress automaticity of the sinus node and prolong AV conduction.[7,8]

Although the Vaughan Williams classification system had served as an effective means to group antiarrhythmic agents, its initial intent was aimed at classifying the antiarrhythmic actions, not the agents themselves. In 1991, a new approach, "The Sicilian Gambit," was proposed by the Task Force of the Working Group on Arrhythmias of the European Society of Cardiology to classify antiarrhythmic drugs based on their actions on arrhythmogenic mechanisms in terms of channels, receptors, and pumps.[9] This classification system is not typically used in the clinical setting, as many arrhythmia mechanisms remain unknown and targets such as receptors or channels may be unclear.[10]

Specific Agents Used in Children

Although there are many antiarrhythmic agents used for the treatment of tachyarrhythmias, there are specific agents that are used more commonly than others in children. The following antiarrhythmic agents used in children are discussed with respect to their actions/uses, dosing and administration, implications for clinicians, and patient and family considerations: digoxin, quinidine, procainamide, mexiletine, phenytoin, flecainide, propafenone, propranolol, atenolol, sotalol, amiodarone, and verapamil. More specific information regarding serum concentrations, adverse effects, and drug interactions can be found in Appendix 5–1. Several of the less commonly used agents, i.e., moricizine, nadolol, and metoprolol, are included in the table but not in the text.

Digoxin

Actions and Uses

Digoxin is commonly administered as an inotropic drug for the treatment of CHF. At slightly higher doses, digoxin has antiarrhythmic properties as well, partially because of its effects on the autonomic nervous system. Although digoxin falls outside of the Vaughan Williams classification system, it is included in more recent drug classification systems.[9] Digoxin is one of the few agents approved by the FDA for use in children. Digoxin exerts a vaguslike effect by increasing cholinergic receptor sensitivity, which results in slowing of atrial and AV nodal conduction. Digoxin therapy is used for long-term prophylaxis of supraventricular tachycardia (SVT) and conversion of SVT. In addition, digoxin may be administered to slow the ventricular response in atrial flutter/fibrillation or other SVTs. Because digoxin crosses the placenta, it may be given maternally to treat fetal tachycardias. At therapeutic levels, electrocardiographic (ECG) changes may include sinus bradycardia, PR prolongation (first-degree AV block), and possible ST segment and T wave changes, including ST depression and QT interval shortening.

The safety of digoxin use in patients with Wolff-Parkinson-White syndrome (WPW) has long been debated. In approximately one third of patients whose accessory pathways have short refractory periods, digoxin may further enhance preexcitation, predisposing them to ventricular fibrillation (VF) if atrial fibrillation were to occur with rapid AV conduction.[11–13] Because atrial fibrillation is quite rare in children with WPW, some cardiologists continue to use digoxin as first-line therapy to control SVT. If there is concern about VF, a β-blocker may be used, either alone or in combination with digoxin.[14]

Dosing and Administration

Digoxin is available for long-term use as an elixir, tablet, or capsule. The elixir comes prepared as 50 μg/mL, the tablets are available in 125, 250, and 500 μg, and the capsules are available as 50, 100, and 200 μg. Because of its long elimination half-life (20 to 40 hours),[15,16] loading of digoxin is recommended when initiating therapy, followed by maintenance dosing at one fourth the total digitalizing dose. Elimination half-lives tend to be shorter in infants and children due to their greater volume of distribution and more rapid elimination of the drug. Relatively higher doses, therefore, are prescribed for these age groups. Dosing practices vary, but generally fall within the ranges listed in Appendix 5–1. Historically, a twice-daily regimen has been recommended to reduce the potential risk of toxic peak concentrations and subtherapeutic trough concentrations.[16] Recent comparison studies demonstrated that, although peak serum concentrations were significantly higher with once-daily versus twice-daily dosing (2.3 to 2.7 nmol/L versus 1.6 to 1.9 nmol/L, respectively), there were no significant differences in trough concentrations, nor were there differences clinically in terms of heart rate, respiratory rate, or liver size in the children studied.[17,18] Importantly, digoxin toxicity was not observed in any of these study groups, perhaps because the lower limit of toxicity is known to be higher in younger children than in adults.[17] Unless an individual is "digoxin sensitive," once-daily dosing may be used safely in children.[18]

Implications for Clinicians

It is generally recommended that digoxin loading, commonly referred to as digitalization, be performed in the hospital setting. If the maintenance dose is used in lieu of loading, digoxin may be initiated on an outpatient basis. During digitalization, most pediatric cardiologists recommend ECG monitoring to assess digoxin effect and potential toxicity. A baseline ECG should be obtained prior to digitalization and then repeated just before starting the maintenance dose.[19] Digoxin effect may manifest as PR prolongation and ST segment and/or T wave changes, including ST depression and QT interval shortening. Any arrhythmia or more advanced AV block should be assumed to be due to digoxin toxicity until proven otherwise, and preparations for external pacing in the event of AV block secondary to overdose/toxicity should be made in advance. Nurses are taught to measure a full 60-second apical pulse rate prior to administering each dose of digoxin, with the intent of screening for bradycardia or other arrhythmias. The physician should always be notified before a dose of digoxin is withheld, if the heart rate is deemed too slow. Additionally, electrolytes should be monitored carefully. Imbalances, such as hypokalemia, hypomagnesemia, and hypercalcemia, predispose patients to digoxin toxicity even when digoxin serum concentrations fall within the therapeutic range. Concomitant administration of catecholamines, quinidine, calcium channel blockers, amiodarone, or antibiotics (e.g., erythromycin, tetracycline) will cause an increase in serum digoxin concentrations. Certain clinical conditions, including myocardial disease, hypoxemia, alkalosis, renal insufficiency, and hypothyroidism, may also contribute to digoxin toxicity.[15,18]

The utility of monitoring serum digoxin concentrations remains controversial. Clearly, serum concentrations are useful in determining patient compliance, evaluating possible toxicity, and managing cases of overdose. Serum concentrations should be obtained as trough levels at least 6 hours after the last administered dose. Therapeutic concentrations for the treatment of congestive cardiac failure range from 0.8 to 2.0 ng/mL. Electrophysiologic effects occur at slightly higher levels than do inotropic effects, but target digoxin levels are not well defined. Although levels greater than 2.0 ng/mL are typically associated with toxicity, higher levels (up to 3.5 ng/mL) may be tolerated in newborns and young infants due to the presence of endogenous digoxinlike immunoreactive factors which cross-react with some digoxin immunoassays.[8,19–21] Newer assays are much less sensitive to cross-reactivity with these substances; however, the surface ECG remains the preferred method for monitoring digoxin therapy. Digoxin toxicity is rare in patients receiving digoxin on a long-term basis, but can be manifested by second- or third-degree AV block and ventricular arrhythmias. It can be treated with the Class Ib agent phenytoin and with digoxin antibodies, (i.e., Digibind). For more information on Digibind, please refer to chapter 4.

Patient and Family Considerations

Safe administration of digoxin must be emphasized to families. Care should be taken to teach parents how to measure accurately and give digoxin elixir to young children. Decimal point errors can occur (e.g., giving 3.0 mL instead of 0.3 mL), resulting in accidental overdose.

Individualized syringes may be marked for the correct dosage amount by the nurse and given to the family for home use. Parents should also be taught to observe for signs of digoxin toxicity, such as anorexia, nausea, vomiting, diarrhea, blurred vision, and fatigue. These signs may be difficult to evaluate in young children. Because an overdose can be fatal, digoxin must be kept out of the reach of children. In addition, parents of all patients with cardiac arrhythmias should be told that certain decongestants, such as pseudoephedrine and phenylephrine, have the potential to exacerbate tachyarrhythmias and should be avoided in susceptible children.

Quinidine

Actions and Uses

Quinidine is a Class Ia agent that blocks sodium and potassium channels. It prolongs the action potential duration and refractory period in atrial, ventricular, and Purkinje fiber tissue. On the ECG, the QRS and QT intervals become significantly prolonged. Quinidine is effective in the treatment of primary atrial tachycardias and atrial fibrillation. The use of quinidine has declined in recent years due to its high incidence of adverse effects and potential for proarrhythmia. Marked corrected QT (QTc) prolongation, torsades de pointes, syncope, and even death have been associated with the use of quinidine.[22] Newer agents have proven to be more effective with less adverse effects.

Dosage and Administration

Quinidine is formulated as quinidine sulfate or quinidine gluconate and is commercially available as follows: quinidine gluconate sustained release tablets available in 324 mg; quinidine sulfate tablets available in 200 and 300 mg; quinidine sulfate sustained release tablets available in 300 mg; and quinidine polygalacturonate tablets available in 275 mg. The sulfate form is dosed at 30 to 60 mg/kg/day, divided every 6 hours. The gluconate form is usually preferred because its slower absorption allows dosing every 8 to 12 hours; however, quinidine gluconate has 20% less quinidine base than quinidine sulfate, so the dose must be adjusted upward accordingly.[8,23]

When digoxin is used concomitantly with quinidine to control primary atrial tachycardias, the dose of digoxin should be reduced by 50% to avoid digoxin toxicity.[24] Quinidine also interacts with warfarin, causing a significantly increased prothrombin time.

Implications for Clinicians

Quinidine's propensity for proarrhythmia warrants in-hospital initiation of therapy. Changes in the QRS duration can be used to guide dosage adjustments. The QRS duration should be evaluated prior to each dosage and should not exceed the baseline measurement by 30%. The QTc intervals should be monitored closely as well for significant prolongation.[24,25] Therapeutic serum concentrations range from 2 to 6 µg/mL. Serum concentrations greater than 7 µg/mL are associated with toxicity. The most serious adverse effects that occur with quinidine toxicity are the cardiac effects. Early cardiac toxicity can be manifested by QT prolongation and QRS widening. Similar to other Class Ia agents, other arrhythmias associated with quinidine toxicity include bradycardia, AV block, ventricular tachycardia (VT), torsades de pointes, VF, and asystole.[26,27] Because of the sodium channel blocking properties of Class Ia agents, intravenous (IV) administration of sodium bicarbonate may assist in reversing cardiac toxicity.[28]

Immunological reactions have been reported in some patients receiving quinidine. Thrombocytopenia is most common but resolves with discontinuation of therapy. Anemia and agranulocytosis are less common. Quinidine's negative inotropic effects may exacerbate congestive cardiac failure in patients with myocardial dysfunction.[8,25] Finally, the IV form of quinidine should never be given to children because of the incidence of associated severe hypotension and ventricular dysfunction.

Patient and Family Considerations

Patient and family education is important since nearly a third of patients taking quinidine experience side effects. Gastrointestinal complaints, particularly nausea, vomiting, and diarrhea, are most common. Cinchonism, manifested by central nervous system symptoms such as headache, tinnitus, and visual changes, appears to be related to higher plasma levels and is managed by reducing the quinidine dose. Allergic reactions, typically presenting as fever or rash, should be reported as well.

Procainamide

Actions and Uses

Procainamide is a Class Ia agent with electrophysiologic actions similar to quinidine. It decreases automaticity, increases refractory periods, and slows conduction through the atrium, AV node, His-Purkinje system, and ventricles. At therapeutic serum concentrations, ECG changes include PR prolongation and widening of both the QRS duration and QT interval. Procainamide is used orally to treat resistant SVT, atrial flutter, atrial fibrillation, and VT. Procainamide crosses the placenta and may be administered maternally to treat fetal SVT. Fetal plasma levels approximate 80% of maternal levels.[29]

Dosage and Administration

Procainamide is available in a standard release preparation that has a half-life of 3 to 4 hours, or a sustained release form with a longer half-life of 5 to 7 hours. Specifically, procainamide is available in 250-, 375-, and 500-mg capsules, 250-, 375-, and 500-mg tablets, and 250-, 500-, 750-, and 1000-mg sustained release tablets. The daily dose ranges from 40 to 100 mg/kg. In infants, it may be necessary to administer procainamide as often as every 4 hours. Most toddlers can be dosed every 6 hours. Once the child is old enough to swallow pills, the sustained release compound permits dosing up to every 8 hours.[23]

Implications for Clinicians

Therapy with procainamide should be initiated in the hospital setting. Monitoring should include serial ECG measurements of the QTc interval. The drug should be stopped in the event of excessive QTc prolongation (>500 ms) or the development of adverse effects. Procainamide is acetylated in the liver to form the active metabolite N-acetylprocainamide (NAPA), which has some Class III antiarrhythmic properties as well as negative inotropic effects. Metabolism can be quite variable, and whether an individual is a slow, moderate, or fast acetylator is genetically determined.[7] In any case, the contribution of NAPA as an antiarrhythmic agent is minimal given its relatively small concentration; however, when monitoring procainamide therapy, obtaining NAPA levels in addition to procainamide levels is generally advocated. Therapeutic procainamide levels range from 4 to 8 μg/mL, although levels up to 12 μg/mL may be required in some patients to suppress their arrhythmia. NAPA levels greater than 40 μg/mL are associated with toxicity. Unlike with quinidine, serum concentrations do not appear to be affected by concomitant administration of digoxin.

A major limitation to long-term oral therapy with procainamide is the high incidence of a drug-induced lupuslike syndrome, especially in slow acetylators. Positive antinuclear antibodies (ANA) develop in 50% to 90% of patients, but only 20% to 40% develop clinical symptoms of systemic lupus erythematosus.[7,8] Fever, arthralgia, pericardial effusions, and hepatomegaly may develop. These clinical symptoms disappear with discontinuation of the drug. If the patient is asymptomatic, a positive ANA is not necessarily an indication to stop therapy. Other adverse effects include thrombocytopenia and, rarely, neutropenia. Complete blood counts, including platelets, as well as ANA testing for systemic lupus erythematosus should be monitored in these patients at least every 6 months. Procainamide's toxic cardiovascular effects are similar to those previously discussed in regard to quinidine. IV sodium bicarbonate can also be used in these patients for toxicity reversal.

Patient and Family Considerations

Patient compliance may be a problem, because of the frequent dosing required with procainamide. Families must understand the importance of adhering to the prescribed dosing schedule, and health care professionals should assist the family in determining appropriate dosing intervals during the child's waking hours. The most serious adverse effect associated with long-term procainamide therapy is the lupuslike syndrome described above. Parents should be instructed to report any lupuslike symptoms, including arthralgia, myalgia, fever, or rash. Gastrointestinal symptoms such as nausea, vomiting, and diarrhea occur less frequently than with quinidine.

Mexiletine

Actions and Uses

Mexiletine is a Class Ib antiarrhythmic agent with actions similar to lidocaine. It exerts its primary effects on the fast sodium channels to slow conduction and decrease excitability and automaticity. The ECG remains relatively unchanged in patients receiving mexiletine therapy. Mexiletine is useful in the treatment of lidocaine-sensitive ventricular arrhythmias, particularly in children with congenital heart disease (CHD). It has been used successfully to control postoperative arrhythmias in children with tetralogy of Fallot, ventricular tumors, and hypertrophic cardiomyopathy.[30,31] It may become an important drug in the treatment of specific forms of LQTS associated with sodium channel defects.[23]

Dosage and Administration

Mexiletine is available as 150-, 200-, and 250-mg capsules. The starting dose of mexiletine is 6 mg/kg/day, divided every 8 hours. The dose may be gradually increased up to 15 mg/kg/day. Mexiletine crosses the placenta, but reports of its use in managing fetal tachycardias are rare.[23]

Implications for Clinicians

Although reports of proarrhythmia associated with mexiletine administration are few, it is recommended that initiation be done in the hospital setting. Therapeutic serum concentrations range from 0.8 to 2.0 µg/mL but are seldom used to gauge therapy.

Patient and Family Considerations

Adverse effects are common, especially gastrointestinal and neurologic side effects, and are responsible for significant patient noncompliance. Nausea, vomiting, and abdominal pain may be diminished by taking mexiletine with food. Some of the neurologic symptoms associated with mexiletine administration include dizziness, tremors, paresthesias, blurred vision, and headaches.[8,30] A fine, maculopapular rash, particularly on the dorsum of the hands, has been observed as well.[23]

Phenytoin

Actions and Uses

Phenytoin is a Class Ib antiarrhythmic agent with actions similar to the other Class Ib agents. It binds predominately to sodium channels in the inactivated state while shortening action potential duration and prolonging refractory periods. It acts selectively on diseased or ischemic tissue and is thought to interrupt reentry circuits.[32] It has been used successfully in the treatment of ventricular arrhythmias after surgery for CHD,[33,34] but it can be used in patients with arrhythmias secondary to digoxin toxicity as well.

Dosage and Administration

Oral phenytoin is commercially available as follows: 50-mg chewable tablets (known as Infatabs), 30 mg/5 mL and 125 mg/5 mL oral suspensions, 30- and 100-mg capsules, and 30- and 100-mg extended release capsules. Oral phenytoin for ventricular arrhythmias is initiated with a loading dose of 3.75 mg/kg (15 mg/kg/day) given every 6 hours over 24 hours, followed by 1.9 mg/kg (7.5 mg/kg/day) every 6 hours for an additional 24 hours. Maintenance dosing is 5 to 6 mg/kg/day, divided twice daily.[33]

In general, chewable Infatabs are used rather than capsules or suspensions for ventricular arrhythmia management because of the approximate 8% increase in drug content absorption with the chewable formulation. Serum concentrations are generally used to guide therapy and are obtained as a trough level when loading is complete and just prior to administering the first maintenance dose.[35] The half-life of phenytoin varies and can be as long as 72 hours in infants. After 1 year of age, it decreases to 8 hours, but it rises again in adulthood.[10]

Implications for Clinicians

Oral phenytoin for the treatment of ventricular arrhythmias in children is initiated in the hospital setting with continuous ECG monitoring. Twenty-four-hour ambulatory monitoring is used intermittently to assess ectopy as well as tachyarrhythmia suppression. Cardiovascular adverse effects associated with phenytoin administration are rare, but there are other noncardiovascular adverse effects that the clinician must be aware of. Phenytoin can affect the central nervous system, as evidenced by symptoms such as drowsiness, stupor, and ataxia; however, these symptoms can generally be minimized or even eliminated with a reduction in dosage. Skin rashes occur in 10% to 20% of patients and usually occur within 10 days of phenytoin administration.[10] The appearance of a rash requires immediate drug discontinuation in order to avoid Stevens-Johnson syndrome. Gastrointestinal upset can be diminished by taking phenytoin with food. Gingival hyperplasia is a common adverse effect associated with long-term phenytoin therapy, but perhaps the most dangerous adverse effect is that of teratogenicity.

Caution should be used when administering phenytoin and warfarin concomitantly, as phenytoin causes an increase in the patient's prothrombin time and international normalized ratio (INR). Other known drug interactions include isoniazid, diazepam, methylphenidate, chlorpromazine, chlordiazepoxide, and disulfiram, all of which can decrease the metabolism of phenytoin. Metabolism enhancers include phenobarbital and carbamazepine.

Patient and Family Considerations

Patients and families should be counseled regarding the aforementioned adverse effects of oral phenytoin. They should be instructed to inform their cardiologist immediately if a measlelike rash appears or if pregnancy occurs. Gingival hyperplasia can be minimized with good oral hygiene. Additionally, if decreased school performance or any other central nervous system effects are noted, the cardiologist should be notified in order to make a dosage decrease.

Flecainide

Actions and Uses

Flecainide, a Class Ic antiarrhythmic agent, blocks the rapid influx of sodium through its ion channels. It depresses automaticity and delays conduction through the atria, AV node, ventricles, and accessory pathways in both antegrade and retrograde directions. On the surface ECG, increases in the PR interval, QRS duration, and, to a lesser extent, QTc interval may occur. Flecainide is effective in the treatment of SVTs. Zeigler and colleagues[36] reported its success in the control of resistant SVT in 50% of patients who failed an average of three previous antiarrhythmic drugs. In a review of the world literature, Perry and Garson[37] reported efficacy rates for oral flecainide in treating SVT caused by a variety of mechanisms: reentry via accessory pathways (73%), AV nodal reentry (81%), permanent junctional reciprocating tachycardia (100%), chaotic atrial tachycardia (100%), and atrial or junctional ectopic tachycardia (81% and 83%, respectively). Successful management of atrial flutter and ventricular arrhythmias with flecainide was also reported. Flecainide may also be administered maternally to treat fetal tachycardia,[38–40] with fetal levels approximating 70% of maternal serum concentrations.

The Cardiac Arrhythmia Suppression Trial (CAST) report[41] prompted vigorous investigation into the safe use of flecainide in the pediatric population. Oral flecainide appears to be safe and effective in children with SVT and normal hearts. For children with SVT, the overall risk of proarrhythmia is approximately 7%, but for children with structural heart disease or cardiomyopathy, the risk is much greater. Flecainide should be avoided in children with atrial flutter or ventricular arrhythmias and structurally abnormal hearts, in whom the risk for cardiac arrest is significantly higher.[37,42]

Dosage and Administration

Flecainide is available as 50-, 100-, or 150-mg tablets. The dose of flecainide is 50 to 200 mg/m²/day or 1 to 8 mg/kg/day. Dosing based on body surface area has been shown to correlate better with serum concentrations than dosing based on weight alone.[43] Children ages 6 months to 10 years have a mean elimination half-life of 8 hours and may benefit by dosing three times daily. Young infants and adolescents tend to have a longer elimination half-life, permitting twice-daily dosing.[43] Caution should be used in dosing neonates, in whom an elimination half-life as long as 27 hours has been reported.[37] For young patients unable to swallow pills, a 5- or 10-mg/mL oral suspension of flecainide may be compounded by pharmacists. Dairy products have been shown to block flecainide absorption.[44] It is very important, especially in infants and small children, that the dosage be periodically adjusted for the child's rapid weight gain.

Implications for Clinicians

In-hospital monitoring during initiation of flecainide therapy and adjustments in doses is recommended with close supervision of serum concentrations. Trough serum concentrations of 200 to 1000 ng/mL are considered therapeutic. Toxicity and increased proarrhythmia can occur at serum concentrations of greater than 1000 ng/mL. A report of flecainide toxicity in a neonate validates the use of IV sodium bicarbonate for flecainide-induced cardiac toxicity.[45] Combination therapy with digoxin or amiodarone can elevate flecainide serum concentrations. Continuous ECG monitoring of patients is essential because of the associated risk of proarrhythmia. During the first few days of therapy, a slower, incessant SVT may occur in children with paroxysmal SVT. Some centers perform routine intracardiac electrophysiology testing prior to discharging patients receiving flecainide in order to assess the risk of associated proarrhythmia. Individuals with structurally abnormal hearts or cardiomyopathies are at greatest risk for developing life-threatening ventricular arrhythmias. In patients with pacemakers, flecainide has been shown to increase pacing thresholds significantly. Flecainide should be avoided in patients with ejection fractions less than 25% because of its negative inotropic effects.[31]

Patient and Family Considerations

Although gastrointestinal and neurologic symptoms such as nausea, vomiting, headaches, blurred vision, irritability, hyperactivity, and dry mouth have been reported by some adults taking flecainide, these non-cardiac side effects appear to be rare in children.[2,7,36] Dairy products such as milk, infant formula, and, possibly, yogurt interfere with the absorption of flecainide. Flecainide levels have been reported to double with a change in diet from formula to dextrose feedings.[44] Therefore, parents must understand the importance of notifying their child's cardiologist in the event of gastrointestinal illness or when they are ready to embark on weaning their child from formula. Flecainide serum concentrations should be monitored closely for toxicity during such times.

In some centers, parents are instructed to telephone the cardiologist with the child's weight in order for the dosage to be adjusted. Also, children aged 1 year to 18 months may be allowed to "outgrow" the dose in order to assess for spontaneous resolution of the tachyarrhythmia. When using the pharmacy-prepared oral suspension requiring refrigeration, it is imperative that parents be instructed to vigorously shake the bottle prior to administration in order for the flecainide to be equally distributed in the diluent; otherwise, toxic amounts may be contained in the last few doses.

Due to the fact that some pharmacies are unable to prepare a liquid formulation, some centers teach the parents or primary caregivers how to formulate their own suspension. They are instructed by an expert cardiovascular nurse and evaluated by return demonstration. Written instructions are given and they are taught to draw up as many as possible individual doses of the medication in oral syringes. An example of these instructions can be found in Table 2. The oral syringes are labeled and then refrigerated until time of usage.

Propafenone

Actions and Uses

Propafenone is a Class Ic agent with predominantly sodium channel blocking effects. It slows conduction through the atria, ventricles, sinus, and AV nodes. Atrial and ventricular refractory periods are prolonged as well. On surface ECG, dose-related prolongation of the PR and QRS intervals can be observed.[46] Propafenone is useful in the management of a wide spectrum of arrhythmias. It slows antegrade and retrograde conduction through accessory pathways. Complete antegrade conduction block has been observed in patients with WPW.[47] In AV nodal reentrant tachycardia, propafenone has been shown to block the fast pathway.[48] Additionally, due to its weak β-adrenergic blocking activity and weak calcium antagonism, it has been shown to be highly effective in controlling automatic/ectopic SVT, including chaotic atrial tachycardia and junctional ectopic tachycardia.[49] At higher doses, propafenone exerts a negative inotropic effect and, because of this, should be used with caution in patients with depressed ventricular function or asthma. It appears to be

Table 2
Instructions for Making Your Child's Medicine into a Liquid Form—Flecainide

Supplies needed	1. Pills or capsules of your child's medicine 2. A simple syrup provided by your pharmacy or drug store 3. A mortar and pestle (provided by your pharmacy or drug store)* 4. Oral (by mouth) syringes
Mixing instructions	1. Take a 100-mg tablet of flecainide and crush in mortar with pestle into a fine powder 2. Slowly add 10 cc's of simple syrup, mixing well with mortar 3. Once the mixture is cloudy and there are no big pieces of the pill left, the medicine is properly mixed
Drawing up your child's dose	1. The mixture now contains **10 mg** of flecainide for every **1 cc** of liquid: **(10 mg/1 cc)** 2. Your child's dose is **25 mg,** so you will need to draw up **2.5 cc's** into an individual syringe: **25 mg/2.5 cc** 3. Draw up as many single doses for your child as possible from the mixture 4. Refrigerate and use within 2 weeks

*Flecainide does better when a mortar and pestle is used for mixing; with other medications, a bowl and spoon may be used.

Hints for clinicians:

1. Instruct parents how to draw the individual doses with oral syringes and provide prescription for oral syringes for parent to take to pharmacy.
2. Instruct parents to paint clear nail polish on outside of syringes to preserve numbers.
3. Instruct parents to discard syringes when numbers are no longer visible.
4. Instruct parents to use only "pharmacy"-obtained syrup for mixing.
5. Instruct parents to keep this and all medications out of the reach of children.
6. Provide phone numbers for parents to call for questions regarding this procedure after discharge.

a more effective drug for children with normal hearts than for those with structural heart disease or cardiomyopathy.[50]

Dosage and Administration

Propafenone is available in tablets of 150 and 300 mg. Oral loading of propafenone is not recommended because acute toxicity may occur. Dosing starts at 200 to 300 mg/m^2/day, or 8 to 10 mg/kg/day, divided every 6 or 8 hours.[47] Patients vary in their ability to metabolize the drug. The elimination half-life has been reported at anywhere from 4 to 16 hours.[23] In most patients, a steady state is reached in 3 to 4 days. Doses can then be increased in 100 mg/m^2/day increments as needed up to 600 mg/m^2/day or 15 mg/kg/day.

Implications for Clinicians

Initiation of propafenone therapy should be done in the hospital because cardiovascular toxicity is unpredictable and unrelated to serum concentrations, which vary widely. This variation can range anywhere from 100 to 5000 ng/mL and correlates poorly with the drug's dose.[23] Studies have shown that the increase in the PR interval and QRS duration relates more to dosage increments than to serum concentrations.[46] Monitoring these ECG changes rather than trough serum concentrations is helpful in evaluating proper propafenone dosing. Liver enzymes should be monitored closely as well, particularly in patients receiving relatively high doses. Digoxin serum concentrations may increase with concomitant administration of propafenone, and should be monitored closely. Proarrhythmia and other adverse cardiac events appear less frequently with propafenone than with flecainide and, similarly, are found predominantly in the presence of structural heart disease.[51] A baseline echocardiogram should be performed prior to initiating propafenone, to assess ventricular function.

Patient and Family Considerations

Propafenone is best absorbed if taken on an empty stomach but can be taken with food if nausea occurs. Systemic adverse effects are unusual in children but may include nausea, vomiting, headaches, dizziness, and tremors.[8,47] Rarely, a propafenone-induced lupuslike syndrome occurs.[8] Parents should be instructed to report symptoms such as dizziness, lethargy, or syncope to their child's cardiologist.

Propranolol

Actions and Uses

Propranolol is a Class II nonselective β-adrenergic blocking agent. It is the most widely used β-blocker in pediatrics. Propranolol, like all β-adrenergic blockers, decreases the effects of sympathetic activity by competitively blocking β-adrenergic receptors. Clinically, propranolol slows the heart rate, depresses automaticity, and prolongs AV nodal conduction and refractoriness. Aside from a slower heart rate, ECG changes associated with propranolol administration include prolongation of the PR interval and occasional shortening of the corrected QT interval. Propranolol is used most commonly for long-term prophylaxis of supraventricular or ventricular tachyarrhythmias. It is effective in reentrant tachycardias that use the AV node as one of the reentrant pathways, such as AV nodal reentry tachycardia or the permanent form of junctional reciprocating tachycardia. Automatic/ectopic tachycardias respond to propranolol therapy as well. Although it does not convert atrial flutter or fibrillation, propranolol may be used to control the ventricular rate. Propranolol is particularly effective in congenital LQTS. In resistant arrhythmias, propranolol may be used in combination with digoxin, Class Ia, or Ic agents.

Dosage and Administration

Oral propranolol is commercially available as an oral liquid, a standard tablet, or a long-acting tablet or capsule. The specific available preparations of propranolol are as follows: liquid preparation containing 4 mg/mL or 8 mg/mL; concentrated liquid preparation containing 80 mg/mL; tablets of 10, 20, 40, 60, 80, and 90 mg; extended release tablets of 80, 120, and 160 mg; and sustained release capsules of 60, 80, 120, and 160 mg. The starting dose is 1 to 2 mg/kg/day and is increased as needed up to 6 mg/kg/day. The dose is divided every 6 hours, due to its short half-life of 4 to 6 hours. With the long-acting form, twice-daily dosing is used, which helps to improve patient compliance.

Implications for Clinicians

Oral propranolol can be initiated on an inpatient or outpatient basis, depending on the patient's clinical presentation or condition. Serum concentrations of propranolol range from 25 to 150 ng/mL for β-blockade. Higher levels may be required for control of ventricular arrhythmias. Levels vary widely and are more useful in assessing compliance than efficacy. Monitoring of heart rate and blood pressure is important when initiating propranolol therapy. Cardiovascular adverse effects associated with propranolol include hypotension, bradycardia, and worsening of CHF. Raynaud's phenomenon has been reported as well.[7] Significant noncardiac side effects such as depression, lethargy, and headache may occur with propranolol. Because it is a nonselective β-blocker, propranolol can exacerbate bronchospasm and should not be used in patients with asthma. Propranolol can also increase the risk of hypoglycemia in diabetic patients, young infants, patients who are NPO (nothing by mouth) for certain procedures, or in the fetus with maternal administration.[8,23] The efficacy of propranolol can be assessed by evidence of arrhythmia suppression, but also by performing exercise stress testing. Evidence of appropriate "β-blockade" should result in the inability of the patient's maximum heart rate to achieve the predicted response for age and is approximately 75% of normal.

Patient and Family Considerations

Propranolol is commercially available as a 4-mg/mL and an 8-mg/mL oral solution, making it easy to dose in young children. Additionally, the extended release form is available for older patients, permitting dosing at less frequent intervals. Parents should be made aware of the central nervous system effects that may occur with propranolol therapy. Headaches, fatigue, depression, and sleep disturbances are relatively common and school-related problems may also occur. The school-related problems include decreased school performance, difficulty concentrating, and decreased attention span. Propranolol can affect compliance, especially in athletic teens whose endurance/performance may be diminished due to blunting of the heart rate. Teenaged girls may experience depression secondary to weight gain and the difficulty exercising when propranolol-induced fatigue sets in. Due to propranolol's tendency to be associated with hypoglycemia, parents should be informed that viral illnesses associated with nausea and vomiting may precipitate episodes. They should be informed of the signs and symptoms of hypoglycemia and should be instructed to notify the child's cardiologist in the event of prolonged viral illnesses.

Atenolol

Actions and Uses

Atenolol is a long-acting cardioselective β-adrenergic blocking agent. Its indications for use are similar to those of propranolol. Atenolol is used primarily to treat SVT resulting from AV reentrant tachycardias and ventricular arrhythmias exacerbated by exercise or catecholamines.[52,53] In atrial flutter, atenolol may convert the rhythm to sinus rhythm but more often acts to reduce the ventricular response. Atenolol is also used in the management of LQTS, usually in conjunction with device therapy; however, Trippel and Gillette[54] found atenolol to be less effective than propranolol in preventing sudden death in their population of patients with LQTS.

Atenolol may be preferred over nonselective β-adrenergic blocking agents in specific patients, since dosing is required only once daily. Patients experiencing neurologic adverse effects may benefit by switching from propranolol to atenolol. In older children and adolescents, the once-daily dosing of atenolol may improve compliance as well as decrease the incidence of neurologic adverse effects.

Dosage and Administration

Atenolol is available in 25-, 50-, and 100-mg tablets. The recommended dose of atenolol is 1 to 2 mg/kg/day, up to 3 mg/kg/day, given once or, sometimes, twice daily. The elimination half-life of atenolol is 5 to 10 hours, longer in neonates.[8,23] Serum concentrations are not useful since there is little correlation between levels and antiarrhythmic effect. As with propranolol, caution should be used when treating children with structural heart disease or cardiomyopathy, because of its negative inotropic effects as well as its effects on sinus and AV node function.

Implications for Clinicians

Atenolol can be initiated on an inpatient or outpatient basis, again depending on the child's presenting arrhythmia and/or clinical symptomatology. The overall incidence of adverse effects appears to be less with atenolol when compared with propranolol. Patients should be monitored for bradycardia and hypotension when therapy is initiated. Cardiac output and blood pressure typically decrease by 15%.[2] Because of its cardioselectivity, atenolol reduces the risk of bronchospasm, but bronchospasm may still occur in asthmatic patients.[24] Although the incidence of complications is lower than with nonselective β-blockers, glucose levels should be monitored in diabetic patients in whom insulin-induced hypoglycemia is a concern.

Patient and Family Considerations

Most frequently reported adverse effects resemble those of propranolol, particularly neurologic symptoms such as difficulty concentrating, headache, fatigue, and sleep disturbances.[52–54] Changes in school performance may be noted as well. In addition, complaints of cool extremities can be common.[23] Females who become pregnant should notify their physician immediately. Atenolol readily crosses the placenta yet is eliminated slowly, resulting in significant fetal bradycardia.[8,31]

Sotalol

Actions and Uses

Sotalol is a Class III antiarrhythmic agent with Class II nonselective β-blocker properties as well. At lower doses β-blockade occurs, while at higher doses Class III effects dominate. Sotalol prolongs the action potential throughout the heart. It decreases automaticity, slows AV conduction, and prolongs AV refractoriness by blocking both potassium channels and β-adrenergic receptors.[25] On surface ECG, sotalol slows the resting heart rate and causes a dose-dependent increase in the QT interval.[7,55] Studies have shown sotalol to be very effective in the treatment of various forms of reentrant SVT, both with and without preexcitation.[55–58] Sotalol is also useful in treating atrial flutter, particularly in children after surgery for CHD, with effective control reported in 48% to 66% of patients.[56–60] Varying results have been reported describing sotalol's efficacy in children with VT. The success rate for achieving control in VT compared to SVT appears to be much lower in the relatively small number of cases cited.[55–58] Sotalol may be preferred over amiodarone in many cases because of the relatively fewer long-term noncardiac adverse effects seen in comparison, but because of its β-blocking properties it should be used cautiously in patients with depressed ventricular function.

Dosage and Administration

Sotalol should be initiated in the hospital setting with continuous ECG monitoring. Sotalol is available in 80-, 160-, and 240-mg tablets. The recommended starting dose of sotalol is 2 mg/kg/day, or 90 to 100 mg/m²/day, divided into two daily doses. The dosage may be increased in 1- to 2-mg/kg increments at 2- to 3-day intervals up to a maximum dose of 8 mg/kg, or 200 mg/m²/day.[23,55] The elimination half-life ranges from 7 to 12 hours in adults. Data concerning pharmacokinetics in children are currently unavailable. Sotalol may be used in combination with digoxin but not with other antiarrhythmic agents that cause QT prolongation.

Implications for Clinicians

Oral sotalol therapy is associated with a significant risk of proarrhythmia. The rate of proarrhythmic events has been reported to be as high as 10%, with most events occurring within 3 to 5 days after initiation of sotalol treatment.[57] The risk is greater in the presence of hypokalemia or hypomagnesemia.[7] Sotalol should be initiated in the hospital setting in order to monitor for prolongation of the QTc interval, which is linearly proportional to the dose administered. The drug should be stopped if the QTc interval becomes greater than 500 ms. Severe bradycardia has been reported in children who receive sotalol with sinus node dysfunction following intracardiac repair of CHD.[56,57] AV block, ventricular ectopy, and torsades de pointes are other early-occurring adverse reactions that warrant close resting ECG and 24-hour ambulatory monitoring. Because of its β-blocking properties, it is advised that patients undergo baseline echocardiography prior to sotalol initiation. After discharge, follow-up with serial ambulatory ECG monitoring, as well as echocardiograms, is recommended.

Patient and Family Consideration

For administration in young children, sotalol can be compounded as a 5-mg/mL oral suspension. The drug is best absorbed when taken 1 hour before meals or 2 hours after meals. Sotalol appears to be well tolerated by children. Dizziness, fatigue, hypotension, and syncope are adverse effects observed with a relatively low (3% to 6%) incidence in pediatric patients.[55]

Amiodarone

Actions and Uses

Amiodarone is recognized as a potent Class III antiarrhythmic agent with β-blocking properties. Additional blocking actions on sodium channels and calcium channels render amiodarone the one drug to exert electrophysiologic effects representative of all four antiarrhythmic classes.

The principal effect of amiodarone is prolongation of the action potential duration in the atria and ventricles and prolongation of the effective refractory period in the atria, ventricles, AV node, and His-Purkinje system. Amiodarone has also been shown to increase refractoriness of accessory pathways in both antegrade and retrograde directions.[7] Additionally, automaticity is suppressed. ECG changes reflecting amiodarone's effects include slowing of the resting heart rate with prolongation of the PR interval, QRS duration, and QT interval.[61]

Amiodarone is useful in the long-term management of atrial and ventricular arrhythmias that are refractory to other agents. It is extremely effective in the treatment of atrial flutter, VT, and resistant SVT.[61,62] In two small series, atrial ectopic tachycardia and junctional ectopic tachycardia were also successfully managed with amiodarone therapy.[61,63] Because it causes little myocardial depression, amiodarone is useful in the management of rhythm disturbances in patients with CHD and/or congestive cardiac failure.[62]

Dosage and Administration

Oral amiodarone is available as 200-mg tablets and therapy should be initiated in the hospital setting. The loading dose of amiodarone is 10 to 15 mg/kg/day, divided twice daily (to avoid gastrointestinal side effects) for 7 to 14 (mean, 10) days followed by 5 to 7 mg/kg/day given once daily. Doses of digoxin, warfarin, and cyclosporine should be reduced by one third to one half and their serum concentrations monitored closely during amiodarone administration because of the propensity of concomitant administration to result in increased serum concentrations of these particular drugs. The half-life of amiodarone is extremely long and variable, but averages approximately 1 to 2 months. Every-other-day administration or preparation of a suspension are options to simplify dose calculations when tablets must be broken.

Implications for Clinicians

In-hospital monitoring for proarrhythmia, particularly bradycardia and torsades de pointes, is essential during loading. Prolongation of the QTc interval with subsequent torsades de pointes has been reported in less than 1% of pediatric patients.[23,61] Prior to initiation of amiodarone, patients with known or suspected sinus or AV node dysfunction may require permanent pacemaker implantation.[62] Therapeutic levels range from 1.0 to 2.5 μg/mL but correlate poorly with efficacy because of active metabolites and peripheral storage.[23] Serum concentrations are helpful only in assessing compliance.

Most adverse effects associated with amiodarone are dose related. Hyperthyroidism, hypothyroidism, and elevated liver enzymes are among the most common. Baseline thyroid and liver function tests should be performed prior to starting amiodarone and repeated every 6 months during therapy. Within 4 months of initiating therapy, many patients will present with corneal microdeposits, but few have actual visual disturbances. Ophthalmologic examinations are indicated if visual symptoms occur. In adults, pulmonary complications are the most serious adverse effects attributed to long-term therapy.[64] Only one recent case of pulmonary fibrosis related to amiodarone therapy has been reported in the pediatric population.[65] Baseline and periodic chest x-rays and pulmonary function testing may be warranted, particularly in the adolescent and young adult population.

Amiodarone can cause a decrease in cardiac output in severe congestive cardiac failure or in patients being weaned from cardiopulmonary bypass. The drug should be stopped 1 to 3 weeks prior to surgery that requires cardiopulmonary bypass.[31] Overall, the incidence of adverse effects in children has been shown to be far less than in adults. These observations have contributed to the increasing popularity of amiodarone in the pediatric population.

Patient and Family Considerations

A number of other adverse effects are associated with amiodarone use. Photosensitivity occurs in more than half of children taking this drug. Patients (and families) should be instructed to apply high-grade sun block, especially on the face and ears, wear sun-protective clothing (hat, long sleeves), and avoid sun exposure whenever possible. Due to the prolonged elimination half-life of amiodarone, these efforts must be continued for at least 1 month after the drug is discontinued. Bluish discoloration of the skin or a rash may occur, but can be reversed in most cases by discontinuing the medication. Gastrointestinal effects such as nausea and constipation are common, particularly during initiation of therapy. Nausea may be alleviated by taking the medicine with food. If irritation due to corneal microdeposits occurs, instillation of artificial tears may be of some benefit.

Verapamil

Actions and Uses

Verapamil, a Class IV antiarrhythmic agent, is a calcium channel antagonist. It exerts its greatest effect on the sinus and AV nodes. By inhibiting the slow inward calcium current, verapamil decreases sinus node automaticity and delays AV nodal conduction; therefore, it is particularly useful in the treatment of arrhythmias that use the AV node as part of their tachycardia circuit. In atrial flutter and fibrillation, verapamil is effective in slowing the ventricular response.[66] Verapamil has also been shown to be effective in certain verapamil-sensitive VTs[67] such as left ventricular outflow tract and fascicular tachycardias.

Dosage and Administration

Verapamil is available as 40-, 80-, and 120-mg tablets, 120-, 180-, and 240-mg sustained release tablets, and 360-mg sustained release capsules. The oral dose of verapamil is 4 to 17 mg/kg/day, divided every 8 hours. With the sustained release form, lower doses are used because of its greater bioavailability, and the frequency of administration is reduced to once or twice daily. The elimination half-life is 8 to 12 hours. Verapamil increases digoxin levels by 50% to 70%. Digoxin doses should be lowered in patients receiving combination therapy.[8,31]

Implications for Clinicians

Oral verapamil can be initiated in the hospital or outpatient setting depending on the patient's specific arrhythmia mechanism and clinical presentation. Therapeutic serum concentrations range from 0.1 to 0.4 µg/mL but vary from patient to patient and generally are not useful.[8] Cardiovascular side effects with oral verapamil include bradycardia, AV block, orthostatic hypotension, and worsening of CHF.[23] The myocardium of small infants handles calcium differently than does the more mature myocardium. Because of reports of asystolic cardiac arrest in young infants receiving the IV form of verapamil, this agent should not be given to infants less than 1 year of age.[68]

Patient and Family Considerations

Constipation is probably the most common noncardiac side effect of oral verapamil therapy. Other symptoms may include headaches, dizziness, flushing, rashes, hair loss, and pruritis.[69] In general, verapamil is well tolerated by most children.

Special Considerations

Children comprise a unique population with very special needs. Because most antiarrhythmic medications are developed with the adult arrhythmia patient in mind, oral formulations (i.e., tablet or capsule strength) are not conducive for pediatric administration in many cases. Although some pharmacies will compound a large tablet or capsule into a form suitable for small patients based on published stability studies,[69–73] which can be found in Table 3, many will not. It is necessary for cardiovascular clinicians to educate families and/or primary caregivers in how to formulate the medicine for these children (Table 2). This is usually done by a nurse specializing in pediatric cardiology in a quiet setting, generally before the child is discharged from the hospital. Both oral and written instructions should be given with a return demonstration to evaluate the teaching process.

Table 3
Pediatric Preparations* of Antiarrhythmic Drugs[70–74]

Drug	Compounded as	Stability	Comments
Procainamide	5, 50, or 100 mg/mL oral suspension	180 days refrigerated	Stability declines in room temperature and at 100 mg/mL concentration
Flecainide	5 or 10 mg/mL oral suspension	45 days at room temperature	Must shake vigorously prior to each use
Propranolol	1 mg/mL oral suspension	120 days at room temperature	Is commercially available in 4 mg/mL and 10 mg/mL solutions
Atenolol	2 mg/mL oral suspension	40 days at room temperature	
Sotalol	5mg/mL oral suspension	180 days at room temperature	Best absorbed when taken 1 hr before or 2 hr after meals
Amiodarone	5 mg/mL oral suspension Single-dose packets of crushed amiodarone	91 days refrigerated 56 days at room temperature	• Must shake vigorously prior to each use • Some pharmacists recommend dispensing new aliquots every 7 days • Can mix crushed drug with food (applesauce) • For nasogastric administration, use cool water to flush crushed tablets through the tube • If nausea occurs, give with food

*As compounded by most pharmacists (not commercially available). Oral suspensions are typically compounded using 1% methylcellulose and cherry syrup.

It is also beneficial to both families and prescribers for clinicians to contact the family's local pharmacy to ascertain drug availability prior to hospital discharge for certain medications. For example, although propranolol is a commonly used drug in adults and children, the pharmacy may not stock the liquid preparation and thus may need to order it from a supplier. If this is known in advance, plans can be made ahead of time to provide "take home" doses of the drug in a sufficient quantity to allow drug procurement by the pharmacy.

When providing patient and family education, it is important to stress the intended action of the specific agent as well as the potential adverse effects. Because everyone is human, it is important to determine ahead of time what should be done if a medication dose is inadvertently omitted. For example, if a dose of amiodarone is inadvertently omitted, it is probably okay to wait until the next dose since the half-life of amiodarone is so long. Conversely, if an oral dose of propranolol is omitted and it has been 1 hour or less from the scheduled dosage time, it is probably okay to go ahead and give it. If more than 1 hour passes, it would be better to wait until the next dose in order to avoid a cumulative effect of giving two doses so closely together. Some centers have specific educational guidelines approved by the prescribing cardiologist that can be given to families to take home, one of which can be found in Table 4. Also, parents like to know what to do if the child vomits the drug dose. In most cases, if it has been 10 minutes or less or if the administered dose is clearly visible in the emesis, the dose can be repeated.

It is also important that clinicians ensure that the prescriptions given to families for the antiarrhythmic medications are written properly. Many physicians prefer that the generic brand of certain antiarrhythmics *not* be used, due to inherent differences in bioavailability. This should be reflected on the prescription, especially in centers where there may be multiple providers writing the prescriptions. If the medication is a liquid formulation, the dosage should include both milligram and milliliter amounts. For example, a digoxin prescription for the elixir should read: Give 25 μg/0.5 mL by mouth twice daily. Some patients rely on mail order for their pharmacy needs, and prescriptions may need to be modified to accommodate these needs. In most cases, a 90-day supply is allowed, but two prescriptions are usually required, one for immediate use and one to mail in. It is very helpful for families if clinicians remain cognizant of these issues and assess the specific needs of the family prior to providing their prescriptions.

In summary, the role of antiarrhythmic medications in the pediatric population is changing as newer applications of radiofrequency ablation and device therapy are employed. While drug therapy may be chronically necessary in some patients, in others it will serve as a "bridge" to more definitive or curative treatment with radiofrequency ablation. Combination therapy, employing implantable devices in conjunction with antiarrhythmic agents, has proven to be useful for specific conditions, such as LQTS. Control of fetal tachyarrhythmias via maternally administered drugs will

Table 4
Sample Medication Information Sheet for
Patients and Parents—Atenolol

Name of Medication	Atenolol (Tenormin)
Your child's dose	_____
What it does	Tenormin helps to decrease or stop the episodes of fast or irregular heart rhythms that come from the upper or lower chambers of the heart.
What you need to know	Tenormin is taken once a day. It is best if it is taken at about the same time every day.
Things to watch for (side effects)	Bad headaches, depression, extreme tiredness, or decreased ability to concentrate in school are the most common side effects of this drug. Please call your heart doctor is your child experiences any of these side effects or if your child passes out.
What to do if you MISS a dose	If it has been more than 4 hours since the scheduled time, wait until the next dose. If it has been less than 4 hours, give the medicine.

*KEEP THIS AND ALL MEDICINES OUT OF THE REACH OF CHILDREN.
*CONSULT YOUR PHYSICIAN BEFORE BECOMING PREGNANT WHEN TAKING ANY MEDICINE.
*ASK FOR NEW PRESCRIPTIONS AT YOUR CLINIC VISITS.
*GET YOUR PRESCRIPTION FILLED SEVERAL DAYS BEFORE RUNNING ENTIRELY OUT OF THE MEDICINE.

If you have questions, please call:

Your Pediatric Cardiologist @ _____ or
Your Pediatric Cardiology Nurse @ _____.

likely be improved as we become more knowledgeable about treating this dyad. Finally, new antiarrhythmic agents are continually being developed; therefore, it is important for nurses and other clinicians to remain current in their knowledge of these medications in order to administer them to their pediatric patients safely and educate patients and their families appropriately.

References

1. Garson A Jr.: Dosing the newer antiarrhythmic drugs in children: Considerations in pediatric pharmacology. Am J Cardiol 1986; 57:1405–1407.

2. Case CL, Trippel DL, Gillette PC: New antiarrhythmic agents in pediatrics. Pediatr Clin North Am 1989; 36:1293–1320.
3. Maxwell GM: Principles of Pediatric Pharmacology. New York: Oxford University Press; 1984:55.
4. Roland M, Tozer TM: Clinical Pharmacokinetics: Concepts and Applications. Philadelphia: Lea & Febiger; 1980:218.
5. Vaughan Williams EM: Classification of antiarrhythmic drugs. In Sandoe E, Flensted-Jensen E, Olesen K (eds.): Cardiac Arrhythmias. Sweden: Astra, Sodertalje; 1981:449–472.
6. Vaughan Williams EM: A classification of antiarrhythmic actions reassessed after a decade of new drugs. J Clin Pharmacol 1984; 24:129–147.
7. Colucci RD, Somberg JC: Treatment of cardiac arrhythmias. In Chernow B (ed.): The Pharmacologic Approach to the Critically Ill Patient. 3rd ed. Baltimore: Williams & Wilkins; 1994:445–469.
8. Moak JP: Pharmacology and electrophysiology of antiarrhythmic drugs. In Gillette PC, Garson A Jr. (eds.): Pediatric Arrhythmias: Electrophysiology and Pacing. Philadelphia: WB Saunders Company; 1990:37–98.
9. Rosen MR, Camm AJ, Fozzard HA, et al: The Sicilian Gambit: A new approach to the classification of antiarrhythmic drugs based on their actions on arrhythmogenic mechanisms. Circulation 1991; 84:1831–1851.
10. Perry JC: Medical antiarrhythmic therapy. In Gillette PC, Garson A Jr. (eds.): Clinical Pediatric Arrhythmias. 2nd ed. Philadelphia: WB Saunders Company; 1999:231–248.
11. Shahar E, Barzilay Z, Shem-Tov AA, et al: Pre-excitation syndrome in infants and children. Effect of digoxin, verapamil, and amiodarone. Arch Dis Child 1983; 58:207–211.
12. Sellers TD Jr., Bashore TM, Gallagher JJ: Digitalis in the pre-excitation syndrome. Analysis during atrial fibrillation. Circulation 1977; 56:260–267.
13. Gillette PC, Garson A Jr., McNamara DG: Wolff-Parkinson-White syndrome in children: Natural history and clinical spectrum. Circulation 1980; 62(suppl III):271. Abstract.
14. Luedtke SA, Kuhn RJ, McCaffrey FM: Pharmacologic management of supraventricular tachycardias in children. Part 1: Wolff-Parkinson-White and atrioventricular nodal reentry. Ann Pharmacother 1997; 31:1227–1243.
15. Park MK: Use of digoxin in infants and children, with specific emphasis on dosage. J Pediatr 1986; 108:871–877.
16. Cree JE, Coltart DJ: Plasma digoxin concentration in children with heart failure. Br Med J 1973; 2:550.
17. Zalzstein E, Koren G, Levy M, et al: Once-daily versus twice-daily dosing of digoxin in the pediatric age group. J Pediatr 1990; 116:137–139.
18. Bakir M, Bilgic A: Single daily dose of digoxin for maintenance therapy of infants and children with cardiac disease: Is it reliable? Pediatr Cardiol 1994; 15:229–232.
19. Park MK: Pediatric Cardiology for Practitioners. 3rd ed. St. Louis: Mosby-Year Book, Inc.; 1996:405–409.
20. Phelps SJ, Kamper CA, Bottorff MB, et al: Effect of age and serum creatinine on endogenous digoxin-like substances in infants and children. J Pediatr 1987; 110:136–139.
21. Pudek MR, Seccombe DW, Whitfield MF, et al: Digoxin-like immunoreactivity in premature and full-term infants not receiving digoxin therapy. N Engl J Med 1983; 308:904–905.
22. Webb CL, Dick M II, Rocchini AP, et al: Quinidine syncope in children. J Am Coll Cardiol 1987; 9:1031–1037.
23. Perry JC: Pharmacologic therapy of arrhythmias. In Deal BJ, Wolff GS, Gelband H (eds.): Current Concepts in Diagnosis and Management of Arrhyth-

mias in Infants and Children. Armonk, NY: Futura Publishing Company, Inc.; 1998:267–308.

24. Artman M: Pharmacologic therapy. In Emmanouilides GC, Riemenschneider TA, Allen HD, Gutgesell HP (eds.): Moss and Adams Heart Disease in Infants, Children, and Adolescents. 5th ed. Baltimore: Williams & Wilkins; 1995: 375–398.

25. Roden DM: Antiarrhythmic drugs. In Hardman JG, Goodman-Gilman A, Limbird LE (eds.): Goodman & Gilman's The Pharmacological Basis of Therapeutics. 9th ed. New York: McGraw-Hill; 1996:839–874.

26. Kim SY, Benowitz NL: Poisoning due to class IA antiarrhythmic drugs. Quinidine, procainamide, and disopyramide. Drug Safety 1990; 5:393–420.

27. Hoffman BF, Rosen MR, Witt AL: Electrophysiology and pharmacology of cardiac arrhythmias: VII. Cardiac effect of quinidine and procaine amide. Am Heart J 1975; 90:117–122.

28. Witman JK, Furbee RB: Class IA antiarrhythmics: Quinidine, procainamide, and disopyramide. In Haddad LM, Shannon MW, Winchester JF (eds.): Clinical Management of Poisoning and Drug Overdose. 3rd ed. Philadelphia: WB Saunders Company; 1998:1055–1063.

29. Dumesic DA, Silverman NH, Tobias S, et al: Transplacental cardioversion of fetal supraventricular tachycardia with procainamide. N Engl J Med 1982; 307:1128–1131.

30. Moak JP, Smith RT, Garson A Jr.: Mexiletine: An effective antiarrhythmic drug for treatment of ventricular arrhythmias in congenital heart disease. J Am Coll Cardiol 1987; 10:824–829.

31. Strasburger JF: Antiarrhythmic drugs. In Garson AJ, Bricker JT, McNamara DG (eds.): The Science and Practice of Pediatric Cardiology. Philadelphia: Lea & Febiger; 1990:2126–2134.

32. Marcus FI, Opie LH: Antiarrhythmic agents. In Opie LH, Chatterjee K, Frishman W, et al. (eds.): Drugs for the Heart. 4th ed. Philadelphia: WB Saunders Company; 1995:207–246.

33. Garson A Jr., Kugler JD, Gillette PC, et al: Control of late postoperative ventricular arrhythmias with phenytoin in young patients. Am J Cardiol 1980; 46:290–294

34. Garson A Jr.: Ventricular arrhythmias. In Gillette PC, Garson A Jr. (eds.): Pediatric Arrhythmias: Electrophysiology and Pacing. Philadelphia: WB Saunders Company; 1990:427–500.

35. Morse TG, Zeigler V: Phenytoin: It's not just for seizures anymore. Mat Child Nurs 1994; 19:33–37.

36. Zeigler V, Gillette PC, Hammill B, et al: Flecainide for supraventricular tachycardia in children. Am J Cardiol 1988; 62:41D-43D.

37. Perry JC, Garson A Jr.: Flecainide acetate for treatment of tachyarrhythmias in children: Review of world literature on efficacy, safety, and dosing. Am Heart J 1992; 124:1614–1621.

38. van Engelen AD, Weijtens O, Brenner JI, et al: Management outcome and follow-up of fetal tachycardia. J Am Coll Cardiol 1994; 24:1371–1375.

39. Perry JC, Ayres NA, Carpenter RJ Jr.: Fetal supraventricular tachycardia treated with flecainide acetate. J Pediatr 1991; 118:303–305.

40. Wren C, Hunter S: Maternal administration of flecainide to terminate and suppress fetal tachycardia. Br Med J Clin Res Ed 1988; 296:249.

41. The Cardiac Arrhythmia Suppression Trial (CAST) Investigators: Preliminary report: Effect of encainide and flecainide on mortality in a randomized trial of arrhythmia suppression after myocardial infarction. N Engl J Med 1989; 321:406–412.

42. Fish FA, Gillette PC, Benson DW Jr.: Proarrhythmia, cardiac arrest and death in young patients receiving encainide and flecainide. J Am Coll Cardiol 1991; 18:356–365.

43. Perry JC, McQuinn RL, Smith RT, et al: Flecainide acetate for resistant arrhythmias in the young: Efficacy and pharmacokinetics. J Am Coll Cardiol 1989; 14:185–191.
44. Russell GAB, Martin RP: Flecainide toxicity. Arch Dis Child 1989; 64:860–862.
45. Zeigler VL, Peterson J: Flecainide toxicity in a neonate with supraventricular tachycardia. Heart Lung 1991; 20:689–691.
46. Janousek J, Paul T, Reimer A, et al: Usefulness of propafenone for supraventricular arrhythmias in infants and children. Am J Cardiol 1993; 72:294–300.
47. Paul T, Janousek J: New antiarrhythmic drugs in pediatric use: Propafenone. Pediatr Cardiol 1994; 15:190–197.
48. Musto B, D'Onofrio A, Cavallaro C, et al: Electrophysiological effects and clinical efficacy of propafenone in children with recurrent paroxysmal supraventricular tachycardia. Circulation 1988; 78:863–869.
49. Reimer A, Paul T, Kallfelz HC: Efficacy and safety of intravenous and oral propafenone in pediatric cardiac dysrhythmias. Am J Cardiol 1991; 68:741–744.
50. Guccione P, Drago F, Di Donato RM, et al: Oral propafenone therapy for children with arrhythmias: Efficacy and adverse effects in midterm follow-up. Am Heart J 1991; 122:1022–1027.
51. Janousek J, Paul T: Safety of oral propafenone in the treatment of arrhythmias in infants and children (European retrospective multicenter study). Am J Cardiol 1998; 81:1121–1124.
52. Trippel DL, Gillette PC: Atenolol in children with supraventricular tachycardia. Am J Cardiol 1989; 64:233–236.
53. Mehta AV, Subrahmanyam AB, Anand R: Long-term efficacy and safety of atenolol for supraventricular tachycardia in children. Pediatr Cardiol 1996; 17:231–236.
54. Trippel DL, Gillette PC: Atenolol in children with ventricular arrhythmias. Am Heart J 1990; 119:1312–1316.
55. Pfammatter JP, Paul T: New antiarrhythmic drug in pediatric use: Sotalol. Pediatr Cardiol 1997; 18:28–34.
56. Maragnes P, Tipple M, Fournier A: Effectiveness of oral sotalol for treatment of pediatric arrhythmias. Am J Cardiol 1992; 69:751–754.
57. Pfammatter JP, Paul T, Lehmann C, et al: Efficacy and proarrhythmia of oral sotalol in pediatric patients. J Am Coll Cardiol 1995; 26:1002–1007.
58. Tanel RE, Walsh EP, Lulu JA, et al: Sotalol for refractory arrhythmias in pediatric and young adult patients: Initial efficacy and long-term outcome. Am Heart J 1995; 130:791–797.
59. Beaufort-Krol GC, Bink-Boelkens MT: Effectiveness of sotalol for atrial flutter in children after surgery for congenital heart disease. Am J Cardiol 1997; 79:92–94.
60. Beaufort-Krol GC, Bink-Boelkens MT: Sotalol for atrial tachycardias after surgery for congenital heart disease. Pacing Clin Electrophysiol 1997; 20: 2125–2129.
61. Guccione P, Paul T, Garson A Jr.: Long-term follow-up of amiodarone therapy in the young: Continued efficacy, unimpaired growth, moderate side effects. J Am Coll Cardiol 1990; 15:1118–1124.
62. Garson A Jr., Gillette PC, McVey P, et al: Amiodarone treatment of critical arrhythmias in children and young adults. J Am Coll Cardiol 1984; 4:749–755.
63. Shuler CO, Case CL, Gillette PC: Efficacy and safety of amiodarone in infants. Am Heart J 1993; 125:1430–1432.
64. Jafari-Fesharaki M, Scheinman MM: Adverse effects of amiodarone. Pacing Clin Electrophysiol 1998; 21:108–120.
65. Bowers PN, Fields J, Schwartz D, et al: Amiodarone induced pulmonary fibrosis in infancy. Pacing Clin Electrophysiol 1998; 21:1665–1667.
66. Porter CJ, Garson A Jr., Gillette PC: Verapamil: An effective calcium blocking agent for pediatric patients. Pediatrics 1983; 71:748–755.

67. Ohe T, Shimomura K, Aihahra N, et al: Idiopathic sustained left ventricular tachycardia: Clinical and electrophysiologic characteristics. Circulation 1988; 77:560–568.
68. Epstein ML, Kiel EA, Victorica BE: Cardiovascular decompensation following verapamil therapy in infants with supraventricular tachycardia. Pediatrics 1985; 75:737–740.
69. Hesslein PS, Finlay CD, Garson A Jr., et al: Chronic oral verapamil: Pediatric experience. Circulation 1986; 74(suppl 2):176.
70. Garner SS, Wiest DB, Reynolds ER Jr.: Stability of atenolol in an extemporaneously compounded oral liquid. Am J Hosp Pharm 1994; 51:508–511.
71. Henry DW, Repta AJ, Smith FM, et al: Stability of propranolol hydrochloride suspension compounded from tablets. Am J Hosp Pharm 1986; 43:1492–1495.
72. Metras J, Swenson C, McDermott M: Stability of procainamide hydrochloride in an extemporaneously compounded oral liquid. Am J Hosp Pharm 1992; 49:1720–1724.
73. Nahata MC: Stability of amiodarone in an oral suspension stored under refrigeration and at room temperature. Ann Pharmacother 1997; 31:851–852.
74. Wiest DB, Garner SS, Pagacz LR, et al: Stability of flecainide acetate in an extemporaneously compounded oral suspension. Am J Hosp Pharm 1992; 49:1467–1470.

Appendix 5–1

Pharmacologic Agents Used for Long-Term Arrhythmia Management in Children

Drug	Uses	Route/Dose	Serum Concentrations	Adverse Effects/Comments	Drug Interactions
Class I: Sodium channel blockers					
Ia					
Quinidine, (Quinaglute, Quinidex)	SVT	PO: 30–60 mg/kg/day sulfate q 6 hr gluconate q 8–12 hr	2–6 µg/mL Peak: 1–2 hr (sulfate) Half-life: 6–8 hr (gluconate)	Hypotension, syncope, headache, tinnitus, nausea, vomiting, diarrhea, rash, thrombocytopenia	Digoxin, phenytoin, amiodarone, cimetidine, propranolol, coumadin, rifampin
Procainamide (Pronestyl. Procan SR)	AVRT, AVNRT, post-op AFL/ AF, ventricular ectopy	PO: 40–100 mg/kg/day q 6 hr SR q 8 hr	4–8 µg/mL (Procainamide) NAPA: 10–24 µg/mL Peak: 1–2 hr Half-life: 3–4 hr	Negative inotropy, nausea, vomiting, diarrhea, rash, Drug-induced SLE; Contraindicated in myasthenia gravis	Amiodarone, digoxin, propranolol, cimetidine
Ib					
Mexiletine (Mexitil)	Ventricular ectopy	PO: 6–15 mg/kg/day q 8 hr	0.8–2.0 µg/mL Peak: 1–4 hr Half-life: 6–12 hr	Nausea, vomiting, headache, tremors, dizziness, drowsiness, paresthesia, rash, hepatitus	Cimetidine, phenytoin, rifampin

Appendix 5-1
Pharmacologic Agents Used for Long-Term Arrhythmia Management in Children (*cont.*)

Drug	Uses	Route/Dose	Serum Concentrations	Adverse Effects/Comments	Drug Interactions
Phenytoin (Dilantin)	Digoxin-induced arrhythmias, Post-op PVCs, VT, prolonged QT	PO: Day 1, 15 mg/kg q 6 hr Day 2, 7.2 mg/kg q 6 hr Maint: 4–8 mg/kg/day q 8–12 hr	10–25 µg/mL Peak: 1.5–3 hr (Infatabs) Half-life: 7–40 hr (75 hr in preemies)	Gingival hyperplasia, ataxia, hypotension, drowsiness, nystagmus, drug-induced SLE; Teratogenic	Coumadin, verapamil, amiodarone, phenobarbital
Moricizine (Ethmozine)	AET, ventricular ectopy	PO: 5–15 mg/kg/day q 8 hr (200–600 mg/m²/day)	Levels not useful Peak: 1–2 hr Half-life: 2–5 hr	Headache, vertigo, tinnitus, nystagmus, paresthesia, rash	Cimetidine
Ic					
Flecainide (Tambocor)	Newborn SVT, AVRT, AVNRT, JET, PJRT, AET, CAT, VT	PO: 1–8 mg/kg/day q 8–12 hr (100–225 mg/m²/day)	200–1000 µg/mL Peak: 1.5–3 hr Half-life: 7–12 hr	Negative inotropy, worsens CHF, nausea, vomiting, headache, blurred vision, irritability, hyperactivity, dry mouth; proarrhythmia; Increases pacing thresholds	Digoxin, amiodarone, propranolol, verapamil, disopyramide
Propafenone (Rhythmol)	Newborn SVT, AVRT, AVNRT, JET, PJRT, AET, CAT	PO: 8–15 mg/kg/day q 6–8 hr (200–600 mg/m²/day)	Levels not useful Peak: 2–3 hr Half-life: 5–17 hr	Worsens CHF, hypotension, blurred vision, dizziness, fatigue, bitter taste, nausea, constipation, elevated	Digoxin, amiodarone

Class II: β-adrenergic blockers

Drug	Indications	Dose	Levels/Pharmacokinetics	Side effects	Drug interactions
Propranolol (Inderal)	Newborn SVT, AVNRT, JET, PJRT, AET, CAT, VT, prolonged QT	PO: 2–6 mg/kg/day q 6 hr; SR q 12 hr	25–150 ng/mL (150–1000 ng/mL for VT)	Hypotension, bradycardia, worsens CHF, fatigue, insomnia, depression, hypoglycemia, bronchospasm; Contraindicated in asthma; liver enzymes, drug-induced SLE; proarrhythmia; Side effects less common in children than in adults	Verapamil, furosemide, lidocaine, cimetidine, insulin, aminophylline
Metoprolol (Lopressor)	Prolonged QT, SVT	PO: 50 mg twice daily (Adult dose)	Not defined; Peak: 2–4 hr; Half-life: 3–4 hr	Hypotension, bradycardia, worsens CHF, dizziness, fatigue, insomnia, depression, headache, dry skin/mouth, bronchospasm; Contraindicated in asthma	Insulin, theophylline, indomethacin, prazosin, hydralazine
Atenolol (Tenormin)	AVRT, AVNRT, JET, PJRT, AET, CAT, VT, prolonged QT	PO: 1–2 mg/kg/day q 12–24 hr	Not useful; Peak: 2–3 hr; Half-life: 5–10 hr (16 hr in neonates)	Fewer than propranolol; Less bronchoconstriction; Bradycardia, hypotension, fatigue	Verapamil, diltiazem, insulin

Appendix 5–1

Pharmacologic Agents Used for Long-Term Arrhythmia Management in Children (cont.)

Drug	Uses	Route/Dose	Serum Concentrations	Adverse Effects/Comments	Drug Interactions
Nadolol (Corgard)	Prolonged QT, SVT	PO: 1–2 mg/kg/day q 24 hr	Not useful Peak: 3–4 hr Half-life: 12–24 hr	Bronchoconstriction in asthmatics, headache, sleep disturbances, abdominal pain	—
Class III: Agents that prolong cardiac refractoriness					
Sotalol (Betapace)	Newborn SVT, AVRT, AVNRT, PJRT, AET, CAT, post-op AFL/AF, post-op PVCs, VT	PO: 2–8 mg/kg/day q 12 hr (90–200 mg/m²/day)	Not defined Half-life: 7–12 hr	Bradycardia, hypotension, fatigue, headache, dizziness; Proarrhythmia	Verapamil and other antiarrhythmics
Amiodarone (Cordarone, Pacerone)	Newborn SVT, AVRT, JET, PJRT, AET, CAT, post-op AFL/AF, PVCs, VT	PO: Load: 10 mg/kg/day q 12 hr ×1–2 weeks (max. 1.2 g/day) Maint: 5–10 mg/kg/day q 24 hr	>1.0 µg/mL (Toxicity common at >2.5 µg/mL) Peak: 5–6 hr (PO) Half-life: 8–107 days (average 1 month)	Bradycardia, hypotension, corneal microdeposits, nausea, ataxia, rash, photosensitivity, skin discoloration, thyroid dysfunction, constipation, pulmonary fibrosis; Side effects less common in children than in adults	Digoxin, quinidine, procainamide, phenytoin, flecainide, coumadin, cyclosporine

Class IV: Calcium channel blockers

Drug	Indications	Dose	Level/Half-life	Side effects	Interactions
Verapamil (Calan, Verelan, Isoptin)	Newborn SVT, AVRT, AVNRT, LVOT/ fascicular tachycardias	PO: 4–17 mg/kg/day q 8 hr SR q 12–24 hr	0.1–0.4 µg/mL Half-life: 8–12 hr	*IV administration is not recommended in infants* Hypotension, bradycardia, atrioventricular block, asystole, CHF, flushing, constipation	β-blockers, digoxin, quinidine, disopyramide, coumadin

Other

Drug	Indications	Dose	Level/Half-life	Side effects	Interactions
Digoxin (Lanoxin)	Newborn SVT, AVRT, AVNRT, PJRT, AET, CAT	PO: TDD: Premature infant: 20 µg/kg Full-term newborn: 30 µg/kg Infant <2 years: 40–50 µg/kg Children >2 years: 30–40 µg/kg Maint: 25% of TDD daily divided q 12 hr	1–2 ng/mL, up to 3.5 ng/mL in infants Half-life: Preemie: 61 hr Newborn: 35 hr Infant: 18 hr Children: 37 hr	Digoxin toxicity: anorexia, nausea, vomiting, lethargy, visual changes, headache, seizures, gynecomastia, atrioventricular block, SVT, PVCs, VT, VF (treat digoxin-induced arrhythmias with Digibind or phenytoin)	Quinidine, amiodarone, verapamil, phenytoin, coumadin, erythromycin, spironolactone

AET = atrial ectopic tachycardia; AF = atrial fibrillation; AFL = atrial flutter; AVNRT = atrioventricular nodal reentry tachycardia; AVRT = atrioventricular reentry tachycardia; CAT = chaotic atrial tachycardia; CHF = congestive heart failure; JET = junctional ectopic tachycardia; Load = loading dose; LVOT = left ventricular outflow tract; Maint. = maintenance dose; PJRT = permanent junctional reciprocating tachycardia; PO = by mouth; PVC = premature ventricular contraction; SLE = systemic lupus erythematosus; SR = sustained release; SVT = supraventricular tachycardia; VF = ventricular fibrillation; VT = ventricular tachycardia.

TDD = total digitalizing dose: initially give half of TDD, then in 8 hours, give one quarter of TDD; 8 hours later, give last one quarter of TDD.

Chapter 6

Radiofrequency Catheter Ablation

Dianne Marlow, RN, BSN, CLNC and
Paul C. Gillette, MD

The advent of radiofrequency current for catheter ablation has dramatically changed the practice of pediatric electrophysiology. Rather than providing only detailed analysis of a child's arrhythmia for medical or surgical management, combining the intracardiac electrophysiology study with radiofrequency catheter ablation (RFCA) permits the electrophysiologist to offer a cure with a cardiac catheterization procedure. This has transformed the focus of the invasive electrophysiology study from diagnostic to therapeutic.

There are many variables to consider when offering RFCA to children. One must understand the natural history of arrhythmias and congenital anomalies and be able to provide child- and family-centered nursing care and support services, such as pediatric cardiac surgeons and pediatric anesthesiologists. The electrophysiologist must possess a high level of catheter manipulation skill for movement in smaller and more challenging chamber dimensions. This chapter presents a brief historical perspective of ablation in children, the use of radiofrequency current for lesion generation, the indications for RFCA in children, sedation/analgesia considerations for children undergoing RFCA, mapping and ablation of specific arrhythmogenic substrates, potential complications of RFCA, implications for clinicians, patient and family considerations, and, finally, future issues in pediatric catheter ablation.

From Zeigler VL, Gillette PC: *Practical Management of Pediatric Cardiac Arrhythmias.* Armonk, NY: Futura Publishing Co., Inc.; ©2001.

Historical Perspective

Before the development of RFCA, an intracardiac electrophysiology study was a diagnostic test performed to obtain information about a patient's conduction system as well as characteristics of the specific arrhythmia mechanism. The degree of risk for an adverse event (i.e., syncope or sudden death) revealed by the electrophysiology study was of interest when considering medical therapy versus surgical ablation as well as activity restrictions for the child. If the risk of injury was significant, the surgical approach was undertaken,[1] and in this situation, the location of the abnormality documented by electrophysiology study became a useful piece of preoperative data. Many arrhythmias examined by electrophysiology study were not deemed to be dangerous, and parents found it difficult to send their children for an open heart procedure to cure a "bothersome" rhythm disturbance.

An early attempt at curing cardiac rhythm disturbances with catheter ablation used direct current as an energy source. At many centers, this therapy was used primarily to treat life-threatening arrhythmias in patients who were not good surgical candidates or for those in whom previous surgical ablation had failed. An electrode catheter was placed in the desired location in the heart and connected to a standard defibrillator. The defibrillator was discharged, and the resulting explosion destroyed tissue in the vicinity of the catheter tip. Direct current ablation carried somewhat of a high risk, including cardiac perforation and ventricular fibrillation (VF) as well as the potential for late development of ventricular arrhythmias and sudden death.[2] Needless to say, direct current ablation did not achieve widespread use by pediatric electrophysiologists.

Radiofrequency current received global attention in 1987, when Huang and colleagues[3] described this method for ablation of the atrioventricular (AV) junction. Pediatric electrophysiologists began using RFCA in 1990, and clinical experience reported since that time has shown it to be safe and effective.[4-7] Much of the data published regarding pediatric ablation procedures has been collected by means of the Pediatric Radiofrequency Ablation Registry,[4,6,8,9] which was founded in 1990 by members of the Pediatric Electrophysiology Society.

Use of Radiofrequency Current for Lesion Generation

Radiofrequency current has been used in various types of surgical procedures for many decades. Bovie developed the most recognized use in 1928 in the form of an electrocautery unit for surgery.[10] Current models of radiofrequency generators allow the operator to control the amount of energy used or the catheter tip temperature and the impedance of the system. These factors are extremely important for ensuring the success and safety of every ablation procedure.

Radiofrequency current generated for ablation procedures is a continuous, unmodulated sinusoidal waveform in the 100- to 750-kHz range.[11] The generator is connected to an active electrode (the tip of the ablation catheter) and a ground electrode (the grounding pad placed on the back or thigh of the patient). When radiofrequency current sent through the catheter flows into the tissue, local ions are accelerated and heating of the tissue occurs. This increase in temperature at the site drives water from the cells, causing desiccation and necrosis, thus making the tissue unable to conduct electrical current. Because power density decreases the further it moves from the tissue contact site, surrounding areas of tissue are not destroyed. The result is a well-demarcated, circular or oval shaped lesion. Chronic lesions appear as localized whitish, thickened scars.[12]

While the mechanics appear relatively safe and simple, there are aspects to lesion generation that one must bear in mind. Destruction of tissue results at approximately 45°C to 50°C,[13] and lower temperatures may only temporarily damage the tissue and allow for conduction properties to return early on (i.e., during postprocedure electrophysiology testing) or at a later time (i.e., days or weeks) following the ablation procedure. For successful lesion generation, there must be stable catheter-tissue contact in order to provide an adequate temperature to destroy the targeted area. This can be somewhat of a challenge in many areas of the pediatric heart, because of differences in size and angle of structures. Setting the maximum power output does not guarantee that the target tissue will receive that amount of energy. The catheter tip must be in firm contact with the heart tissue in order to generate the degree of temperature necessary for tissue destruction. Ideally, firm catheter contact will enable the system to heat to the desired temperature with lower output settings. For example, a catheter position with only the right side of the electrode touching tissue may use the maximum 50 W of output and only achieve a temperature of 40°C, while moving the catheter to a more stable position might use 15 W, generating a temperature of 60°C, which would be more likely to secure a permanent lesion. If temperatures are being monitored during lesion placement, one can see fluctuations that signal unstable contact and the need to reposition the catheter. Other methods for improvement in catheter-tissue contact include the use of a catheter with a different size or shape of its distal curve or the use of a long sheath over the catheter for stability.[14]

Another important variable to monitor during lesion placement is the impedance of the system. If the catheter tip temperature exceeds 100°C, blood and tissue may desiccate and coat the tip of the catheter.[15] This coagulum must be removed immediately to prevent thrombus formation. The impedance will sharply rise during coagulum formation, which is the indication to turn off the power output if the generator model in use does not have an automatic safety shut-off and remove the catheter for cleaning. This is an important consideration in any case, whether the patient is an adult or a child.

Indications

A common saying in pediatric practice is "children aren't just little adults." True to fashion, the indications for ablation in children are relatively different than those for adults. Even when considering ablation for a relatively "benign" arrhythmia such as concealed AV reentry tachycardia (AVRT), also known as a concealed accessory pathway, the natural history of the mechanism must be considered, as should the risk-benefit ratio for ablation in a patient with a small heart.

For the adult population, Wolff-Parkinson-White (WPW) and/or AVRT (also known as supraventricular tachycardia or SVT) are indications to perform RFCA at any age. However, infants born with WPW syndrome and SVT may have spontaneous resolution of their tachycardia,[16] with a chance of recurrence at, on average, 8 years of age.[17] With this in mind, WPW or AVRT in an infant would be more likely to be managed medically for the first year. The incidence of spontaneous resolution is lower if the WPW is associated with significant congenital heart disease (CHD).[18] Since sustained tachycardia is not well tolerated in this particular population, because of their potentially compromised ventricular function, RFCA would be indicated for elimination of the arrhythmogenic substrate before the child undergoes surgery for the congenital heart defect.

WPW syndrome can be a life-threatening situation if the accessory pathway is capable of conducting rapidly, especially in the instance of atrial fibrillation, which could easily degenerate into VF. The development of atrial fibrillation in children is considered to be less frequent than in the adult population, but one study of patients with WPW[19] found a 2.3% incidence of sudden death in children, which is similar to that seen in the adult literature. The family of a child with a "slick" accessory pathway should be counseled that their child is in a higher risk category and deserves consideration for ablation as a first-line treatment versus medical management.

Another situation that requires serious consideration for ablation as opposed to medical management is the presence of tachycardia-induced cardiomyopathy. Depressed cardiac function may develop from incessant rapid ventricular rates, such as those found with atrial ectopic tachycardia (AET), the permanent form of junctional reciprocating tachycardia (PJRT), and junctional ectopic tachycardia (JET). In addition, these arrhythmias tend to be difficult, if not impossible, to control medically. Elimination of the mechanism of tachycardia has been shown to permit the ventricular function to return to normal.[20]

The presence of an arrhythmia substrate amenable to catheter ablation can serve as an indication for RFCA in the young child and adolescent. With current records for safety and efficacy of ablation in a variety of tachyarrhythmias, both with and without concomitant CHD, many children prefer a trip to the electrophysiology laboratory rather than life-long medications and the obligatory visit to the cardiologist and/or emergency department. A recent study[21] demonstrated that catheter ablation generates a lower cost and less mortality and morbidity than either medical management or surgery; thus, the authors recommend RFCA as the treatment of choice for children 5 years or older with WPW and SVT.

There are lifestyle considerations that must be taken into account when dealing with the pediatric population, especially adolescents. Many teenagers are adamant that they will not take medication and may be noncompliant with the treatment regimen. Some wish to compete in sports programs in which coaches may have little understanding of how their "heart condition" may limit them—that is if the side effects of their medications do not limit their endurance first. Even a simple sleepover at a friend's house can seem overwhelming to both sets of parents when plans have to be made for the possibility of a tachycardia episode. Health insurance can be difficult to find and often costly for a child with a cardiac diagnosis. Many families simply prefer a cure for their child rather than using medications to prevent tachycardia episodes. It is interesting to observe the changes over time of the indications for ablation of paroxysmal SVT from the Pediatric Radiofrequency Ablation Registry. In the first year of data collection, "medically refractory tachycardia" was the primary indication for 44% of the cases and "patient choice" for 33%. The 1995 to 1996 data listed 58% of the cases as patient choice and 29% were performed for refractory tachycardia.[6]

Sedation/Anesthesia Considerations

One of the questions most frequently heard from children before a procedure is "Will I be asleep?" Those who care for pediatric patients must remember that it is nearly impossible for a child of any age to remain still and cooperative for what he or she perceives to be a frightening, uncomfortable, and often lengthy procedure. Common choices for sedation have included diazepam, midazolam, or meperidine with promethazine given in doses measured for body weight. Over the past several years, intravenous propofol appears to have increased in popularity because it can be dosed for deep sedation or anesthesia and it is associated with a quick recovery with fewer side effects such as nausea and vomiting.[22] Pediatric Radiofrequency Ablation Registry data published in 1994 indicated that deep sedation was used for 68% of the procedures and general anesthesia for 36% (some received sedation initially and progressed to general anesthesia).[4] Whether deep sedation administered by the nursing staff or anesthesia administered by an anesthesiologist is used, care must be taken that the agents given do not alter cardiac conduction properties or suppress the target tachyarrhythmia, especially when dealing with an ectopic focus that must occur spontaneously and cannot be induced. Nurses with pediatric experience are valuable for providing emotional support and comfort, which may lead to less sedative use and possibly less chance for sedative overdose.[23]

Mapping and Ablation of Specific Arrhythmogenic Substrates

The mapping and ablation of specific arrhythmogenic substrates requires specific knowledge of basic electrophysiologic principles. In many instances, electrophysiologists no longer perform complete electrophysiology studies in patients undergoing radiofrequency ablation. For this reason, the basics of electrophysiology testing are discussed in chapter 1 of this text. Some of the protocols discussed in chapter 1 are performed during RFCA procedures and may be required for arrhythmia induction and/or for postablation assessment of the procedure's success. The following discussion focuses on the mapping and subsequent ablation of specific arrhythmogenic substrates responsible for tachyarrhythmias in pediatric patients. These substrates include AVRT, AV nodal reentry tachycardia (AVNRT), intraatrial reentry tachycardia (IART) in patients with CHD, ventricular tachycardia (VT), and other substrates such as PJRT, Mahaim fibers, JET, and deliberate ablation of the AV node or bundle of His.

Atrioventricular Reentry Tachycardia

AVRT is an arrhythmia that has been known by a variety of names. Paroxysmal atrial tachycardia and SVT were used as broad, former terms for AVRT, but they did not address the nature of the mechanism other than the involvement of the atrium. The new title, "atrioventricular" indicates that the ventricles are also involved in the tachycardia circuit and "reentrant" specifies the mechanism for the tachycardia. Although current literature is moving toward using the term "AVRT," one can still find SVT used synonymously.

As previously delineated in chapter 2, AVRT involves an accessory pathway, which is a muscle fiber that traverses the fibrous annulus of the mitral or the tricuspid valve allowing electrical conduction between the atrium and the ventricle in a retrograde and/or antegrade fashion. Knowing this information, one can anticipate that the mapping procedure will involve pinpointing the location of the accessory pathway on the annulus of one of these valves and that this involves observation of ventriculoatrial (VA) conduction intervals and possibly mapping using the delta wave (if present). There are mapping challenges inherent in each of these areas.

The tricuspid valve on the right side of the heart usually presents the greater challenge. There is a larger circumference to map on the tricuspid annulus (12 cm as opposed to 5 to 6 cm of mitral annulus), and approximately 10% of patients with a right-sided accessory pathway may have multiple accessory pathways. An association between some congenital anomalies and WPW has been well documented for years.[24] Ebstein's anomaly of the tricuspid valve can make mapping difficult, due to the displaced annulus and abnormal intracardiac electrograms.[25] For this reason, all patients with WPW should have a preablation echocardiogram. The acute angle and height of attachment of the tricuspid valve alone make it difficult to get sufficient catheter-tissue contact for an adequate radiofrequency lesion. This is especially difficult in the smaller heart, when achieving a tight curve to the ablation catheter is necessary and seemingly impossible at times. One of the most delicate areas for lesion placement lies in the right septal region. Accessory pathways in this location may lie close to the AV node or His bundle, and carry a higher risk for AV block, especially in the smaller heart. Accessory pathways found in the posteroseptal region can be mapped to the right side, but in some cases successful ablation may require lesion placement on the left side of the septum. These are but a few of the formidable obstacles to mapping and ablation on the right side of the heart.

As previously stated, the mitral annulus has less circumference to map. Because no muscular tissue exists from the left midseptal to the left anterior area, there is no substrate for an accessory pathway. The coronary sinus (CS), accessed from the right side of the heart and passing posterior along the AV groove to the left side, provides a source for electrode catheter placement and recording of atrial and ventricular electrograms from the left side of the heart. The challenge of ablation on the left side is the need to advance the ablation catheter to the mitral annulus. This can be achieved using a transseptal puncture in the absence of a patent foramen ovale or by a retrograde arterial approach. The transseptal approach has not been shown to increase the risk of valve damage[26] and has long been used by pediatric cardiologists in patients with CHD. The retrograde approach has been found to be associated with a greater risk of complications, including coronary artery perforation and mitral valve injury.[27,28] Regardless of the specific approach used, there is a theoretical risk of thrombus and embolic complications with lesion placement in the left heart. For this reason, heparin is administered with serial activated clotting times drawn periodically during the case, followed by oral aspirin therapy for several days to weeks following the ablation. The activated clotting time is maintained at greater than 300 seconds throughout the case when heparin is administered.

Special consideration should be given to the patient with an accessory pathway and CHD. If at all possible, RFCA should be performed before repair of the congenital anomaly. Tachycardia can be difficult for these patients to tolerate in the postoperative period, and access to the necessary chamber for ablation may be obstructed by the surgical procedure.[29]

A simple technique for differentiating a right-sided accessory pathway from a left-sided accessory pathway during the electrophysiology study involves pacing the ventricle or inducing AVRT and observing the retrograde activation sequence on the CS catheter. The distal electrodes (usually starting with CS1 and CS2) record electrograms from the left heart and the proximal electrodes (the larger numbers on the CS catheter) closest to the mouth of the CS record those from the right heart. The electrodes near the accessory pathway will have the shortest VA times (Figs. 1 and 2). If during ventricular pacing, accessory pathway conduction fuses

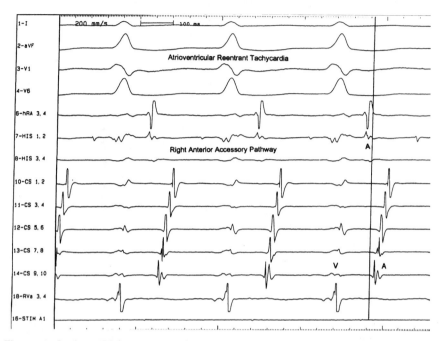

Figure 1. Surface ECG leads I, aVF, V_1, and V_6 with the following intracardiac electrograms: high right atrium (HRA) ×1 His bundle (HIS) ×2, coronary sinus (CS) ×5, and right ventricular apex (RVa) ×1. During an episode of atrioventricular reentry tachycardia, the atrial electrogram on the HIS catheter (electrodes 1 and 2) is earlier than the atrial electrogram on the proximal CS catheter (electrodes 9 and 10) indicating a right anterior accessory pathway.

with retrograde AV nodal conduction, it may be somewhat confusing; therefore, evaluation of retrograde accessory pathway conduction is best assessed during AVRT.

Mapping the precise location of an accessory pathway by retrograde conduction is accomplished by positioning the ablation catheter on the annulus in the region of the shortest VA time during tachycardia or ventricular pacing. The catheter is moved in small increments until the earliest retrograde atrial electrogram is found locally at the distal electrode of the ablation catheter (Fig. 3). The atrial insertion site of an accessory pathway can be identified by a local VA time of 40 ms or the surface QRS to local atrial electrogram of 80 ms during tachycardia.[30] Once the accessory pathway's insertion site has been identified, radiofrequency energy may be applied. Placement of a successful lesion will result in VA dissociation, also known as retrograde block (Fig. 4). It is permissible to ablate during tachycardia, but the possibility exists that when the tachycardia breaks due to accessory pathway destruction, the dramatic change in

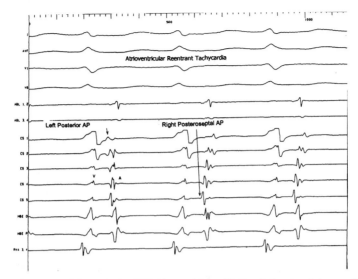

Figure 2. Surface ECG leads I, aVF, V_1, and V_6 with the following intracardiac electrograms: ablation (ABL) x2, coronary sinus (CS) ×5, His bundle electrogram (HBE) ×2, and right ventricular apex (RVA) ×1. The two distinct pathways are delineated by a comparison of the retrograde activation sequences: the earliest ventriculoatrial (VA) time for the left-sided accessory pathway (AP) can be seen on distal CS electrodes 1 and 2, whereas the earliest VA time for the second complex is more proximal (CS5) delineating an AP location in the right posteroseptal region.

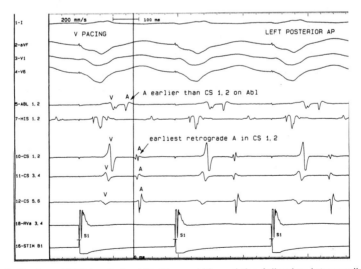

Figure 3. Surface ECG leads I, aVF, V_1, and V_6 and the following intracardiac electrograms: ablation (ABL) x1, His bundle (HIS) ×1, coronary sinus (CS) ×3, right ventricular apex (RVa) ×1, and stimulation catheter (STIM) x1. Retrograde mapping using ventricular pacing illustrates that the atrial electrogram on the ablation catheter (ABL 1 and 2) is earlier than the retrograde atrial electrogram on CS 1 and 2, indicating that the ablation catheter is close to the accessory pathway.

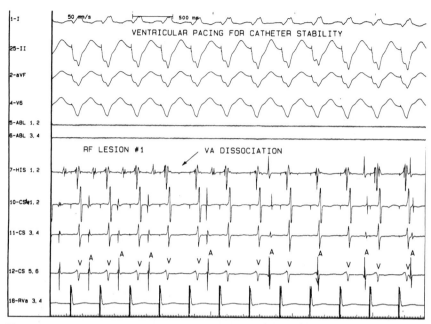

Figure 4. Surface ECG leads I, II, aVF, and V$_6$ with the following intracardiac electrograms: ablation (ABL) ×2, His bundle (HIS) ×1, coronary sinus (CS) ×3, and right ventricular apex (RVa) ×1. A successful radiofrequency lesion is placed during retrograde mapping using ventricular pacing for catheter stability. The labeling of the atrial and ventricular electrograms on CS 5 and 6 is used to delineate ventriculoatrial (VA) dissociation which occurs with the fourth V which is not followed by a retrograde A. The VA dissociation indicates that the accessory pathway can no longer conduct in a retrograde fashion.

rhythm may cause the catheter to lose firm contact with the tissue and fail to provide an adequate lesion. Occasionally, a patient will lose rhythm may cause the catheter to lose firm contact with the tissue and fail to provide an adequate lesion. Occasionally, a patient will lose retrograde conduction through the accessory pathway but will continue to demonstrate VA conduction up the AV node. The VA time will prolong but not dissociate, and it is possible to document the retrograde decremental conduction of the AV node. Loss of accessory pathway conduction less than 2.3 seconds after the beginning of radiofrequency application has been shown to be predictive of the permanence of a successful radiofrequency application and may be an indicator of anatomic proximity of the catheter tip to the accessory pathway.[31] If no effect is noted in 15 seconds, it is unlikely that a permanent effect will occur with prolonged application of radiofrequency energy.[32]

Delta wave mapping is a technique in which antegrade conduction of the accessory pathway can be mapped. Because the accessory pathway preexcites a specific site in the ventricle, mapping efforts will be aimed at finding the earliest local ventricular activation, usually 20 to 40 ms in advance of the earliest surface delta wave (Fig. 5). Ablation may be per-

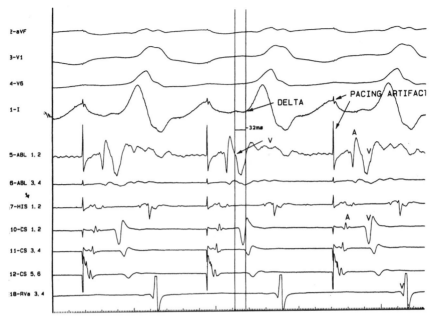

Figure 5. Surface ECG leads aVF, V_1, V_6, and I with the following intracardiac electrograms: ablation (ABL) $\times 2$, His bundle (HIS) $\times 1$, coronary sinus (CS) $\times 3$, and right ventricular apex (RVa) x1. The mapping for this accessory pathway (AP) is being performed with atrial pacing to enhance the delta wave in a patient with manifest Wolff-Parkinson-White syndrome. Electrodes 1 and 2 on the ablation catheter reveal a ventricular electrogram that occurs 32 ms before the surface delta indicating proximity to the AP.

formed in sinus rhythm or with atrial pacing. Atrial pacing may be accomplished using the CS catheter while using the ablation catheter for radiofrequency energy delivery. It is important to pace faster than any anticipated junctional ectopy in order to confirm continued AV node function during radiofrequency application, especially when ablating an accessory pathway in close proximity to the AV node. A successful radiofrequency lesion will result in a narrowing of the QRS due to the loss of preexcitation by the accessory pathway indicating the inability of the accessory pathway to conduct in an antegrade fashion (Fig. 6).

Occasionally, an accessory pathway is encountered that resists destruction. It is important that a variety of methods are attempted, including remapping to a different location for lesion placement or exchange of the ablation catheter to one with a different length or type of curve. For example, if a lesion on the atrial side does not produce results, it may be necessary to place a lesion on the ventricular side of the annulus. Posteroseptal accessory pathways can be ablated from the right side, but sometime require an approach from the left side. A recent case study[33] reported successful ablation of a posteroseptal accessory pathway via the middle cardiac vein in a 6-year-old child. It is important to remember that persistence and ingenuity can produce results.

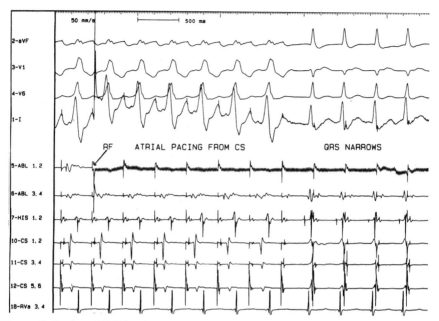

Figure 6. Surface ECG leads aVF, V₁, V₆, and I with the following intracardiac electrograms: ablation (ABL) ×2, His bundle (HIS) ×1, coronary sinus (CS) ×3, and right ventricular apex (RVa) ×1 in a patient with manifest Wolff-Parkinson-White syndrome. Atrial pacing is being performed via the coronary sinus as evidenced by the atrial pacing artifact noted on many of the electrograms. Radiofrequency energy is delivered through electrodes 1 and 2 on the ablation catheter with subsequent narrowing of the QRS complex delineating successful ablation of the pathway.

Endpoints for successful accessory pathway ablation are absence of antegrade and retrograde conduction of the accessory pathway, as well as the inability to induce AVRT. Many electrophysiologists place consolidation or "insurance" lesions at the site of successful lesion placement to further ensure permanent destruction of the accessory pathway. It is common to wait 20 to 30 minutes or longer after successful lesion placement and then test for return of accessory pathway conduction. Selected parts of the electrophysiology study can be repeated during this time to document postablation function and test for a second accessory pathway. A single atrial extrastimulus protocol may be performed to reveal the presence of dual AV nodal physiology. Ventricular pacing will demonstrate VA dissociation. Administration of adenosine will block the AV node and show the lack of antegrade conduction (Fig. 7). Success rates of accessory pathway ablation from the Pediatric Radiofrequency Ablation Registry data are 95% success for the left free wall, 86% for the right free wall, and 87% for septal accessory pathways.[6]

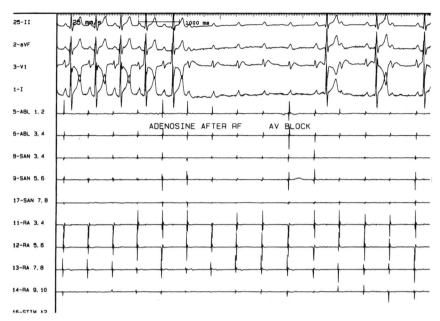

Figure 7. Surface ECG leads II, aVF, V$_1$, and I with the following intracardiac electrograms: ablation (ABL) ×2, sinoatrial node (SAN) ×3, and right atrium (RA) ×4. Adenosine was administered after successful ablation of an accessory pathway (AP) to demonstrate the absence of antegrade AP conduction. The adenosine results in temporary atrioventricular block.

Atrioventricular Nodal Reentry Tachycardia

Although AVNRT is more prevalent in adults, ablation in children has been shown to be both safe and effective.[7] As discussed in chapter 2, AVNRT often occurs in the presence of dual AV nodal physiology. This can be documented during the electrophysiology study using the single atrial extrastimulus protocol by measuring the atrial electrogram to His electrogram on the His catheter for each extrastimulus. Dual AV nodal physiology becomes evident when there is an "AH jump," or a 50-ms increase in the A$_2$-H$_2$ interval with a 10-ms decrease in atrial extrastimulus cycle length (Fig. 8). Induction of AVNRT usually occurs during atrial extrastimulus protocols but occasionally requires the administration of isoproterenol.

The mapping procedure for AVNRT involves identification of known anatomic landmarks as well as optimal electrogram appearance on the ablation catheter. The fast pathway lies anterior on the septum, close to where the His potential is recorded. The slow pathway lies more posterior near the mouth of the CS. There tends to be a higher incidence of AV node damage with fast pathway ablation, prompting most centers to attempt slow pathway ablation. Data from the Pediatric Radiofrequency Ablation

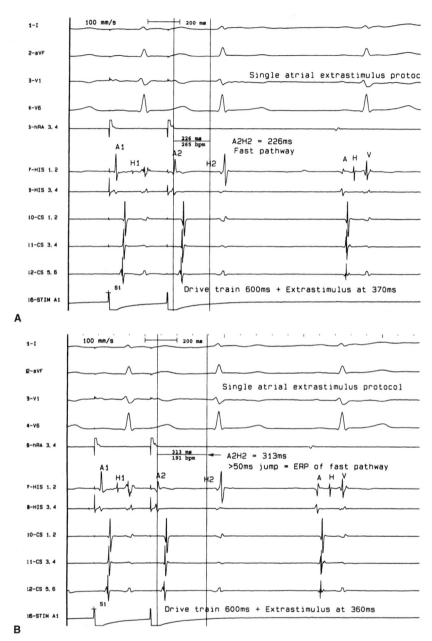

Figure 8. A. Surface ECG leads I, aVF, V_1, and V_6 with the following intracardiac electrograms: high right atrium (hRA) ×1, His bundle (HIS) ×2, coronary sinus (CS) ×3, stimulation catheter (STIM) ×1. A single atrial extrastimulus is delivered at 370 ms into a paced atrial rhythm (drive train) at 600 ms. The A-H interval of 226 ms indicates lack of conduction through the fast atrioventricular (AV) nodal pathway, thus indicating its refractoriness. **B.** ECG recording from the same patient in **A**. A single atrial stimulus is now delivered 10 ms earlier at 360 ms and the A-H interval increases to 313 ms, which is a greater than 50 ms "jump" indicating dual AV nodal pathways.

Registry regarding 920 AVNRT ablations revealed that the slow pathway was the target of choice in 889 cases.[6] The appearance of an electrogram on the distal ablation catheter with an atrial-to-ventricular ratio of approximately 0.45 and an M-shaped pattern to the atrial electrogram have been considered important for successful lesion placement.[34]

The aim of AVNRT ablation is to destroy an AV nodal pathway that allows perpetuation of a reentrant atrial tachycardia. Some electrophysiologists accomplish this by dragging the catheter to form a linear lesion, and some choose a "spot welding" approach by placing several lesions in a row. It is wise to perform either type of ablation during atrial pacing from the CS catheter to document continuing AV nodal function. Junctional ectopy can be anticipated during radiofrequency application, and has been linked with successful slow pathway ablation as well as impending AV block during fast pathway ablation[35] (Fig. 9).

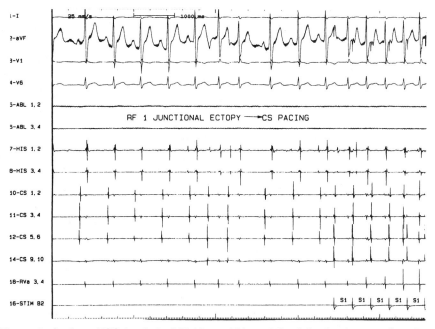

Figure 9. Surface ECG leads I, aVF, V_1, and V_6 and the following intracardiac electrograms: ablation (ABL) ×2, His bundle (HIS) ×2, coronary sinus (CS) ×4, right ventricular apex (RVa) ×1, and stimulation catheter (STIM) ×1. Ablation of the slow atrioventricular (AV) nodal pathway is being performed during normal sinus rhythm. Junctional ectopy can be seen on the sixth and seventh complex followed by atrial pacing in the coronary sinus (S1 on STIM) confirming intact AV nodal conduction of the fast pathway.

There are two endpoints for a successful AVNRT ablation procedure. The primary endpoint is the inability to induce tachycardia both with and without isoproterenol. A second possible endpoint is the lack of an AH jump with an atrial extrastimulus protocol. It is common to place a radiofrequency lesion and then perform a quick atrial extrastimulus protocol to check for inducibility or the presence of dual AV nodal physiology. If it remains present, additional lesions may be placed. It is not necessary to continue ablating if the patient has residual single echo beats. The Pediatric Radiofrequency Ablation Registry data indicate a 96% success rate for slow pathway ablation.[6]

Atrial Ectopic Tachycardia

AET can prove difficult for primary care practitioners to diagnose because it is often incessant at a rate faster than sinus rates and slower than reentrant tachycardias. Twenty-four-hour ambulatory monitoring may show little heart rate variability. Drug therapy is often unsuccessful in controlling AET,[34] and the incessant nature can lead to a tachycardia-induced cardiomyopathy. RFCA has been shown to be safe and effective in the treatment of drug-resistant AET and may be considered first-line therapy for those with depressed ventricular function.[36] There is usually one focus for the AET, but it is possible to have multiple foci.

In the setting of AET, since the mechanism is automatic in nature and the ventricle does not play a part in sustaining the tachycardia, placement of a ventricular electrode catheter is not required for mapping. Because AET is caused by an ectopic focus, it cannot be induced with pacing protocols and must occur spontaneously. Unfortunately, this type of tachycardia is subject to suppression with sedation and anesthetic agents, so patients must often remain conscious during the procedure. Isoproterenol may be infused to sustain tachycardia for ease of mapping and to document successful radiofrequency ablation during lesion placement.

Mapping of AET is similar to mapping of AVRT in that the target must be found using incremental catheter movements. The atrial electrogram on the ablation catheter is measured against the surface P wave, which is a stable marker for comparative analysis. A desirable location for ablation will have the atrial electrogram before the surface P wave by 30 ms or more[37] (Fig. 10). Care must be taken when moving the catheter, as mechanical trauma to the focus may cause resolution of tachycardia that may last for hours, thus preventing further mapping and destruction by radiofrequency ablation at that time.

Successful ablation of the ectopic focus will result in a change in the activation sequence to that of an atrial electrogram from the sinus node region (Fig. 11). Acceleration of the AET focus within 5 seconds of radiofrequency application and lasting 2 to 4 seconds has been shown to be a predictor for successful lesion placement.[38] The endpoint for a successful AET ablation procedure is the lack of spontaneous ectopic tachycardia both with and without isoproterenol infusion. One report of pediatric ablation experience with AET related a 100% success rate in simple cases (a single automatic focus with frequent sustained tachycardia), but cases involving multiple foci or AET "not reliably present during the procedure"

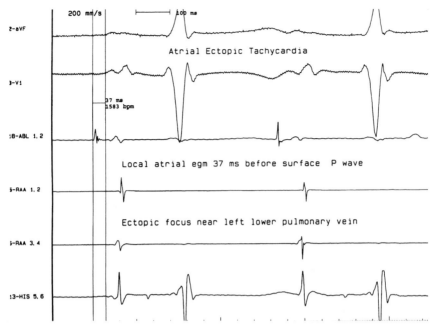

Figure 10. Surface ECG leads aVF, V$_1$, and the following intracardiac electrograms: ablation (ABL) ×1, right atrial appendage (RAA) ×2, and His bundle (HIS) ×1 at 200 mm/s paper speed. A measurement is made from the beginning of the surface P wave to the beginning of the atrial electrogram on the ablation catheter. The local atrial electrogram on the ablation catheter is 37 ms earlier than the surface P wave indicating a left atrial ectopic focus that was found to be near the left lower pulmonary vein.

resulted in success in only 1 out of 7 cases.[5] Of note, 55% of patients in this study with AET had ventricular dysfunction before the procedure, and all who had successful ablation of the ectopic focus eventually exhibited normal ventricular function.[5]

Intraatrial Reentry Tachycardia in Patients with Congenital Heart Disease

IART (also known as atrial flutter) is noted to be a common problem after repair of many forms of CHD and may be the single largest cause of late morbidity and mortality after surgery.[39–42] IART is uncommon in children as a primary arrhythmia, but is usually associated with congenital disease repairs such as the Mustard or Senning operation for transposition of the great arteries and the Fontan procedure for single ventricle.[43] Studies show a 50% prevalence of IART at 12 years after the Fontan operation.[42,44] Factors that predispose this patient population to IART include atrial scarring, high atrial wall stress and hypertrophy, abnormal atrial anatomy, changes in atrial refractoriness, and sinus node dysfunction.[39] IART and loss of AV synchrony is poorly tolerated in this patient

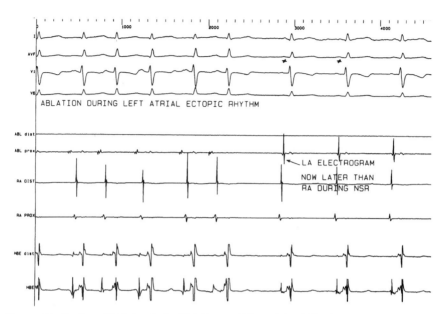

ABLATION DURING LEFT ATRIAL ECTOPIC RHYTHM

LA ELECTROGRAM
NOW LATER THAN
RA DURING NSR

Figure 11. Surface ECG leads I, aVF, V$_1$, and V$_6$ and the following intracardiac electrograms: ablation (ABL) ×2, right atrium (RA) ×2, and His bundle electrogram (HBE) ×2. The ablation is being performed for left atrial ectopic tachycardia. Prior to successful lesion placement, the left atrial electrogram (as seen on the proximal ABL catheter) is earlier than the right atrial electrogram (as seen on the distal RA catheter). Upon successful lesion placement, the patient exhibits normal sinus rhythm with the left atrial electrogram now later than the right atrial electrogram.

population, due to hemodynamic alterations/consequences, and proves difficult to manage medically, especially in the likely presence of sinus node dysfunction. There appears to be an increased risk of right and left atrial thrombosis with chronic IART similar to that of the adult population with chronic atrial fibrillation.[45] These are but a few of the complex issues that have compelled pediatric electrophysiologists to investigate the possibility of IART ablation.

Ablation of atrial flutter in patients with normal cardiac anatomy interrupts a zone of slow conduction found inferior and posterior to the mouth of the CS and anterior to a narrow isthmus of tissue between the inferior vena cava and the tricuspid annulus.[46] Ablation of IART involves the identification of a zone of slow conduction as well. This zone is critical to the maintenance of the tachycardia circuit, and exists between barriers that may be natural or surgically created. For this reason, one publication[47] suggests that IART be renamed "incisional reentry" tachycardia. It is important to review the patient's anatomy and operative summaries to become familiar with the location of atrial suture lines and scars around which the circuit may move before attempting the ablation procedure. Mapping the zone of slow conduction in IART involves a technique known as concealed entrainment. This is accomplished by pacing the atrium to accelerate the IART to the pacing cycle length without altering the P wave morphology or the endocardial activation sequence and without terminating the tachycardia when pacing is stopped.[48] The sites associated with the best rates of success are those that demonstrate a local atrial electrogram 20 to 45 ms before the surface P wave, concealed entrainment with a stimulus to P wave interval of 20 to 30 ms (suggesting exit from the IART circuit), and termination of IART within 5 seconds of radiofrequency application.[48] Deep, linear radiofrequency lesions are placed by dragging the ablation catheter to transect this zone of slow conduction from one anatomic barrier to another.

The extensive surgery involved in the atrial baffle procedures of the Senning and Mustard operations create barriers to impulse propagation and establish potential routes for IART.[49] The site of successful radiofrequency lesion placement in one series of Senning/Mustard ablation patients was most frequently the area of the mouth of the CS, which may drain to the systemic or pulmonary venous atrium.[49] Other locations identified in postoperative patients were at or near the site of the Fontan anastomosis, at the lateral junction of the right atrium and the superior vena cava, at the lateral junction of the right atrium and the inferior vena cava, and near the triangle of Koch.[50] The endpoint for successful ablation of IART is the inability to induce the tachycardia, as well as documentation of a zone of block in the area of lesion placement.

The success rate for ablation of IART is not as impressive as that for other tachycardias. Reasons for lower success rates may be the presence of multiple reentrant circuits, the width of the lesion required to connect the two fixed obstructions, and the depth needed to achieve a transmural lesion in the often-hypertrophied atrial myocardium.[34] Recurrence of IART in postoperative patients is often a result of new reentrant circuits.[43,51] Patients with recurrence of IART after an initially successful ablation procedure did show a decrease in subsequent events compared with the 2 years preceding the RFCA.[51]

The focus for many current innovations in the subspecialty of pediatric electrophysiology involves methods for improving the success rate of IART ablation in patients with CHD. Multielectrode basket catheters enable the operator to rapidly obtain high-density atrial activation maps that may be played in a movielike fashion over the fluoroscopy image, while intravascular ultrasound imaging further clarifies anatomic structures. Additional energy sources may be investigated to provide deeper transmural lesions.[39] One recently released analysis system provides arrhythmia mapping in a single beat, which is of great value in the patient who cannot tolerate sustained runs of tachycardia. This system uses a noncontact balloon with 64 electrodes that sense the changes in voltage (isopotentials) signaling the rapid spread of depolarization so that one can observe the beat on a three-dimensional map as it travels through the chamber. A navigation feature tracks the mapping catheter relative to the balloon position, thus enabling the operator to position the catheter to the point of interest with minimal fluoroscopy. One of the most promising innovations may well involve improvement in surgical techniques for prevention of the formation of IART substrates in this patient population.

Ventricular Tachycardia

The diagnosis of VT has historically engendered feelings of helplessness for families and health care professionals alike. This tachyarrhythmia carries a high risk for life-threatening events, and antiarrhythmic medications are not guaranteed to be effective. Polymorphic VT may involve a diffuse area of excitability or damage that does not lend to correction with catheter ablation techniques. For children with VT that is monomorphic, there is a chance for a cure with RFCA. It is important to differentiate monomorphic VT from aberrantly conducted AVRT, antidromic AVRT, or Mahaim tachycardia. Furthermore, the presence of arrhythmogenic right ventricular dysplasia should be ruled out.[52] There are three main types of VT that may be amenable to correction with catheter ablation in the pediatric population.

Idiopathic VT is often exercise related and occurs in patients without structural heart disease.[34] This type of VT usually originates from the right ventricular outflow tract or from the posteroseptal aspect of the left ventricle,[53] the precise location of which must be further delineated with mapping techniques. Mapping of the VT focus includes documentation of the endocardial ventricular electrogram 10 to 50 ms before the surface QRS, with pace mapping performed to pinpoint the target more accurately.[53] Pace mapping is done by pacing different spots in the region of the focus until the 12-lead electrocardiogram (ECG) of the paced beats matches the 12-lead ECG of the tachycardia. When these criteria are met, radiofrequency lesions may be placed in the area of the focus (Fig. 12).

RFCA of bundle branch reentrant VT has been shown to be a safe and effective treatment.[54] This type of VT is defined as one in which a deflection occurs before each QRS complex, a spontaneous change in His-to-His intervals precedes a change in VT cycle length, and AV dissociation is present. Baseline intervals will often reflect a prolonged HV interval in sinus rhythm. Cure for this type of reentrant VT is RFCA of the right bundle branch.[34]

A current area of interest to pediatric electrophysiologists is the possibility of ablating the VT that often occurs after repair of tetralogy of Fallot. The ventriculotomy scar is hypothesized to be similar to the scarring in postmyocardial infarction patients in the arrhythmogenesis of VT. The use of concealed entrainment to locate the exit site from a zone of slow conduction may prove to be the most successful approach for ablation of this type of VT.[34]

Other Substrates

PJRT occurs predominantly in infants and young children. This "long RP" tachycardia (the RP interval is greater than the PR interval) has an-

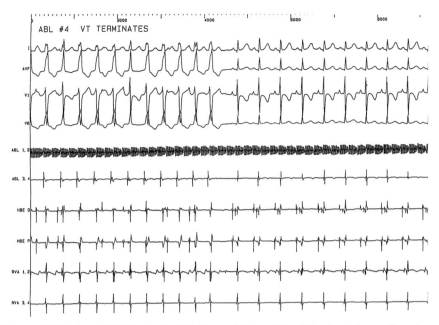

Figure 12. Surface ECG leads I, aVF, V$_1$, and V$_6$ and the following intracardiac electrograms: ablation (ABL) ×2, His bundle electrogram (HBE) ×2, and right ventricular apex (RVA) ×2. The ablation is being performed for right ventricular outflow tract (RVOT) tachycardia, which can be seen in the first half of the recording. The atrioventricular dissociation frequently seen with ventricular tachycardia can be seen on the HBE catheter. With successful lesion placement, the rhythm converts to normal sinus rhythm with normal A-V activation as seen on the HBE catheter.

tegrade and retrograde decremental properties as well as variable rates. PJRT is difficult to control medically and, due to the often incessant nature of the tachycardia, it often results in ventricular dysfunction, occasionally to the point of cardiomyopathy. Although most PJRT pathways are found in the right posteroseptal area just inside the mouth of the CS, some pathways have been ablated in the right atrial free wall, the right anterior septum, and the left posterior region.[55]

Occasionally, a patient with Mahaim conduction is given a diagnosis of WPW, as there may be a slight ventricular preexcitation pattern on a resting ECG. However, these AV or atriofascicular fibers differ from AVRT accessory pathways in that they have antegrade decremental properties and no retrograde conduction. They may be involved in sustaining a tachycardia or they may exist as an innocent bystander.[56] During tachycardia, the earliest ventricular activation is usually mapped to the right ventricular apex near the distal insertion of the right bundle branch.[57] These fibers tend to have a distal arborization, so ablative efforts may be more effective toward the proximal insertion.[58]

Congenital JET is associated with a high rate of mortality in infants and is difficult to control medically. Considering the diminutive size of an infant's heart, only skilled pediatric electrophysiologists should attempt RFCA of JET. Attempts to provide relief from this arrhythmia include ablation of the His bundle with permanent pacemaker implantation[59] or ablation of the focus without damage to AV nodal function.[60]

Ablation of the AV node or His bundle can be performed to create intentional complete AV block in order to protect a patient from life-threatening conduction of rapid atrial arrhythmias that cannot be controlled by any other means. Implantation of a permanent pacemaker prior to the RFCA is advised, as adequacy of the native intrinsic ventricular rate after loss of AV node conduction cannot be guaranteed. In addition, most candidates for AV junction ablation have CHD with less than optimal hemodynamics and cannot tolerate slow junctional rates or loss of AV synchrony. Ablation can be performed from the right or left side of the septum, but patients with septal hypertrophy may be more amenable to the left-sided approach.[34]

Potential Complications

Complications are to be anticipated when performing any invasive procedure, and, fortunately, they are relatively uncommon in the pediatric ablation experience. Potential complications associated with any RFCA procedure are listed in Table 1. Data published in 1997 from the Pediatric Radiofrequency Ablation Registry revealed 118 complications in 3653 cases, or a 3.2% complication rate.[6] The most frequently noted were AV block (n=25), perforation and/or pericardial effusion (n=24), brachial plexus injury (n=10), emboli (n=8), and pneumothorax (n=7). The mortality rate was 0.11%, with 1 death at the time of the procedure and 3 late deaths.[6]

Inadvertent AV block may occur during the procedure or late after RFCA. It is associated with ablation of anterior and midseptal accessory pathways, ablation for AVNRT, and relative institutional inexperience.[9] Another risk factor that has been identified is a body weight of ≤15 kg.[6] The safety and efficacy of RFCA in infants and small children has been doc-

Table 1
Potential Complications of Radiofrequency Catheter Ablation

Pleural/pericardial effusion
Hemorrhage
Infection
Hematoma
Cardiac perforation/tamponade
Pulmonary embolism
Stroke
Atrioventricular block
Coronary artery occlusion
Valve dysfunction
Death

umented in a report with an average patient body weight of 6 kg,[61] but a separate report of RFCA in 10 children less than 18 months of age included 1 patient death.[62] The authors of this report highlight two important factors for consideration: the typical radiofrequency lesion size is larger relative to the heart of an infant compared to that in an adult, and lesions that were placed in infant sheep ventricles appeared to grow with time.[62]

Regardless of the skill of the electrophysiologist, it should be obvious that any institution that offers RFCA to children must have pediatric emergency services in house, not just "in the vicinity." The staff caring for children undergoing RFCA should be vigorously trained in the resuscitation of children and should possess an excellent rapport with any and all support services involved in caring for pediatric patients.

Implications for Clinicians

The responsibilities of health care providers caring for children undergoing RFCA begin once the decision has been made to pursue this particular treatment modality. The clinician has certain specific responsibilities depending on the particular phase of the procedure that the child is in. The following implications for clinicians are reviewed in the context in which they appear—that is, prior to, during, and immediately after the ablation procedure. The implications for those involved in the child and family's follow-up care are also discussed. The implications for clinicians regarding patient and family education are covered in the section on patient and family considerations.

Prior to the Procedure

The team of clinicians caring for children undergoing RFCA is multifaceted with ongoing specific responsibilities. While some clinicians are responsible for ensuring certain elements regarding the patient, others have specific tasks related to the catheterization/electrophysiology laboratory. The following discussion regarding preprocedural tasks is presented relative to the patient considerations, and is followed by a discussion of laboratory considerations.

Patient Considerations

Since many ablation procedures are now performed as outpatient or 23-hour observational stays, the clinician has much to accomplish in a small amount of time, including but not limited to specific preprocedural tests ordered by the physician performing the procedure. The authors recommend that this and other preparations be done at a preoperative or work-up visit on the day prior to the procedure. At this time, the clinician should ensure that the specific preprocedural tests are completed. The authors routinely perform pregnancy tests in all females 12 years and older, as well as echocardiograms in all patients with CHD. Other preprocedural tests that may (or may not) be required include blood work, such as hemoglobin/hematocrit, clotting studies, and type and cross-match for blood products, 12-lead ECG, 24-hour ambulatory monitor, exercise stress test, chest radiograph, and magnetic resonance imaging. It is imperative that the responsible clinician make sure that all tests are completed and readily available on the day of the procedure.

In the authors' institutions, a specific nurse is generally the coordinator of these activities, and orchestrates the work-up day. If the child will be receiving general anesthesia for the procedure, the clinician must ensure that the child and family meet with anesthesia personnel to discuss anesthesia and sedation issues, including when to withhold food and fluids. Many centers have separate consent forms for anesthesia, which should be signed and on the patient's chart in order to prevent unnecessary delays on the day of the procedure. If sedation is to be administered by catheterization/electrophysiology laboratory personnel, these issues should be discussed with the patient and family by the electrophysiologist.

In most cases, the child and family will meet with the physician performing the procedure at this time, to review the risks and benefits of the procedure and to sign the consent form for the RFCA. A history and physical is also generally performed and any last minute issues or questions are clarified. Once completed, the clinician should reiterate when and why food and fluids are to be withheld and the patient and family should be told exactly when and where they are to report on the day of the procedure as well as what (or what not) to bring with them.

Laboratory Considerations

Cardiovascular clinicians directly involved in the RFCA procedure have distinctly different responsibilities. A major responsibility is to assure the safety of the patient. This requires specific knowledge of the procedure itself as well as the equipment used for or available for use throughout the procedure. All electrical equipment should be properly grounded and in excellent working order as evidenced by frequent evaluations by the institution's biomedical department.

The clinician working in the catheterization/electrophysiology laboratory should have an adequately stocked diagnostic and ablation catheter supply for any and all patient sizes and clinical situations. Smaller catheters (e.g., 5 Fr or 6 Fr ablation catheters) as well as catheters with closer electrode spacing are a must when caring for pediatric patients. The radiofrequency generator used varies from one laboratory to another. Regardless of the specific generator, the clinician must be knowledgeable regarding the use and misuse of that generator. Some generators are battery-powered, in which case the clinician must assure that the batteries (absolutely more than one) are fully charged prior to the ablation procedure. As in any electrophysiology laboratory, whether RFCA is performed or not, two external defibrillators should be available, preferably with a least one of them having the capability to provide external pacing. The clinician should ensure that the procedure room is fully equipped with all necessary drugs and equipment needed for cardiopulmonary resuscitation as well.

Once the child has been brought into the catheterization/electrophysiology laboratory, certain preparations are necessary prior to the start of the procedure. The adequacy of surface ECG electrode placement as it relates to the quality of the displayed ECG must be verified. If there are problems with ECG electrode placement, they should be addressed early on rather than waiting until the patient is prepped and draped. The grounding pad for the radiofrequency generator should be properly placed on the patient's back or thigh. Adequate body temperature for the individual patient should be maintained by either manipulating the room temperature or by using an additional external temperature-regulating apparatus. Adequate radiation safety precautions should be made for the patient (as well as the staff) to reduce radiation exposure, such as the use of thyroid drapes and/or gonad shields.

During the Procedure

The most important task of the clinician during the RFCA procedure is an ongoing assessment of the child's overall hemodynamic status. If conscious or deep sedation is used, the nurse managing the care of the patient should have no other responsibilities during the procedure, in order to ensure that the patient is always attended and constantly monitored.[63] The inherent responsibilities for clinicians involved in the use of conscious/deep sedation in children is beyond the scope of this chapter, but the implications are vast and should be initiated prior to the procedure, maintained during the procedure, and adhered to after the procedure.[64] The clinician should always be aware of the patient's response to his or her tachyarrhythmia, and should be prepared to assist with any emergency interventions. Knowledge of pediatric drug dosages is critical for nurses and other clinicians involved in RFCA in children. The clinician should constantly monitor the patient for any signs and symptoms of complications associated with RFCA. It is imperative that clinicians working in cardiac catheterization/electrophysiology laboratories be trained in basic and advanced pediatric cardiac life support. Because of the high level of parental anxiety and the variable lengths of the RFCA procedure, the authors have a designated clinician that speaks with the family once every hour, giving them an update on their child's condition.

After the Procedure

The average length of the pediatric RFCA procedure from sheath insertion to removal is 257 ± 157 minutes.[6] Postablation intracardiac intervals are documented and a 12-lead ECG is obtained. Pressure is held over the puncture sites until bleeding has stopped and a pressure dressing is applied. Depending on whether the procedure is performed on an outpatient, 23-hour observational, or inpatient basis, as well as the type of sedation/anesthesia used, will dictate whether the patient is transferred from the procedure room to the postanesthesia care unit, other outpatient observation area, or inpatient hospital bed. Regardless of where the patient recovers, the clinician now plays a vital role in the patient's care.

The clinician assuming care for the patient after RFCA must obtain specific information regarding the procedure from the cardiac catheterization/electrophysiology laboratory personnel. This is typically termed "report," and should include the following: the specific substrate ablated (e.g., WPW or AVNRT), whether the procedure was deemed successful, whether heparin was used (increased risk of bleeding), the type and amount of sedation/anesthesia used, any problems or unusual circumstances encountered during the procedure, and the number and condition of the puncture sites and dressings at the end of the procedure. The clinician should perform an overall clinical assessment of the patient upon assuming care. The catheterization site(s) should be inspected for presence of hemorrhage, swelling, or hematoma and the affected extremity evaluated for warmth, color, capillary refill, and palpable pulses. The child's level of consciousness (LOC) should be documented, as should the heart rate and rhythm, blood pressure, respiratory rate (including presence of any nasal flaring, use of accessory muscles, grunting, or retractions), and temperature.

Instead of the customary sandbag used in adults, the dressing over the puncture sites in children is generally a pressure dressing. The child's leg is generally kept straight for several hours following the procedure, although log rolling from side to side is permissible to change positions. If bleeding at the puncture site should occur, the clinician should hold firm pressure and have someone else notify the child's physician. In most cases, holding pressure will stop the bleeding and a new dressing will be applied.

Depending on the type of sedation/anesthesia used for the procedure, the child's LOC will vary. An intravenous line may be left in place with or without fluids attached. Diet progression from clear liquids to a full diet is dependent on the type of sedation used, the degree of nausea and vomiting, and the child's degree of somnolence. With the "push" to get patients in and out of the hospital environment quickly, patients are often "rushed" to wake up before they are ready in order to take fluids prior to discharge. This can increase the risk of aspiration and may promote avoidable nausea and vomiting. The authors advocate ice chips, followed by clear liquids with progression to full liquids when the child is fully awake and alert.

Regardless of the type of sedation used for the procedure or where the patient recovers after the procedure, the clinician has the distinct responsibility of ensuring the patient a safe return to his or her presedation state.[64] This includes the monitoring of the aforementioned vital signs, LOC, and patency of the child's airway. Also, knowledge of the specific agents used (and their elimination half-life) will aid the clinician in discharge planning, especially for patients who are discharged the day of the procedure.

Regardless of the patient's location following the procedure, continuous ECG monitoring should be performed. The clinician should obtain a baseline recording for initial assessment but also for comparison with subsequent recordings. The clinician should evaluate the ECG for heart rate, rhythm, and intervals as well as any signs of AV block, tachycardia recurrence, ventricular ectopy, or recurrence of a delta wave. Any changes from the postablation baseline ECG should be immediately reported to the child's physician for further evaluation. If tachycardia recurs, the clinician should immediately assess the child's hemodynamic status and be prepared to assist with any maneuvers deemed appropriate by the child's physician, including administration of antiarrhythmic or other medications, cardioversion/defibrillation, and/or institution of temporary pacing measures. More than one half of AVRT recurrences occur within the first 24 hours and the remainder are generally within 2 months post ablation.[65,66]

A 24-hour ambulatory monitor may be placed to document cardiac rhythm for the period immediately after the ablation. Patients are requested to remain quiet overnight, but may visit the bathroom as needed with assistance. Ambulation may be restricted overnight in patients who received heparin according to the particular physician's discretion.

Discharge Planning

Many institutions discharge routine ablation patients a few hours after the procedure, while some will keep them for 23 hours or longer. Children with CHD may require an inpatient stay for further observation or to restart anticoagulation medications. The electrophysiologist may prefer a longer observation period for patients who have had RFCA of a life-threatening arrhythmia. Regardless of when the patient is discharged, the clinician must ensure that proper plans are made. A major component of discharge planning is that of patient and family education, which is discussed in the following section on patient and family considerations.

The clinician's primary responsibility is to ensure an adequate return to the individual patient's baseline status. The child's vital signs should be stable, hemostasis and respiratory status should be returned to the preprocedure state, the child should take an adequate amount of fluids, and the child should have urinated. In regard to patients who undergo RFCA on an outpatient basis, the clinician must be able to document that specific discharge criteria are met, especially when conscious/deep sedation is used. The American Academy of Pediatrics (AAP) has established specific discharge criteria for patients undergoing diagnostic and therapeutic procedures in which sedation is used,[67] which can be found in Table 2. The AAP specifically recommends that before the procedure, a responsible person is identified to care for the child after discharge.[67]

Table 2
Recommended Discharge Criteria

1. Cardiovascular function and airway patency are satisfactory and stable.
2. The patient is easily arousable, and protective reflexes are intact.
3. The patient can talk (if age appropriate).
4. The patient can sit up unaided (if age appropriate).
5. For a very young or handicapped child, incapable of the usually expected responses, the presedation level of responsiveness or a level as close as possible to the normal level for that child should be achieved.
6. The state of hydration is adequate.

From American Academy of Pediatrics, Committee on Drugs: Guidelines for monitoring and management of patients during and after sedation for diagnostic and therapeutic procedures. Pediatrics 1992; 89:1110, with permission.

If specific tests have been ordered after the procedure, the clinician should ensure that they have been completed and reviewed by the discharging physician. These tests may include blood work, 12-lead ECG, or an echocardiogram. The clinician should provide oral and written instructions including puncture site care, prescribed medications (if applicable), subacute bacterial endocarditis (SBE) prophylaxis (if applicable), signs and symptoms to report to the physician, activity restrictions, phone numbers for problems or questions, and follow-up care. Additionally, if patients are discharged the day of the procedure, they should be instructed regarding food and fluid intake and when to remove the puncture site dressing (usually the next morning), and told that they are to remain quiet overnight (but they may visit the bathroom as needed, with assistance). At this nurse author's institution, most ablation procedures are performed on an outpatient basis and the children are given their ablation catheter and a fluoroscopy film picture showing the catheter position for successful lesion placement as souvenirs.

Follow-Up Care

Follow-up is necessary for ablation patients, in order to document cardiac rhythm and investigate the possibility of recurrence. ECGs are helpful for children who previously had WPW, IART, or AV node or His bundle ablation, but will not show evidence for recurrence of concealed accessory pathways or AVNRT unless the patient is in tachycardia. Exercise tests and 24-hour ambulatory monitors may be ordered for children after VT ablation. A thorough history from the child and family will provide information regarding absence or return of symptoms. Many children may have premature ventricular contractions (PVCs) after RFCA, and are often concerned that their tachycardia has returned. They may feel that their tachycardia is starting, but it doesn't feel as fast. This may be due to the feeling of a PVC, which used to initiate tachycardia, and the child's anxiety then causes sinus tachycardia. It may be necessary to issue a transtelephonic event monitor to document the cardiac rhythm during symptoms, for reassurance.

Although long-term follow-up is often left to the family's discretion (with the assumption that an appointment will be made if symptoms recur), it is important for pediatric electrophysiologists to document the long-term safety of radiofrequency lesions in children. In addition to evaluating the efficacy of the procedure, follow-up is necessary for evaluating issues regarding enlargement of chronic lesions resulting from cardiac growth as well as the potential for a stretched lesion to become arrhythmogenic. The authors recommend a 2-month follow-up after the ablation procedure, with annual follow-up for several years, followed by intervals of 2 to 3 years depending on the arrhythmogenic substrate.

Patient and Family Considerations

In this rapidly changing health care environment, health care professionals involved in the care of children (and their families) undergoing RFCA must remember to take the time to educate the child and family about the procedure. This journey of education should begin as soon as the decision to perform RFCA has been made. Many patients and families misconstrue the procedure as "heart surgery" and must be corrected early on in order to avoid unnecessary anxiety for both the child and the family. The insistence of third party payers to perform "outpatient" procedures often leaves little time for patient/family education; nevertheless, clinicians must "find the time" to provide this extremely important service. The patient and family education consists primarily of that provided before the RFCA and after the procedure as part of the discharge planning process.

Prior to the Procedure

Although the Pediatric Radiofrequency Ablation Registry data describe "patient choice" as a reason for ablation, "family choice" might be a more suitable term to use when dealing with pediatric patients. In most instances, the decision to proceed with an elective procedure is a collaborative effort between the parents, the child, and the electrophysiologist. The weight of the decision often falls on the shoulders of the parents of a minor. In order to make the best choice for their child and family, the parents must have a thorough knowledge base, not only about the risks, benefits, and details of the electrophysiology study and ablation, but the arrhythmia mechanism, natural history, and other treatment options as well. This information can be presented initially by the electrophysiologist and reinforced by the pediatric electrophysiology nurse in further detail.

The child should receive education at an age-appropriate level by a pediatric nurse. Knowledge of developmental levels (cognitive, intellectual, and psychosocial stages) is recognized as essential in caring for the child and family.[68,69] Customized brochures to be taken home with the family reinforce the content of the teaching and can serve as a valuable reference after the initial educational session. Other teaching tools include a heart model, videotapes, and play therapy.

Content of the teaching session will vary among families, depending on the level of interest and the ability to understand technical details. Regardless of the family's sophistication, or lack thereof, some details must be covered in order for the child to be prepared for the experience and the parents to be cognizant of their responsibilities before and after admission. The remainder of this section presents a framework of basic information to which details can be added accordingly.

Most patients will be required to discontinue their antiarrhythmic medications before the RFCA to allow for arrhythmia induction and mapping. Exceptions to this rule might be the patient with hemodynamically unstable VT or IART that conducts rapidly to the ventricle. These patients may need to continue their medications in order to slow rates or conduction and permit adequate mapping. Discontinuing antiarrhythmic medications almost always generates a high parental stress level, as many parents are certain that their child will have tachycardia within minutes of missing one dose. It is important to provide these families with a written plan designating the last dose, as well as steps to follow if tachycardia should occur. Some families feel more comfortable restricting the children from strenuous physical activities and caffeine during this period.

Routine ablation procedures are commonly performed as day surgery or outpatient admissions. Directions regarding when to withhold food and fluids (i.e., NPO [nothing by mouth] orders) and time of admission should be clarified, as should the anticipated discharge time. It is helpful for families to be familiar with the "when, where, and why" of routines such as admitting, intravenous line insertion, and sedation or anesthesia induction. Older children and adolescents may appreciate a tour of the electrophysiology laboratory before the admission so that they are not as overwhelmed by the staff and equipment when they "wheel in" on the day of the ablation. It is ideal if the parents can stay with the child until he or she is asleep. Most children want to hear that they will not wake up until the procedure is over and the catheters are out. Recovery room routines should be discussed to make the child aware that his or her parents may not be with them initially, but are close by in a waiting area until visitation is permitted. The child should know that there will be catheter insertion sites in the groins and possibly the neck with tight bandages over them. It is somewhat comforting to the child and parents that these are not incisions with stitches, but "poke marks." The child should be told that he or she will need to lay flat and still for a few hours to prevent bleeding at the sites, and that the parents' assistance in this endeavor will be expected. In some institutions, the patients are discharged after 4 hours of observation in the postanesthesia care unit. Before the procedure is scheduled, the family should receive information regarding the types of restrictions that will be imposed after the discharge, such as no tub baths or swimming until the puncture sites are healed. This will allow the family to make necessary plans for time off from school or work and will hopefully avoid the scheduling of vacations to the beach immediately after discharge.

Home Care Instructions

Home care instructions after RFCA should be given to the responsible person (usually the child's parents) in a quiet, relaxed, and unrushed atmosphere. In addition to oral instructions, it is helpful for most families to receive written instructions, such as those found in Table 3. Individuals

Table 3
Home Care Instructions After Radiofrequency Catheter Ablation

Activity	Light activity for 3 days following the procedure
	No swimming, running, or hard exercise for 3 days
	May return to school 1–2 days after hospital discharge
	May resume full activities (as determined by physician) 3 days after procedure
Bathing	No tub baths for 3 days following the ablation
	May shower immediately
Care of puncture site(s)	Keep the area(s) clean and dry
	A bandaid may be used if clothing or underwear irritates the area
	Clean with soap and water
When to call the cardiologist	Tachycardia comes back
	Fever over 101°F within 3 days after the procedure
	Pus from the puncture site(s)
	Blood flow from the puncture site(s)
	Leg(s) or arm where catheters were placed becomes cooler or more pale than when you left the hospital
Subacute bacterial endocarditis prophylaxis	Endocarditis prophylaxis is to prevent infection in your child's heart
	Your doctor or nurse will inform you if you need to observe these precautions
Medications	_____
	_____
	_____
Return Appointment:	_____
	_____
	_____
Phone Numbers:	Cardiologist: _____
	Cardiology Nurse: _____
	Cardiology Clinic: _____

who develop patient and family education materials should be cognizant of reading and readability concepts when preparing these materials.[70]

Patients and their families should be instructed to keep the catheterization/puncture sites clean and dry. A bandaid may be used (but is not necessary) if clothing or underwear irritate the site. In order to prevent infection and promote healing, showers should be substituted for tub baths for 3 days following the RFCA. If the child is discharged with the dressing intact, parents should be instructed as to when to remove the dressing (usually the next morning), how the site should look once the dressing is removed, and that a small amount of blood-tinged drainage at this time is normal but blood flow is not. If the dressing is removed prior to hospital discharge, patients and parents should be asked to look at the site (or sites) at this time in order to have a comparison for later assessment. They should be instructed to inspect the site daily for 3 days and to notify the cardiologist for any purulent drainage, swelling, redness, or hematoma.

Limitations or restrictions from various activities vary from physician to physician. General recommendations include light activity for 3 days following the RFCA to allow healing of the puncture sites—specifically no swimming, running, or vigorous exercise during this time. In most cases, children can return to school 1 to 2 days following the procedure. Most children with anatomically normal hearts and a successful ablation are allowed to resume full activity after 3 days, including varsity and other competitive athletics as well as unlimited physical education. Patients with concomitant CHD will probably have limitations imposed by their structural heart defect that are essentially the same after RFCA as they where before. Patients on long-term anticoagulant therapy may have more specific activity restrictions.

After discharge, many children continue aspirin therapy for days, weeks, or even months following the procedure. The exact dose and dosing schedule should be reviewed with the patient and parents, as should the availability of enteric-coated brands that decrease stomach irritation. If the patient is taking other medications at the time of discharge, prescriptions for those medications should be given in addition to education regarding the drugs' intended actions, potential adverse effects, and issues that require physician notification.

Some centers request that patients adhere to SBE prophylaxis following RFCA. In this physician author's institution, it is suggested for 1 year post ablation in patients with structurally normal hearts. Patients with CHD may need continued SBE prophylaxis for life. If SBE prophylaxis is recommended, instructions should indicate the reason it is being used, and SBE cards should be provided to the patient and family.

Many patients experience PVCs after the procedure and become concerned that their arrhythmia has recurred. In many cases, the anxiety about the PVC leads to sinus tachycardia, which the child (or family) often mistakes as tachycardia. Home care instructions should include an explanation regarding this phenomenon so that patients and families can be prepared for its potential occurrence. If there is some doubt regarding the success of the procedure, the cardiologist may prescribe a transtelephonic monitor. Instructions regarding the use of transtelephonic monitors can be found in chapter 1, and should include both oral and written instructions as well as a return demonstration to determine the adequacy of their technique.

Patients and families should be instructed as to when to call the cardiologist or cardiology office once discharged from the hospital setting. Obviously, they should call if the child experiences tachycardia recurrence, but also for any of the following: fever higher than 101°F, purulent drainage from the puncture site(s), blood flow from the puncture site(s), or if the affected extremity becomes cooler or more pale than at the time of discharge.

The provision of patient and family education is an important part of the RFCA experience and should not be overlooked. Patients and families will have less anxiety and feel more informed about the child's care if they receive information before, during, and after catheter ablation, and this will hopefully result in a positive interaction with the health care system.

Future Issues in Pediatric Catheter Ablation

It is easy to appreciate how far electrophysiologists have come in understanding not only the mechanisms for arrhythmias, but also how to eliminate them with a therapeutic catheterization. Add to this the challenge of destroying targets in the often-confusing anatomy of complex CHD and you will find a puzzle that few pediatric electrophysiologists can resist. Unfortunately, technology seems to develop more slowly than do the scientists' imaginations.

Several advances in science and technology have been presented thus far in this chapter. Enhanced mapping programs, various types of catheter configurations, and different types of energy delivery are being investigated in many institutions at the time of this writing. Surgeries for congenital disease are being modified in an attempt to prevent these arrhythmias from occurring at all.

Regardless of how exciting the science and technology of RFCA may be, we must keep in mind the primary objective for this procedure. We are charged with a commitment to curing children with cardiac arrhythmias in an attempt to provide as normal a childhood as possible. An experienced pediatric ablation program will make the effort to ensure that although the catheters may leave scars on the body, the adventure will not leave a scar on the soul.

References

1. Crawford FA Jr., Gillette PC: Surgical treatment of cardiac dysrhythmias in infants and children. Ann Thorac Surg 1994; 58:1262–1268.
2. Perry JC, Kearney DL, Freidman RA, et al: Late ventricular arrhythmia and sudden death following direct-current catheter ablation of the atrioventricular junction. Am J Cardiol 1992; 70:465–468.

3. Huang SK, Bharati S, Graham AR, et al: Closed chest catheter desiccation of the atrioventricular junction using radiofrequency energy: A new method of catheter ablation. J Am Coll Cardiol 1987; 9:349–358.
4. Kugler JD, Danford DA, Deal B, et al: Radiofrequency catheter ablation for tachyarrhythmias in children and adolescents. N Engl J Med 1994; 330:1481–1487.
5. Tanel RE, Walsh EP, Triedman JK, et al: Five-year experience with radiofrequency catheter ablation: Implications for management of arrhythmias in pediatric and young patients. J Pediatr 1997; 131:878–887.
6. Kugler JD, Danford DA, Houston K, et al: Radiofrequency catheter ablation for paroxysmal supraventricular tachycardia in children and adolescents without structural heart disease. Am J Cardiol 1997; 80:1438–1443.
7. Silka MJ, Halperin BD, Hardy BG, et al: Safety and efficacy of radiofrequency modification of slow pathway conduction in children ≤10 years of age with atrioventricular node reentrant tachycardia. Am J Cardiol 1997; 80:1364–1367.
8. Danford DA, Kugler JD, Deal B, et al: The learning curve for radiofrequency ablation of tachyarrhythmias in pediatric patients. Am J Cardiol 1995; 75:587–590.
9. Schaffer MS, Silka MJ, Ross BA, et al: Inadvertent atrioventricular block during radiofrequency catheter ablation. Results of the Pediatric Radiofrequency Ablation Registry. Circulation 1996; 94:3214–3220.
10. McLean A: The Bovie electrosurgical current generator. Arch Surg 1929; 18:1863.
11. Kalbfleish SJ, Langberg JJ: Catheter ablation with radiofrequency energy: Biophysical aspects and clinical applications. J Cardiovasc Electrophysiol 1992; 3:173–186.
12. Huang SK: Advances in applications of radiofrequency current to catheter ablation therapy. Pacing Clin Electrophysiol 1991; 14:28–42.
13. Haines DE: The biophysics of radiofrequency catheter ablation in the heart: The importance of temperature monitoring. Pacing Clin Electrophysiol 1993; 16:586–591.
14. Saul JP, Hulse JE, De W, et al: Catheter ablation of accessory atrioventricular pathways in young patients: Use of long vascular sheaths, the transseptal approach and a retrograde left posterior parallel approach. J Am Coll Cardiol 1993; 21:571–583.
15. Haines DE, Verow AF: Observations on electrode-tissue interface temperature and effect on electrical impedance during radiofrequency ablation of ventricular myocardium. Circulation 1990; 82:1034–1038.
16. Deal BJ, Keane JF, Gillette PC, et al: Wolff-Parkinson-White syndrome and supraventricular tachycardia during infancy: Management and follow-up. J Am Coll Cardiol 1985; 5:130–135.
17. Perry JC, Garson A Jr.: Supraventricular tachycardia due to Wolff-Parkinson-White syndrome in children: Early disappearance and late recurrence. J Am Coll Cardiol 1990; 16:1215–1220.
18. VanHare GF: Indications for radiofrequency ablation in the pediatric population. J Cardiovasc Electrophysiol 1997; 8:952–962.
19. Russell MW, Dorostkar PC, Dick M II: Incidence of catastrophic events associated with the Wolff-Parkinson-White syndrome in young patients: Diagnostic and therapeutic dilemma. Circulation 1993; 88:I-484. Abstract.
20. Lashus AG, Gillette PC: Catheter ablation treatment of supraventricular tachycardia-induced cardiomyopathy. Arch Pediatr Adolesc Med 1997; 151:264–266.
21. Garson A Jr., Kanter RJ: Management of the child with Wolff-Parkinson-White syndrome and supraventricular tachycardia: Model for cost effectiveness. J Cardiovasc Electrophysiol 1997; 8:1320–1326.
22. Lebovic S, Reich DL, Steinberg LG, et al: Comparison of propofol versus ket-

amine for anesthesia in pediatric patients undergoing cardiac catheterization. Anesth Analg 1992; 74:490–494.

23. Kugler JD: Catheter ablation in pediatric patients. In Zipes DP, Jalife J (eds.): Cardiac Electrophysiology: From Cell to Bedside. Philadelphia: WB Saunders Company; 1995:1524–1537.

24. Scheibler GL, Adams P, Anderson RC: The Wolff-Parkinson-White syndrome in infants and children: A review and a report of 28 cases. Pediatrics 1959; 24:585–603.

25. VanHare GF, Lesh MD, Stanger P: Radiofrequency catheter ablation of supraventricular arrhythmias in patients with congenital heart disease: Results and technical considerations. J Am Coll Cardiol 1993; 22:883–890.

26. Lau YR, Case CL, Gillette PC, et al: Frequency of atrioventricular valve dysfunction after radiofrequency catheter ablation via the atrial approach in children. Am J Cardiol 1994; 74:617–618.

27. Calkins H, Langberg J, Sousa J, et al: Radiofrequency catheter ablation of accessory atrioventricular connections in 250 patients. Circulation 1992; 85: 1337–1346.

28. Greene TO, Huang SK, Wagshal AB, et al: Cardiovascular complications after radiofrequency catheter ablation of supraventricular tachyarrhythmias. Am J Cardiol 1994; 74:615–616.

29. VanHare GF: Radiofrequency ablation of accessory pathways associated with congenital heart disease. Pacing Clin Electrophysiol 1997; 20:2077–2081.

30. Swartz JF, Tracy CM, Fletcher RD: Radiofrequency endocardial catheter ablation of accessory atrioventricular pathway atrial insertion sites. Circulation 1993; 87:487–499.

31. Laohaprasitiporn D, Walsh EP, Saul JP, et al: Predictors of permanence of successful radiofrequency lesions created with controlled catheter tip temperature. Pacing Clin Electrophysiol 1997; 20:1283–1291.

32. Chen X, Borggrefe M, Hindricks G, et al: Radiofrequency ablation of accessory pathways: Characteristics of transiently and permanently effective pulses. Pacing Clin Electrophysiol 1992; 15:1122–1130.

33. O'Connor BK, Case CL, Gillette PC: Radiofrequency ablation of a posteroseptal accessory pathway via the middle cardiac vein in a six-year-old child. Pacing Clin Electrophysiol 1997; 20:2504–2507.

34. Fenrich AL, Friedman RA, Ott DA: Nonpharmacologic treatment of arrhythmias: Radiofrequency ablation and surgery. In Garson A Jr., Bricker JT, Fisher DJ, Neish SR (eds.): The Science and Practice of Pediatric Cardiology. Baltimore: Williams & Wilkins; 1998:2471–2488.

35. Epstein LM, Lesh MD, Griffin JC, et al: A direct midseptal approach to slow atrioventricular nodal pathway ablation. Pacing Clin Electrophysiol 1995; 18:57–64.

36. Walsh EP, Saul JP, Hulse JE, et al: Transcatheter ablation of ectopic atrial tachycardia in young patients using radiofrequency current. Circulation 1992; 86:1138–1146.

37. Pappone C, Stabile G, De Simone A, et al: Role of catheter-induced mechanical trauma in localization of target sites of radiofrequency ablation in automatic atrial tachycardia. J Am Coll Cardiol 1996; 27:1090–1097.

38. Perry JC, Fenrich AL, LeGras MD, et al: Acceleration of atrial ectopic tachycardia as a guide to successful radiofrequency ablation. Pacing Clin Electrophysiol 1993; 16:2007–2011.

39. Saul JP, Triedman JK: Radiofrequency ablation of intraatrial reentrant tachycardia after surgery for congenital heart disease. Pacing Clin Electrophysiol 1997; 20:2112–2117.

40. Garson A Jr., Bink-Boelkens M, Hesslein PS, et al: Atrial flutter in the young: A collaborative study of 380 cases. J Am Coll Cardiol 1985; 6:871–878.

41. Flinn CH, Wolff GS, Dick M II: Cardiac rhythm after the Mustard operation for complete transposition of the great arteries. N Engl J Med 1984; 310:1635–1638.
42. Fishberger SB, Wernovsky G, Gentles TL, et al: Factors that influence the development of atrial flutter after the Fontan operation. J Thorac Cardiovasc Surg 1997; 113:80–86.
43. Kanter RJ, Garson A Jr.: Atrial arrhythmias during chronic follow-up of surgery for complex congenital heart disease. Pacing Clin Electrophysiol 1997; 20:502–511.
44. Gelatt M, Hamilton RM, McCrindle BW, et al: Risk factors for atrial tachyarrhythmias after the Fontan operation. J Am Coll Cardiol 1994; 24:1735–1741.
45. Feltes TF, Friedman RA: Transesophageal echocardiographic detection of atrial thrombi in patients with nonfibrillation atrial tachyarrhythmias and congenital heart disease. J Am Coll Cardiol 1994; 24:1365–1370.
46. Feld GK, Fleck RP, Chen PS, et al: Radiofrequency catheter ablation for the treatment of human type I atrial flutter. Identification of a critical zone in the reentrant circuit by endocardial mapping techniques. Circulation 1992; 86:1233–1240.
47. Kalman JM, VanHare GF, Olgin JE, et al: Ablation of 'incisional' reentrant atrial tachycardia complicating surgery for congenital heart disease. Use of entrainment to define a critical isthmus of conduction. Circulation 1996; 93:502–512.
48. Chen SA, Chiang CE, Yang CJ, et al: Radiofrequency catheter ablation of sustained intraatrial reentrant tachycardia in adult patients. Identification of electrophysiological characteristics and endocardial mapping techniques. Circulation 1993; 88:578–587.
49. Van Hare GF, Lesh MD, Ross BA, et al: Mapping and radiofrequency ablation of intraatrial reentrant tachycardia after the Senning or Mustard procedure for transposition of the great arteries. Am J Cardiol 1996; 77:985–991.
50. Triedman JK, Saul JP, Weindling SN, et al: Radiofrequency ablation of intraatrial reentrant tachycardia after surgical palliation of congenital heart disease. Circulation 1995; 91:707–714.
51. Triedman JK, Bergau DM, Saul JP, et al: Efficacy of radiofrequency ablation for control of intraatrial reentrant tachycardia in patients with congenital heart disease. J Am Coll Cardiol 1997; 30:1032–1038.
52. O'Connor BK, Case CL, Sokoloski MC, et al: Radiofrequency catheter ablation of right ventricular outflow tachycardia in children and adolescents. J Am Coll Cardiol 1996; 27:869–876.
53. Coggins KL, Lee RF, Sweeney J, et al: Radiofrequency catheter ablation as a cure of idiopathic tachycardia of both left and right ventricular origin. J Am Coll Cardiol 1994; 23:1333–1341.
54. Cohen TJ, Chien WW, Lurie KG, et al: Radiofrequency catheter ablation for treatment of bundle branch reentrant ventricular tachycardia: Results and long-term follow-up. J Am Coll Cardiol 1991; 18:1767–1773.
55. Ticho BS, Saul JP, Hulse JE, et al: Variable location of accessory pathways associated with the permanent form of junctional reciprocating tachycardia and confirmation with radiofrequency catheter ablation. Am J Cardiol 1992; 70:1559–1564.
56. Kusumoto FM, Lesh MD: Radiofrequency catheter ablation of an atriofascicular connection guided by direct recording of a Mahaim potential. Am Heart J 1995; 129:614–616.
57. Klein LS, Hackett FK, Zipes DP, et al: Radiofrequency catheter ablation of Mahaim fibers at the tricuspid annulus. Circulation 1993; 87:738–747.
58. Haissaguerre M, Cauchemez B, Marcus F, et al: Characteristics of the ventricular insertion sites of accessory pathways with anterograde decremental conduction properties. Circulation 1995; 91:1077–1085.

59. Van Hare GF, Velvis H, Langberg JJ: Successful transcatheter ablation of congenital junctional ectopic tachycardia in a ten-month-old infant using radiofrequency energy. Pacing Clin Electrophysiol 1990; 13:730–735.

60. Rychik J, Marchilinski FE, Sweeten JT, et al: Transcatheter radiofrequency ablation for congenital junctional ectopic tachycardia in infancy. Pediatr Cardiol 1997; 18:447–450.

61. Case CL, Gillette PC, Oslizlok PC, et al: Radiofrequency catheter ablation of incessant, medically resistant supraventricular tachycardia in infants and small children. J Am Coll Cardiol 1992; 20:1405–1410.

62. Erickson CC, Walsh EP, Triedman JK, et al: Efficacy and safety of radiofrequency ablation in infants and young children less than 18 months of age. Am J Cardiol 1994; 74:944–947.

63. Association of Operating Room Nurses: Proposed recommended practice: Monitoring the patient receiving IV conscious sedation. AORN J 1992; 56:316–324.

64. Zeigler VL, Brown LE: Conscious sedation in the pediatric population: Special considerations. Crit Care Nurs Clin North Am 1997; 9:381–394.

65. Langberg JJ, Calkins H, Kim YN, et al: Recurrence of conduction in accessory atrioventricular connections after initially successful radiofrequency catheter ablation. J Am Coll Cardiol 1992; 19:1588–1592.

66. Wagshal AB, Pires LA, Mittleman RS, et al: Early recurrence of accessory pathways after radiofrequency catheter ablation does not preclude long-term cure. Am J Cardiol 1993; 72:843–846.

67. American Academy of Pediatrics, Committee on Drugs: Guidelines for monitoring and management of pediatric patients during and after sedation for diagnostic and therapeutic procedures. Pediatrics 1992; 89:1110–1115.

68. Zeigler VL, Corbett KS: Psychosocial aspects of caring for pediatric pacemaker recipients and their families. In Gillette PC, Zeigler VL (eds.): Pediatric Cardiac Pacing. Armonk, NY: Futura Publishing Company, Inc.; 1995:181–203.

69. Zeigler VL: Care of adolescents and young adults with cardiac arrhythmias. Prog Cardiovasc Nurs 1995; 10:13–21.

70. Owen PM, Johnson EM, Frost CD, et al: Reading, readability, and patient education materials. Cardiovasc Nurs 1993; 29:9–13.

Chapter 7

Permanent Pacemakers

Sherry J. Taylor, RN, BSN, Vicki L. Zeigler, RN, MSN, and John M. Clark, MD

Permanent cardiac pacing was originally used in the pediatric population to keep children alive after attempted repair of congenital heart defects.[1] The indications for cardiac pacemakers in children and young adults have evolved over the past few decades to include a variety of patients, including those with anatomically normal hearts. This is due to an improved understanding of the mechanisms, hemodynamic consequences, and natural history of bradyarrhythmias in children. The pulse generators and pacing leads have also dramatically improved technologically and now, in addition to prolonging a patient's life, they can improve the patient's quality of life as well.[2-6]

The rapid changes in pacemaker technology and function that occur almost daily require that the clinician caring for these patients become and remain knowledgeable not only about the specific patient but about the nuances of pacemaker technology as well. An extremely organized approach is necessary for optimal outcomes in the pediatric pacemaker recipient, and requires not only expertise in caring for children and families but a working knowledge of congenital heart disease (CHD) as well. This chapter includes an overview of the pacing indications in children, pacing system selection, implantation technique (endocardial and epicardial as well as intraoperative testing), implications for clinicians, follow-up care, patient and family considerations, and related issues.

Indications

The *American College of Cardiology/American Heart Association Guidelines for Implantation of Cardiac Pacemakers and Antiarrhythmia*

From Zeigler VL, Gillette PC: *Practical Management of Pediatric Cardiac Arrhythmias.* Armonk, NY: Futura Publishing Co., Inc.; ©2001.

Devices were published in 1984,[7] revised in 1991,[8] and recently updated[9] to reflect the advances in pacemaker technology as well as an increased knowledge level regarding the natural history of bradyarrhythmias and tachyarrhythmias that may benefit from device therapy.

The specific indications for permanent cardiac pacing in children and adolescents can be found in Table 1. Class I conditions include patients in whom there is general agreement that the device will be beneficial, Class II conditions include patients in whom the device may or may not be beneficial, and Class III conditions include patients in whom there is agreement that the device will *not* be useful. An addition to the 1998 guidelines is a "level of evidence" ranking.[9] Level A is assigned if the literature reports data from multiple, randomized clinical trials involving many subjects. Level B is assigned if the literature reports data from a small number of trials with a limited number of subjects. Level C is assigned when the indication was derived by expert consensus. The pediatric indications include no assignments of Level A, in part because of the small number of pediatric patients who require permanent cardiac pacemakers.

Although the general indications for pacemaker implantation in children are similar to those in adults, there are several important issues to be considered in the pediatric and young adult pacemaker population.[10] Generally, the child, adolescent, or young adult requiring a permanent cardiac pacemaker will fit into one of four main categories: 1) surgical/acquired advanced second- or third-degree atrioventricular (AV) block; 2) congenital complete AV block (CCAVB); 3) symptomatic bradycardia; or 4) recurrent bradycardia-tachycardia.[9]

The most common pacing indication in children undergoing permanent cardiac pacemaker implantation is surgically acquired AV block, which accounts for nearly 30% to 60% of patients.[11–16] These patients may receive permanent devices for Mobitz Type II second-degree, fixed 2:1, or complete AV block if it persists up to 10 days after surgery for CHD. Serwer and colleagues[17] report that surgical repair of an AV septal defect results in the greatest incidence of surgically acquired AV block, with a 17% incidence over the past 12 years according to the Midwest Pediatric Pacemaker Registry. Other congenital cardiac defects associated with surgically acquired AV block include Mustard/Senning repair for d-transposition of the great arteries, levo-transposition of the great arteries, tetralogy of Fallot, aortic valve replacement (usually associated with subaortic membrane resection), and ventricular septal defect.

CCAVB is the next most common pacemaker indication in children and young adults and may occur in the presence of an anatomically normal heart or may be associated with structural heart disease. The specific indications for these two subsets of patients are different because of the high mortality rate in patients with concomitant structural heart disease and congestive heart failure who do not receive permanent pacemakers by the age of 2 years.[18] The published guidelines recommend pacemaker place-

Table 1
Indications for Permanent Pacing in Children and Adolescents

Class I
1. Advanced second- or third-degree AV block associated with symptomatic bradycardia, congestive heart failure, or low cardiac output. (Level of evidence: C)
2. Sinus node dysfunction with correlation of symptoms during age-appropriate bradycardia. The definition of bradycardia varies with the patient's age and expected heart rate. (Level of evidence: B)
3. Postoperative advanced second- or third-degree AV block that is not expected to resolve or that persists at least 7 days after cardiac surgery. (Level of evidence: B, C)
4. Congenital third-degree AV block with a wide QRS escape rhythm or ventricular dysfunction. (Level of evidence: B)
5. Congenital third-degree AV block in the infant with a ventricular rate <50 to 55 bpm or with congenital heart disease and ventricular rate <70 bpm. (Level of evidence: B, C)
6. Sustained pause-dependent VT, with or without prolonged QT, in which the efficacy of pacing is thoroughly documented. (Level of evidence: B)

Class IIa
1. Bradycardia-tachycardia syndrome with the need for long-term antiarrhythmic treatment other than digitalis. (Level of evidence: C)
2. Congenital third-degree AV block beyond the first year of life with an average heart rate <50 bpm or abrupt pauses in ventricular rate that are two to three times the basic cycle length. (Level of evidence: B)
3. Long QT syndrome with 2:1 AV, or third-degree AV, block. (Level of evidence: B)
4. Asymptomatic sinus bradycardia in the child with complex congenital heart disease with resting heart rate <35 bpm or pauses in ventricular rate >3 seconds. (Level of evidence: C)

Class IIb
1. Transient postoperative third-degree AV block that reverts to sinus rhythm with residual bifascicular block. (Level of evidence: C)
2. Congenital third-degree AV block in the asymptomatic neonate, child, or adolescent with an acceptable rate, narrow QRS complex, and normal ventricular function. (Level of evidence: B)
3. Asymptomatic sinus bradycardia in the adolescent with congenital heart disease with resting heart rate <35 bpm or pauses in ventricular rate >3 seconds. (Level of evidence: C)

Class III
1. Transient postoperative AV block with return of normal AV conduction within 7 days. (Level of evidence: B)
2. Asymptomatic postoperative bifascicular block with or without first-degree AV block. (Level of evidence: B)
3. Asymptomatic Type I second-degree AV block. (Level of evidence: C)
4. Asymptomatic sinus bradycardia in the adolescent with longest R-R interval <3 seconds and minimum heart rate >40 bpm. (Level of evidence: C)

From: Gregoratos G, Cheitlin MD, Conill A, et al: ACC/AHA guidelines for implantation of cardiac pacemakers and antiarrhythmia devices. J Am Coll Cardiol 1998; 31:1175–209, with permission.

ment in the neonate with CCAVB and a normal heart with a ventricular rate of ≤55 beats per minute (bpm) AND in the neonate with CCAVB and structural heart disease and respiratory distress with a ventricular rate ≤70 bpm.[9]

The neonate with a structurally normal heart may not require immediate pacemaker placement in the absence of symptoms, but should be followed closely on an outpatient basis for indications that a permanent device should be implanted. These symptoms include syncope, congestive heart failure, ventricular ectopy, increased heart size on chest radiograph, and decreased ventricular function. Recently, Michaelsson and colleagues[19] suggested that, regardless of symptoms, children with CCAVB should receive permanent cardiac pacemakers prior to adolescence in order to avoid syncope, irreversible myocardial dysfunction, and/or death.

Symptomatic bradycardia and/or recurrent bradycardia-tachycardia syndrome can theoretically fall into the category of sick sinus syndrome, which is the next most common pacing indication in children. In general, sick sinus syndrome is acquired, although in rare cases it can be congenital.[20] The operation that most commonly results in sick sinus syndrome in children is the Mustard/Senning repair for d-transposition of the great arteries, with the need for a permanent pacemaker increasing with time from the initial repair.[21] The presence of concomitant tachyarrhythmias in these patients is common, often necessitating treatment with antiarrhythmic drugs that can further compromise sinus node function and AV node function as well.

Other less common indications for permanent pacemakers in children include advanced symptomatic second-degree AV block, 2:1 AV block due to a markedly prolonged QT interval, and hypertrophic obstructive cardiomyopathy. Patients with hypertrophic cardiomyopathy receive permanent pacemakers to decrease aortic outflow tract gradients by preexcitation of the right ventricular apex. This has resulted in improved hemodynamics and decreased symptomatology in some pediatric patients.[22]

Pacing System Selection

The choice as to the most appropriate pulse generator, pacing mode, and pacing leads for a specific patient as well as the pacing indication for that patient is multifaceted. Such determining factors include the specific electrophysiologic indication (i.e., sinus bradycardia or AV block), the patient's overall cardiac condition, the size of the patient, the percentage of time that the device will be required to stimulate (versus sensing), and the need for battery longevity. The goal of the pacing system should be to "mimic" the normal conduction system as much as possible in order to improve the patient's overall hemodynamics, since an abnormal pattern of myocardial activation has been shown in recent animal studies[23] to contribute to the long-term development of myocardial changes.

Pulse Generator

The specific pulse generator should match the patient's pacing indication as closely as possible. The chosen device should be capable of pacing in a variety of modes, which are comprised using the pacemaker mode code found in Table 2. In the patient with complete AV block and normal sinus node function, a pacemaker capable of atrial synchronous (DDD) pacing would be most appropriate. In the patient with complete AV block and existing or a predisposition to sinus node dysfunction, the addition of a sensor (DDDR) is preferred.

In patients with sinus node dysfunction with intact AV nodal conduction, atrial pacing (AAICO) is the mode of choice.[21] Some physicians recommend that AV node function be evaluated by electrophysiology testing prior to permanent atrial pacing because AV node disease is not always apparent in the resting state.[17] If there is chronotropic incompetence in the aforementioned patient, rate adaptation in the single chamber mode (AAIRO) is most appropriate and if there is documented intraatrial reentry tachycardia (IART) or suspicion that the patient may develop it in the future, atrial antitachycardia pacing (AAICP) is the pacing mode of choice.[24–26]

Table 2
Revised NASPE/BPG Pacemaker Code

Position Category	I Chamber(s) paced	II Chamber(s) sensed	III Response to sensing modulation	IV Program-mability;rate function	V Antitachy-arrhythmia
	0 = none A = atrium	0 = none A = atrium	0 = none T = trig-gered	0 = none P = simple program-mable	0 = none P = pacing (antitachy-arrhythmia)
	V = ventricle	V = ventricle	I = inhib-ited	M = multi-program-mable	
	D = dual (A + V)	D = dual (A + V)	D = dual (T + I)	C = com-municating R = rate modulation	S = shock D = dual (P + S)
Manufactur-ers' designa-tion only	S = single	S = single (A or V)	(A or V)		

Positions I through III are used exclusively for antibradyarrhythmia function.
NASPE = North American Society of Pacing and Electrophysiology; BPG = British Pacing Group.
From: Gillette PC, Garson A, Jr.: Pediatric Arrhythmias: Electrophysiology and Pacing. Philadelphia: WB Saunders Company; 1990, with permission.

Single chamber, fixed-rate ventricular pacemakers are being used less frequently in the pediatric population. The patient requiring infrequent pacing might be best suited for a single chamber ventricular pacemaker, without rate adaptation (VVICO). A postoperative patient with intermittent (i.e., 10 to 20 min/day) AV block 7 to 10 days after open heart surgery would be the most likely candidate for this type of device. Patients with extremely poor venous access may benefit from single chamber pacing with rate adaptation (VVIRO).

Rate-adaptive devices are used when there is a need for a sensor that the cardiac conduction system is no longer capable of providing.[27] These sensors include activity-triggered devices such as those with a piezoelectric crystal or accelerometer, or minute ventilation, which uses impedance pneumography. There are several current devices that are capable of providing both types of sensors, either alone or in combination. Since the healthy child is capable of a linear heart rate increase with increasing exercise intensity,[28] the sensor should be capable of allowing an appropriate rate increase to exercise, but also a slower rate of decrease following exercise.

The availability of certain programming options is very important for pediatric pacemaker recipients. In many patients, an upper tracking limit of 180 pulses per minute (ppm) is desired, so the device must be capable of providing high upper rate limits. Adaptive AV intervals that shorten with increasing atrial rates are important in the pediatric pacemaker recipient, as are short post ventricular atrial refractory periods (PVARPs) that allow Wenckebach, rather than 2:1 block, at the upper rate limit. Because many postoperative CHD patients are at risk for developing atrial tachycardia, a device capable of mode switching or providing the DDI pacing mode is an attractive option. Other desirable features include high outputs (especially for use with epicardial leads), higher lower rates (for newborns, infants, and postoperative patients), and the option to decrease the lower pacing rate at night when the patient is sleeping.

Lead Selection

When choosing the pacing lead(s) most appropriate for each individual patient, the first decision is to determine which implant technique, epicardial versus endocardial, will be used.[29-31] Since the epicardial technique is more invasive, often results in higher stimulation thresholds and/or lead fractures, and results in decreased pacemaker longevity,[32] it is generally reserved for those few cases in which endocardial pacing is contraindicated.[33-35] These contraindications include weight of less than 5.0 kg, intracardiac shunts, a superior vena cava that does not connect at the atrial level, an anatomy that does not allow venous access to the chamber requiring lead placement, such as that of the Fontan patient with complete AV block, and right-sided prosthetic valves.

When using the epicardial implant technique, the choice of pacing leads is somewhat limited.[36-39] Although there have been some reports of placing endocardial bipolar pacing leads transatrially,[40] the placement of unipolar, epicardial pacing leads is more commonplace. The three most commonly used unipolar leads include the stab-on (or fish hook), the screw-in, and the steroid-eluting suture-on electrode. The latter has become the epicardial pacing lead of choice at the authors' institutions, because of its small contact surface area, low chronic pacing thresholds, excellent sensing characteristics, and applicability to both the atria and ventricles for chronic cardiac pacing.[33,41,42] This type of lead may not be ideal in a patient with severe epicardial fibrosis, in which case a fishhook or screw-in lead might be more optimal for epicardial penetration. This suture-on lead has recently become available in a bipolar configuration as well.

When using the endocardial or transvenous implant technique, bipolar pacing leads are preferable to unipolar leads.[43] Although they are minimally larger than their unipolar counterparts, they are less likely to sense skeletal muscle and cause stimulation of that muscle, due to the close interelectrode spacing. The type of lead fixation is variable as is the length of the lead. For atrial placement in small children as well as those postoperative for CHD, an actively fixated, screw-in lead is clearly preferred, although some authors recommend using all active fixation leads in children because they are easily repositioned and/or extracted.[44] Passively fixated, tined leads can be considered for placement in the ventricle. Overall, silastic insulation has proven to last longer than polyurethane and is favored for pediatric use where longevity is highly desirable.

Steroid-eluting leads, both actively and passively fixated, have proven to result in increased longevity due to lower acute and chronic pacing thresholds.[6,35] A fixed screw-in, steroid-eluting, silastically insulated lead is the bipolar pacing lead of choice in the authors' institutions. Chronic pacing leads must be extremely flexible and have a short interelectrode distance for optimal sensing capabilities. Leads with extendable/retractable screws tend to irritate the child's heart due to their inherent stiffness. Single pass (VDD) leads have been used in children.[45,46] These leads were designed with the gallant intent of providing AV synchrony with the use of one lead versus two, but problems with the spacing of the atrial electrode from the electrode tip, the inability to atrial pace, and the increased potential for electrode failure have limited their use in the pediatric population.

The length of the lead is also an important consideration in children. It is not preferable, even in the smallest of infants, to use extremely short epicardial pacing leads. If the chronic pacing thresholds are low, the potential for the device to last more than 3 years is high. With the amount of growth experienced from the newborn to preschool years, a very short lead may become taut enough to fracture. In very young patients requiring epicardial pacing lead placement, a 35-cm lead is preferred. In older patients, a 50-cm lead is used.

For endocardial placement, the size of the child at the time of lead placement is important. The use of an absorbable suture at the site of lead tie-down allows inward migration of the pacing lead as the child grows.

Again, a medium length is preferable to a shorter one in order to get as much use from the original lead as possible. In the authors' institutions, in children who have not yet reached adolescence, a 45-cm and 52-cm lead are used for the atrium and ventricle, respectively. In adolescents and young adults, especially those who are very tall or who are expected to become very tall, a 52-cm lead is used in each chamber.

Implant Technique

As previously discussed, the implant technique is determined by the size of the child, the presence of intracardiac shunts, superior vena cava obstruction, lack of a connection at the atrial level, or structural anatomy that precludes endocardial lead placement.[30,47,48] All pertinent noninvasive data should be reviewed prior to system implantation including 12-lead electrocardiogram (ECG), 24-hour ambulatory monitor, exercise stress testing (if applicable), previous operative/catheterization reports, current medications, and, importantly, an echocardiogram. All efforts to determine the presence of intracardiac shunting should be undertaken prior to pacemaker placement, since the incidence of embolic events is increased in these patients.[49] In some cases, this may require contrast or transesophageal echocardiography. The following discussion includes descriptions of the transvenous/endocardial technique of pacemaker placement, the variable approaches for epicardial placement, and, importantly, intraoperative testing.

Endocardial/Transvenous Technique

The endocardial or transvenous implant technique is generally performed in the pediatric catheterization/electrophysiology laboratory by a team consisting of individuals who routinely care for children and who have a working knowledge of caring for children with CHD. The optimal laboratory is one that implants more than 20 pacemakers per year and is also used for other major interventional procedures.[50] Sterility and air handling/filtration standards should be consistent with the operating room, and staff must remain cognizant of maintaining strict sterile technique.

Most patients undergoing transvenous pacemaker implantation receive general anesthesia. Once adequate anesthesia has been obtained, the authors require groin preparation in order to place an indwelling arterial line for invasive blood pressure monitoring and blood gas analysis throughout the procedure. Additionally, a venous catheter (which can also be used as a temporary pacing catheter) is placed via the femoral vein all the way into the subclavian vein for a hand contrast injection to demonstrate venous anatomy (Fig. 1). Preapplied self-adhesive pacing/defibrillation electrodes are placed prior to the procedure in the event that temporary pacing becomes necessary, which occasionally occurs when devices have reached elective replacement.

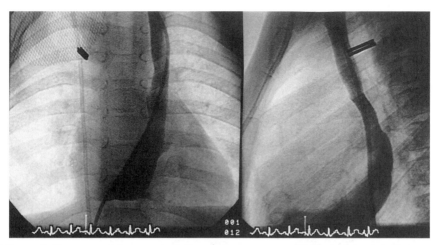

Figure 1. Fluoroscopic image of a left superior vena cava (SVC) draining into the coronary sinus. There is no evidence of a "bridging vein" between the left and right SVCs. It is important to identify this congenital anomaly prior to transvenous pacemaker implantation.

In most pediatric patients, the pacemaker is placed in a pocket in the left shoulder, although some centers place the device on the opposite side of the patient's handedness. An incision of approximately 125% of the pacemaker's diameter is generally made one to two finger breadths below the clavicle to accommodate the pulse generator that is being implanted. In the majority of young patients, the preferred implant site is below the pectoralis major muscle (i.e., subpectoral).[51] This is preferable not only because it looks better cosmetically, but because it tends to protect the device somewhat from injury and/or infection as well.

Once the pocket has been created, the subclavian vein is punctured under fluoroscopy (Fig. 2). A cutdown to the subclavian is generally not performed secondary to the risk of inadvertent arterial or lung puncture. Once access is obtained, a guidewire is placed into the needle and passed to the right atrium or inferior vena cava. A sheath is then positioned over the wire with subsequent removal of the dilator and guidewire. The lead is then inserted into the sheath for positioning in the atrium or ventricle. If two leads are being placed, a second sheath/dilator is used for the second lead, which can be positioned with a second puncture or by the retained guidewire technique utilizing the initial sheath. A second puncture leads to less bleeding and less "drag" when the leads are manipulated. The leads are affixed either actively or passively and the lead stylets and sheaths are removed.

Once the stylets and sheaths are removed, the leads are acutely tested with an external device. Once adequate pacing and sensing thresholds have been obtained, the leads are secured with absorbable suture and attached to the pulse generator. Pocket closure, including the pectoral and

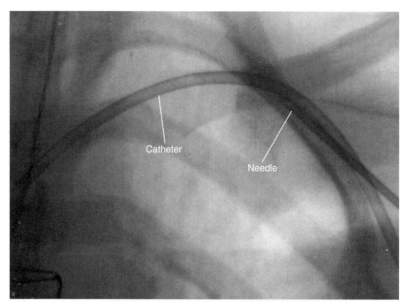

Figure 2. Fluoroscopic images of a radiopaque diagnostic catheter that has been placed from the femoral vein as an "aiming catheter." It passes through the right atrium into the left axillary vein and the needle is then introduced through the subpectoral pocket into the vein with fluoroscopic guidance.

subcutaneous layers, is performed using absorbable sutures also. Steri-strips are placed vertically over the incision to approximate the skin edges, followed by a telfa pad and gauze dressing secured with paper tape. The venous and arterial lines are removed with placement of the usual postcatheterization pressure dressing. The patient is then usually extubated and transferred to the postanesthesia care unit for 1 to 2 hours before being transferred to a telemetry-monitored hospital bed.

Epicardial Technique

Epicardial pacing system implantations are performed in the operating room, with the patient under general anesthesia. Typically, the unipolar pacing configuration is used, with the body of the pulse generator functioning as the indifferent electrode. The current availability of bipolar, steroid-eluting epicardial leads may change this practice in patients who have adequate space on their epicardium for electrode placement. In addition to the usual advantages of using bipolar versus unipolar leads, the former have a higher impedance, which will hopefully lead to increased pacemaker longevity. The specific approach to pacemaker placement must be individualized for each patient and his or her specific clinical situation. Epicardial pacing electrodes can be placed using the following approaches: me-

dian sternotomy, subxiphoid approach, or thoracotomy. The median sternotomy approach is used most often in the authors' institutions due to the
large number of dual chamber implants and the excellent results with the
steroid-eluting epicardial pacing lead. This approach allows better visualization and "pace mapping" for atrial pacing electrode placement.

Median Sternotomy

The median sternotomy approach provides excellent access to the
atrial and ventricular surfaces, especially in neonates and small infants.
Despite the need for sternal division, this approach results in optimum
electrode placement, lower acute and chronic pacing thresholds, excellent
sensing of intrinsic deflections, and extended battery longevity.

After adequate general anesthesia has been obtained, a midline incision is performed and may be extended into the upper abdomen if the generator is to be placed through the same incision. Alternately, a separate
transverse left upper quadrant abdominal incision can be used for creation of the pulse generator pocket. Once a median or partial sternotomy
is performed, the pocket is created. For a subfascial pocket, the anterior
rectus fascia is opened using electrocautery to create the pocket. For a
subrectus pocket, the rectus muscle is retracted laterally from the midline
and the dissection carried out by staying anterior to the posterior rectus
fascia or by splitting the rectus muscle fibers by dissection.

The pericardium is then opened to expose the epicardium and a pericardial well is created with stay sutures. Steroid-eluting leads can then
be used to map the atrial and ventricular surfaces by holding the electrode
firmly against the epicardial surface. Intrinsic deflections can be measured and pacing thresholds performed. Once a suitable site has been selected, the preferred steroid-eluting lead is fixated by securing the surface
of the lead with nonabsorbable suture. The fixation is important to prevent motion of the electrode surface against the epicardium; such motion
could potentially lead to chronic irritation, fibrosis, and elevated chronic
pacing thresholds. It is also important to avoid ischemia of the underlying myocardium with incorrectly or too tightly placed sutures.[52]

After the leads have been sutured in place, intraoperative testing is
performed. If the measurements are acceptable, the leads are tunneled via
a subxiphoid route to the pulse generator pocket. In order to avoid lead
fracture, the leads are not tunneled between or over the ribs. Acute bend-
ing of the lead at the subcostal border must be avoided to prevent the possibility of lead fracture. A loop of electrode is left within the mediastinum
to allow for growth and to prevent stretching of the lead against the rib
cage that leads to potential fracture during movement and/or growth. The
leads are connected to the pulse generator and placed into the abdominal
pocket with the noninsulated aspect of the generator facing away from the
muscle. Redundant lead length is gently looped beneath the pulse gener-

ator. Excessive intrapericardial loops are avoided so that vascular structure or chamber entrapment does not occur.[53–55] The pericardial edges are loosely reapproximated and a temporary drainage catheter is placed within the mediastinum. The sternal edges are subsequently reapproximated and the sternal incision closed in the usual manner.

Subxiphoid Approach

The subxiphoid approach can also be used for epicardial pacemaker implantation, including the placement of dual chamber systems.[56,57] The advantages of this approach include minimal postoperative morbidity and an excellent cosmetic result. Through a single incision the epicardium can be exposed, electrodes placed, and the pulse generator pocket created.[58] A short upper midline abdominal incision is used and the rectus fascia opened to expose the diaphragm and pericardium. With anterior retraction of the sternum, the pericardium is incised and the epicardial surface exposed. Appropriate leads are placed and intraoperative testing is performed. The leads are then tunneled into the pacemaker pocket and, as described previously, additional electrode length is left in the mediastinum and in the pocket. The edges of the fascia are reapproximated and the wound is closed in layers. This approach provides good access to the ventricular epicardium but has limited exposure to the atrium, making placement of the steroid-eluting lead somewhat difficult, especially in small infants. This approach may also be problematic in the patient requiring reoperation in whom there is significant epicardial fibrosis.

Thoractomy

The thoracotomy approach to epicardial pacemaker implantation is being used less frequently than in the past. This approach may be beneficial in patients who have previously undergone cardiac surgery and in very small neonates. Dual chamber pacing is possible with this approach, although left atrial pacing is required when using a left-sided approach. An anterior thoracotomy through the fourth to sixth intercostal space is used to expose the pericardium. The pericardium itself is opened longitudinally with care taken to avoid the phrenic nerve. An appropriate site for lead placement is selected and intraoperative testing is performed. The pulse generator is placed in an abdominal pocket through a separate subcostal incision. The leads are tunneled below the costophrenic angle into the pulse generator pocket. It is important that the leads not be passed above the ribs in order to avoid lead fracture. Again, a gentle loop of lead is left in the mediastinum and the redundant lead looped underneath the pulse generator. Tension on the lead should be avoided as it passes under the costophrenic angle, to prevent rubbing of the lead against the rib cage and making it subject to lead fracture. The thoracotomy incision is then closed in the standard fashion.

General Considerations

Epicardial pacing systems are implanted in patients while they are under general anesthesia, and prophylactic antibiotics are initiated preoperatively and administered for 24 hours postoperatively. The generator pocket is created first so that the use of electrocautery can be minimized once the electrodes have been placed, reducing the potential for "microburns," scarring at the electrode tip, and potential early lead abandonment.[59,60] In most cases, the pulse generators are placed on the left side of the abdomen so as not to impede physical examination of the liver, although generators have been placed on the right side of the abdomen in the presence of a gastrostomy tube. Subcutaneous abdominal pockets should be avoided in children because of the possibility of migration and erosion of the pulse generator. Additionally, subcutaneous placement generally results in a poorer cosmetic result. The subrectus location provides added protection to the generator, lowers the risk of erosion and/or wound infection, and is cosmetically superior in small patients.[61]

Intraoperative Testing

Intraoperative testing is best performed by a clinician with a background in pediatric pacing. When a center has manufacturer representatives assist with pacemaker implantation in children, the center should ensure that specific issues are taken into consideration, since the majority of these representatives have minimal experience with the pediatric population. Intraoperative testing begins long before the leads require evaluation, with the preprogramming of the pulse generator that will be implanted. This is true for initial pacemaker implantation as well as for replacements for pacemaker battery depletion.

Pacemaker Preprogramming

The soon to be implanted device is interrogated and preprogrammed still within its sterile packaging prior to implantation. The lead polarity and pacemaker polarity should be the same, which may or may not require reprogramming. Most devices are programmed to nominal settings prior to implantation, and certain programmed values require reevaluation. Since acute pacing thresholds rise to a peak value in the first few weeks after implant,[62] the authors use a standardized output setting of 5.0 V and 0.5 ms at the time of implant. The rate of the pulse generator should be programmed to meet the individual needs of each patient (i.e. age, hemodynamic benefit, optimal electrophysiologic benefit). In a dual chamber system (DDDCO), the lowest acceptable atrial rate for the patient is chosen as the permanently programmed lower rate. In a rate-adaptive system, the lower rate chosen should be age appropriate, with a higher sensor-driven upper rate. In patients receiving atrial antitachycardia devices (AAICP), a "faster" than normal bradycardia pacing rate is used in an attempt to decrease ectopy and prevent tachycardia episodes that may be bradycardia induced.[63]

The sensitivity can be programmed prior to implantation, but it may require readjustment based on the intrinsic deflections obtained with lead placement. Although a setting of 1.0 mV is acceptable for atrial sensitivity, the authors generally use 0.5 mV due to the fact that the atrial electrogram amplitude decreases with exercise in children.[64] When this setting is used in patients with intraatrial tachycardia, it often results in R wave oversensing on the atrial electrogram; however, less sensitive settings may result in undersensing of the atrial tachycardia.[65] The ventricular sensitivity is programmed from 2.8 to 4.0 mV depending on the intrinsic R wave deflection.

The upper rate limit in a dual chamber device should be programmed to a value that is acceptable for the patient's age and hemodynamic status. It may not always be desirable for postoperative patients to sense the atrium to rates of 180 ppm. Also, the "true tracking limit" must be recognized as the total atrial refractory period, i.e., the sum of the AV delay and the PVARP. If the total atrial refractory period is less than the programmed upper rate limit, the device will exhibit 2:1 AV block *before* Wenckebach, the latter of which is the desired upper rate limit behavior in children.

The AV delay is programmed anywhere from 75 to 100 ms in the neonate to 120 to 150 ms in older patients and in those with postoperative CHD. The availability of rate-adaptive AV delays has been of great benefit in pediatric patients, since it mimics the physiologic adaptation to a shorter PR interval with increasing atrial rates.[66]

The ventricular refractory period, used primarily to prevent T wave oversensing, is generally programmed to 200 ms. Ventricular blanking must be programmed in such a way that premature ventricular events are appropriately sensed and sensing of atrial signals on the ventricular channel is alleviated. For most pediatric patients, this parameter can be programmed to the lowest available setting without unwanted sequelae. Rate-adaptive parameters are generally programmed to the "nominal settings" until postprocedure testing can be performed to ascertain the most appropriate settings for each individual patient.[67] Specific events in the postoperative period, i.e., chest percussion or ventilatory support, may preclude the programming of rate-adaptive parameters at the time of implantation. Antitachycardia functions can be programmed based on the patient's clinical tachycardia in most cases and should be patient and tachycardia specific. In many patients, a detection algorithm of high rate and sudden onset are sufficient for recognizing most IARTs.

Acute Threshold Testing

Once the lead(s) is/are positioned, the sterile test cables are attached to the lead and the pacing system analyzer (PSA). The pacing mode used for acute lead testing depends on how many leads are placed. When using two leads, the authors use the DOO mode for testing in order to obtain a higher atrial pacing rate. Once capture is verified in the patient who is minimally paralyzed with muscle relaxants, a high output of 10.0 V and 2.0 ms is used to evaluate the presence of diaphragmatic or phrenic nerve stimulation. In some cases, this high output setting will result in the atrial lead pacing the ventricle; this is of little clinical significance in this setting. If diaphragmatic pacing or phrenic nerve stimulation occurs, the lead is repositioned. This high output test is not accurate in the patient who is maximally medicinally paralyzed.

Lead resistance (impedance) measurements are obtained at 5.0 V and 0.5 ms and vary according to lead polarity and manufacturer characteristics. An acceptable range for lead resistance in an acute lead is from 250 to 1500 Ω. If an extreme measurement is obtained (e.g., too high or too low), all connections from the PSA to the lead are verified and the measurement repeated. For chronic lead testing in pulse generator replacements, a difference of 200 Ω from the initial measurement is acceptable.[65]

Pacing thresholds are obtained for one or two leads depending on the number of leads implanted. The acute pacing threshold is considered to be the lowest output setting (voltage) that captures the chamber being paced 100% of the time. In the authors' institutions, a voltage threshold is performed at a constant pulse width, but testing can be performed in the opposite manner as well. Acceptable acute pacing threshold ranges are 0.5 to 2.5 V for the atrium and 0.5 to 2.0 V for the ventricle. Again, these voltage thresholds are performed at 0.5 ms.

Intrinsic deflections should be obtained at implant whenever possible. These values should be compatible with the available sensitivity settings of the implanted pulse generator. The intrinsic atrial deflection or atrial electrogram should be at least 1.0 mV, with an acceptable range of 1 to 5 mV. Many postoperative patients have very small atrial signals, which again stresses the importance of available programmable parameters and intrinsic deflection measurement compatibilities. The actual intrinsic deflection measurement can be obtained using the PSA or through a physiologic recorder (Fig. 3). It is preferable to have little to no R wave on the atrial electrogram. The ventricular intrinsic deflection or R wave electrogram should range from 4 to 7 mV and again must be compatible with the available ventricular sensitivity settings within the implanted pulse generator.

Once all acute lead measurements have been obtained, the generator is attached and placed in the pocket and a telemetry measurement is obtained with the sterile programming wand. This will provide baseline impedance measurements through the programmer and will also verify that there are no connector problems prior to pocket closure. A sterile magnet, which forces the device to pace asynchronously, can be used at this time to verify pacing and capture of the implanted device.

In the patient receiving unipolar leads, an indifferent electrode must be

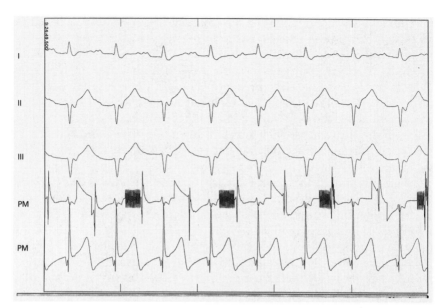

Figure 3. Surface ECG leads I, II, and III with intrinsic deflections from an atrial and ventricular lead, respectively, as seen through a physiologic recorder. A 1-mV calibration mark is seen on the atrial electrogram.

used for testing. This electrode provides a "ground" for the unipolar system. It is placed in the pocket and the terminal end is attached to the positive clip (versus the negative clip) on the test cables. The negative clip is attached to the lead's connector pin in order for testing to be accomplished. Additionally, once the unipolar device is attached to the leads, pacemaker function *cannot* be verified until the device has been placed in the pacemaker pocket.

The clinician should ensure proper documentation in the patient's record, including the model and serial numbers of all implanted components, implant measurements, and programmed pacemaker parameters. The manufacturer's implant record should be accurately and completely filled out, with copies distributed to the manufacturer, the implanting physician, the patient's medical record, and the patient's pacemaker clinic record.

Implications for Clinicians

Nurses and other clinicians caring for pediatric pacemaker recipients are presented with multiple challenges.[68] Children are a unique population who require that a family-centered approach be used to fulfill their needs before, during, and after pacemaker implantation. One of the most critical aspects of caring for the pediatric pacemaker recipient is that of patient and family education. This aspect of the patient's overall plan of care is discussed in detail in the section on patient and family considerations. The following discussion includes, specifically, the implications for clinicians in a variety of roles who care for these patients and their families. It addresses what the clinician must know prior to implementing an educational plan as well as specific issues to consider when planning care before, during, and immediately after pacemaker implantation.

Baseline Knowledge for the Clinician

In order to provide expert care, the clinician must have specific baseline knowledge regarding certain aspects of pediatric pacing. The clinician must be knowledgeable regarding the indications for pacemaker implantation, and should be able to apply these guidelines to each individual patient. Although some pediatric patients may remain asymptomatic from a parent's perspective, the clinician must be able to explain the reason for pacemaker implantation. For example, many children with CCAVB compensate for the lack of AV synchrony and bradycardia, appearing similar to other children their age regarding activity levels; however, upon routine follow-up, the physician will document increasing heart size and decreasing ventricular function indicating the necessity for pacemaker implantation. The clinician must be able to use this knowledge to help the patients and their families understand why implantation is necessary at this time.

Clinicians must also be able to understand and identify the components of the pacing system. The pacemaker itself is a battery-operated pulse generator that houses the device's microcircuitry, battery, and header, and is made of titanium. The microcircuitry or brain of the pacemaker is similar to a computer that is intelligent enough to convert energy from the battery into an electrical impulse. The battery, made of lithium iodide, is housed inside the pacemaker and generates the energy that produces the electrical impulse. The battery's longevity is dependent on many factors which makes it difficult to explain to patients and families "how long the battery will last." The longevity of any given pacemaker battery is dependent on the programmed rate, the number of chambers being paced, the programmed output, the size of the battery, and the percentage of time that the device actually paces. Because of all of these factors and because of the variability from patient to patient, it is difficult to speculate on exactly how long a pacemaker will last; thus, what clinicians involved in the care of children receiving cardiac pacemakers should tell patients and their families about pacemaker battery longevity is that it is nearly impossible to say exactly "how long" the device will last.

The pacemaker header sits atop the pacemaker can and houses a connector for one end of the pacemaker lead. The permanent pacing lead is a thin, insulated wire that contains an electrode (or electrodes) on its end and is generally coated with silicone or polyurethane. The lead is responsible for carrying the electrical impulse from the pulse generator to the heart. The lead tip or electrode is in direct contact with the heart and can be actively (via a screw) or passively (via fins) fixated/attached to the heart.

The third component to the clinician's knowledge base is the differentiation between the epicardial and endocardial/transvenous implant techniques. Since the transvenous technique is generally preferable to the epicardial technique, it is important to be able to explain to patients and families the reason that the epicardial technique is being used. In general, it is chosen because of the patient's size or cardiovascular anatomy. Anatomic reasons for using the epicardial technique include lack of venous access, such as in the patient who has undergone a Fontan repair and has complete AV block, the presence of intracardiac shunts, and/or stenosed or thrombosed veins commonly used for transvenous lead placement.

Prior to the Procedure

The team of clinicians who care for children undergoing permanent pacemaker implantation is multifaceted with ongoing specific responsibilities. While some clinicians are responsible for ensuring certain elements regarding the patient, others will have specific tasks related to the catheterization/electrophysiology laboratory or operating room. The following discussion regarding preprocedural tasks includes patient considerations and laboratory considerations.

Patient Considerations

Although in most centers at which transvenous pacemaker implantation is performed patients are admitted for a least one night after device placement, the push to perform more of these procedures as outpatient or 23-hour observational stays is on the rise. Since nearly all patients are now admitted the day of the procedure, most patients are required to come in the day before for a preprocedural work-up and evaluation. This evaluation generally includes specific preprocedural tests ordered by the implanting physician as well as a history and physical examination.

The clinician should make sure that the patient and family know where to report on this day, and that they have an idea of how long the testing will take and what to expect in regard to the tests that the child will undergo. Potential diagnostic tests that may be ordered by the implanting physician prior to the procedure include blood work, urinalysis, chest radiograph, 12-lead ECG, 24-hour ambulatory monitor, exercise stress test, and echocardiogram. It is the policy in the authors' institutions that all females 12 years and older undergo pregnancy testing prior to the procedure. Blood work may include a complete blood count, clotting studies, and a type and cross-match for one unit of packed red blood cells. The authors rarely obtain a urinalysis or chest radiograph unless particulars of a specific patient's clinical condition deem it necessary. A 12-lead ECG is nearly always obtained and routine 24-hour monitors are seldom obtained again just prior to the procedure unless the physician is trying to ascertain more specific information. An exercise stress test may be undertaken in order to assist the physician in determining the type and mode of the specific pacemaker to be implanted. An echocardiogram is almost always performed in order to obtain a final disposition regarding the presence of intracardiac shunts and in many patients with postoperative CHD it is performed with contrast.

Patients should also be evaluated for the type of anesthesia to be used, with special emphasis on previous sedation/anesthesia experience. Many centers now use general anesthesia for permanent pacemaker implantation outside of the operating room. It is important that the patient and family meet with anesthesia personnel prior to the procedure in order to know what type of sedation agents will be used for the child's procedure as well as when to withhold food and fluids from the child in preparation for the implant procedure. The clinician should provide the anesthesia personnel with any records from previous hospitalizations, procedures, and/or surgeries, especially in children who have congenital anomalies, cardiovascular or otherwise, and those with previous airway problems.

The clinician should also ensure that the patient and family meet with the implanting physician to have answered any further questions about the pacemaker itself as well as about the procedure and recovery period. At this time, consent for the procedure is obtained. After all diagnostic tests are complete and the family has met with the anesthesia personnel, the clinician should review with the patient and family the plans for the day of the procedure. This review should include where to report on the day of the procedure, what to bring on the day of the procedure, the child's NPO (nothing by mouth) orders, and an overview of what to expect on procedure day, including approximately how long the procedure will take, where the family is expected to wait during the procedure, where the child will go after the procedure, and how the family will get messages about their child during the procedure.

Once the preprocedural work-up has been completed, the clinician should ensure the availability of any and all necessary supplies that may be required during the pacemaker implant procedure. If the procedure consists of a generator replacement only, the clinician should be knowledgeable enough about lead connector and pulse generator compatibilities to have the correct supplies available. The fact that most manufacturers have recently made an effort to make the lead connectors universally compatible has made this less of an issue than in the past. A duplicate of each lead and pulse generator should be readily available. In addition, the following items are necessary: PSA with functioning batteries, sterile test cables, extra lead stylets, indifferent electrode (for unipolar implants), appropriate screwdrivers (for generator replacements), sterile magnet, sterile programming wand, and a pacemaker-specific programmer.[65] Collaboration and communication between the implanting physician and the clinician or manufacturer's representative responsible for the technical pacemaker aspects of the procedure is critical.

Laboratory Considerations

Cardiovascular clinicians who are directly involved in the pacemaker implantation itself have more specific responsibilities regarding preparation of the procedure room as well as that of the patient. The major responsibility is to ensure the safest possible environment for the patient as well as for the staff. All electrical equipment should be properly grounded and in excellent working order as evidenced by frequent evaluations by the institution's biomedical department. The clinician working in the implant procedure room should have an adequately stocked supply of pacing system equipment as well as diagnostic and interventional catheters for any and all patient sizes and clinical situations. Specific equipment related to the pacemaker implant itself (Fig. 4) should be readily available,

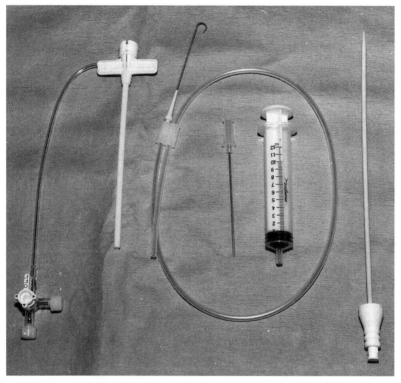

Figure 4. Pacemaker lead introducer kit. The sheath has a bleed back valve and is "tear away." The needle, wire, and dilator are used to introduce the sheath.

and includes surgical instruments, introducers, suture material, electrocautery, headlight, temporary pacing equipment, suction equipment, and resuscitation equipment. An additional tool that was recently adapted at the authors' institutions is an ultrasonic scalpel. In addition to avoiding the problems associated with electrocautery, it causes no interference with surface ECG monitoring and no false inhibition or triggering of the pacemaker in patients with existing pacemakers or defibrillators. It provides adequate cauterization without charring and is clearly cost effective in "redo" patients as well as in patients with permanent devices who are undergoing other surgical procedures.

Once the child has been brought into the laboratory or operating room, certain preparations are necessary prior to the start of the procedure itself. Adequate surface ECG electrode placement as it relates to the quality of the displayed ECG must be verified. If any problems are noted, they should be addressed before the patient is draped. The grounding pad for the electrocautery unit should be properly placed on the patient's thigh. The authors routinely place preapplied self-adhesive pads for temporary pacing as well as cardioversion/defibrillation. A pulse oximeter should also be placed on any extremity, with the exception of the extremity closest to the pacemaker pocket. Adequate body temperature for the individual patient should be monitored and maintained for the duration of the procedure. Adequate sterility procedures and radiation safety precautions should be used at all times.

During Implantation

Clinicians have many roles during the pacemaker implant procedure. Catheterization laboratory or operating room personnel must constantly assess the child's overall hemodynamic status. If conscious or deep sedation is used, the nurse managing the care of the patient should have no other responsibilities during the procedure so that he or she can ensure that the patient is always attended and constantly monitored.[69] The clinician should always be aware of the child's response to his or her bradyarrhythmia and should be able to assist with any emergency maneuvers if necessary. Knowledge of pediatric drug dosages is critical for nurses and other clinicians involved in caring for children undergoing pacemaker implantation. The clinician should constantly monitor the patient for any signs or symptoms of pacemaker- or procedure-related complications.

The clinician performing the intraoperative testing should remain cognizant of the particular phase of the implant procedure and should be ready to provide his or her services. Once the vein has been punctured, the clinician can open the lead's sterile packaging and hand the contents to the physician or his or her assistant in preparation for placement. The sterile test cables can be placed on the sterile field at this time. It is the responsibility of this particular individual to ensure that all documentation of the intraoperative testing is completed at the end of the procedure.

Immediately After Implantation

Once the procedure has been completed, the patient is transferred to the postanesthesia care unit or cardiovascular telemetry unit depending on whether general anesthesia or deep sedation was used, respectively. The clinician assuming care for the pediatric pacemaker recipient must obtain specific information regarding the implant procedure from the cardiac catheterization/electrophysiology laboratory or operating room personnel. This "report" should include the following: the type of pacemaker implanted, the pulse generator pocket location, any complications or problems encountered during the procedure, the type and amount of sedation/anesthesia used, catheter puncture sites (if applicable), the patient's underlying rhythm and pacing indication, and the following pacemaker parameters: pacing mode, pacing rate (upper and lower rates when applicable), output settings, sensitivity settings, refractory periods, rate-adaptive parameters (if applicable), sleep rate (if applicable), and the presence of drainage tubes (e.g., chest tube in epicardial pacemaker recipients).

The clinician assuming care for the patient should perform an overall clinical assessment of the patient immediately upon the patient's arrival to his or her unit. If venous and/or arterial catheters were placed, the puncture site(s) should be inspected for the presence of hemorrhage, swelling, or hematoma and the affected extremity evaluated for warmth, color, capillary refill, and palpable pulses. The child's level of consciousness and airway patency should be documented, as should heart rate and rhythm, blood pressure, respiratory rate (including any signs of difficulty or distress), and temperature. Telemetry should be placed upon the patient's arrival to the telemetry unit and a baseline recording obtained and compared with the pacemaker settings. Care should be taken not to place the electrodes over the pacemaker pocket in any pacemaker patient (acute or chronic) being monitored, because of the increased risk of infection if skin breakdown should occur underneath the electrode or when it is removed.

The postoperative orders should include frequent assessment of vital signs, including temperature in the immediate postoperative period. An intravenous line is left in place for hydration and medication administration, and oral fluids are allowed only when the patient is fully awake and alert. Ambulation is deferred for overnight, but is encouraged the next day. Medications include prophylactic antibiotics (e.g., Ancef 12.5 mg/kg every 6 hours for 8 doses at the authors' institutions for transvenous implants), acetaminophen with codeine for pain, acetaminophen for fever or mild pain, Decadron 1 to 2 mg every 6 hours for elevated acute pacing threshold, Phenergan for nausea and vomiting, and any medications previously prescribed prior to pacemaker implantation. A shoulder immobilizer is used on most patients with new endocardial leads, to decrease possibility of early lead dislodgment. All patients are monitored on telemetry until discharge by personnel knowledgeable about pacemakers, arrhythmias, and monitor artifacts; the risk of monitor failure to detect cardiac arrest in patients with pacemakers is decreased with the use of an "attended" system.[70]

The pacemaker dressing should be inspected frequently (with vital sign assessment), and any drainage noted on the bandage. If excessive drainage or hemorrhage is noted, the clinician should immediately notify the implanting physician. The intravenous site should be inspected for signs of infiltration and/or infection. Parents should be informed that pain medication is given on an "as needed" basis and that it should be requested before the child experiences excruciating pain. Pediatric patients in whom the system was implanted endocardially remain hospitalized for 2 days, and those in whom the system was implanted epicardially remain hospitalized for 4 days. The authors prefer to keep the transvenous implants for 48 hours, but this may change with the push by third party payers to discharge them earlier.

Pacemaker Rhythm Analysis

Clinicians caring for pediatric pacemaker recipients must understand basic pacing concepts and possess specialized knowledge in order to appropriately assess pacemaker rhythm strips. In order to evaluate pacemaker function, the clinician must at the very least know the pacemaker's programmed mode of operation and the pacing rate. There are four basic factors to consider when evaluating pacemaker function: pacing, capture, sensing, and the pacing interval. Specific questions to consider when evaluating these four factors, respectively, are: 1) Is the pacemaker pacing/firing at all and if so, is it at the preset rate? 2) Is a cardiac response elicited when the pacemaker fires? 3) Is the patient's intrinsic rhythm recognized? 4) What is the interval between paced beats (or between paced and intrinsic beats) and does it correlate with the prescribed pacing rate? By answering these basic questions, the clinician should be able to determine whether the pacemaker is functioning properly. Evaluation of pacing rate should always be made using a printed rhythm strip, not by using the heart rate displayed on the cardiac monitor, as the latter can be distorted by artifact or electrode movement.

The single chamber rhythm strip is relatively easy to decipher, although most pediatric patients generally receive dual chamber devices. The rhythm strip should be systematically evaluated by comparing the mode and pacing rate to that which is seen on the rhythm strip. In the VVI mode, (Fig. 5) capture is evident when a pacemaker stimulus/spike is followed by a paced QRS complex (Fig. 6). The paced QRS complex is generally wider than the native QRS complex due to an abnormal depolarization

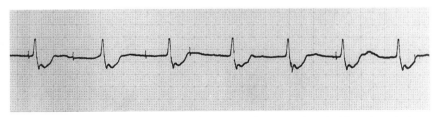

Figure 5. ECG recording of a ventricular demand pacemaker that is not capturing or sensing.

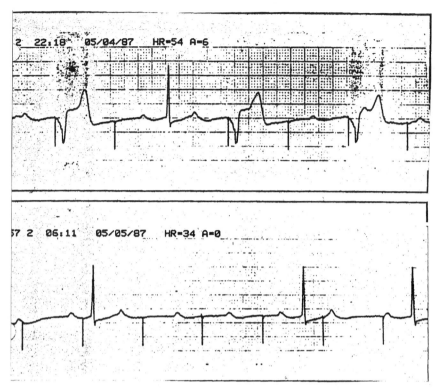

Figure 6. ECG recordings from a hospital telemetry unit on a patient with a ventricular demand pacemaker that is not capturing. Note the QRS duration on the paced versus the intrinsic beats.

pattern. The pacemaker stimulus should only be emitted if the patient's intrinsic ventricular rate is less than the prescribed pacing rate. The pacemaker is sensing appropriately if the child's ventricular rate exceeds that of the prescribed pacing rate and no pacemaker spikes are emitted.

When evaluating a rhythm strip on a child with an atrial demand or AAI pacemaker, the same approach as above is used. The pacing artifact should only be emitted when the child's *atrial* rate falls below that of the programmed pacing rate. If the child's atrial rate is faster than the programmed rate, the pacemaker should not emit a pacing stimulus if indeed it is sensing appropriately (Fig. 7). Depending on where the atrial lead was placed, the paced P wave may be positive or negative and may or may not have a similar appearance to the child's native P wave. It is important for clinicians to know that in the event of AV block in the patient with a functioning atrial pacemaker, the device may continue to pace the atrium with 100% capture *without* conduction to the ventricles.

In patients with single chamber devices with rate adaptation (VVIR or AAIR), the clinician needs additional information for pacemaker analysis. The sensor-driven pacemakers currently respond to physical activity or minute ventilation and allow the patient's heart rate to increase in re-

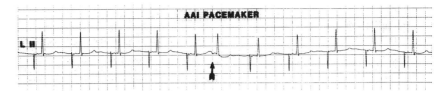

Figure 7. Surface ECG lead II on a patient with an atrial demand pacemaker. The first five beats are atrial paced beats, which are subsequently followed by a premature atrial contraction, which is appropriately sensed by the pacemaker.

sponse to either of these or a combination of both. In these devices, there is a lower and an upper pacing rate which the patient's rate may fluctuate between depending on activity or thoracic impedance. For example, if the lower rate is programmed to 60 ppm and the upper to 150 ppm, the paced rate may vary anywhere from 60 to 150 ppm.

Evaluation of the ECG rhythm strip of a patient with a dual chamber device becomes slightly more complicated. The clinician will need additional information for pacemaker rhythm analysis. The most commonly used dual chamber mode in children is the atrial synchronous or DDD mode. The DDD mode incorporates virtually every other pacing mode and can thus function in a variety of ways (Figs. 8 and 9). Additional parame-

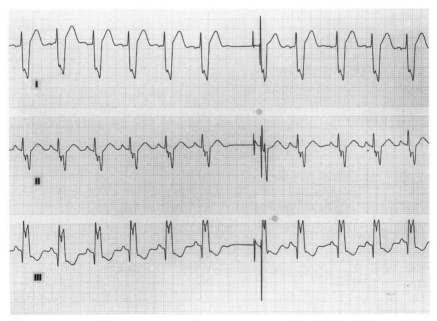

Figure 8. Surface ECG leads I, II, and III from a patient with right bundle branch block and sinus node dysfunction. The first six beats are sinus rhythm with right bundle branch block followed by a sinus pause that meets the lower rate criteria of the dual chamber pacemaker. Although there is a ventricular pacing spike emitted, it is considered a fusion beat because the QRS morphology is unchanged from the previous ones with right bundle branch block.

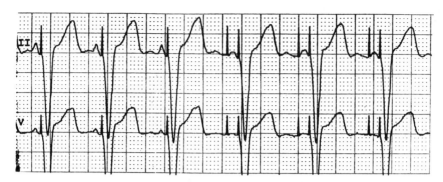

Figure 9. Simultaneous surface ECG leads on a patient with a DDD pacemaker. The first three beats are atrial synchronous with ventricular pacing. The sinus rate then slows to the lower rate limit and atrial and ventricular pacing ensues.

ters that the clinician must be knowledgeable about prior to rhythm strip analysis include lower rate, upper rate, AV delay (paced and sensed), refractory periods, and upper rate limit behavior. These and other terms commonly used when referring to pacemakers can be found in Table 3.

Kleinschmidt and Stafford[71] recommend using the following four steps to evaluate DDD pacemaker function: 1) Assess the presence and morphology of the P wave (sensed or paced), its rate, and its relationship to the rest of the cardiac cycle; 2) Assess/analyze the timing of the AV interval to determine whether an R wave/P wave is sensed and, if so, whether the ventricular and/or atrial output is inhibited; 3) Assess/evaluate the ventricular event in order to determine whether it is paced or sensed and whether or not it reset the ventricle-to-atrium (VA) interval; and 4) Assess the VA interval including its timing, presence of intrinsic cardiac activity, and the pacemaker's response to this activity.[71]

Dual chamber pacemakers can function in a variety of ways. They can sense the atrium and pace the ventricle, sense both the atrium and the ventricle and totally inhibit, pace the atrium and sense the ventricle (rarely), and pace both the atrium and the ventricle. An additional mode used in children with AV block and concomitant atrial reentrant tachycardias is the DDI mode. In this mode, atrial tracking does not occur; therefore, the device functions mostly in an AV sequential or ventricular demand mode in order to avoid the high tracking rates associated with atrial tachycardias. A characteristic behavior seen in dual chamber pacemakers programmed to the DDD mode is that of upper rate limit behavior (Fig. 10). If the pacemaker is programmed appropriately, this type of behavior will occur when the child's atrial rate reaches the programmed upper rate limit and will appear similar to Wenckebach on the surface ECG. This most commonly occurs in the immediate postoperative period when the child is emerging from anesthesia, is febrile, is experiencing pain, or is simply agitated.

Prior to discharge, all patients undergo the following tests: 12-lead ECG, chest radiograph, and noninvasive pacemaker testing. The chest ra-

Table 3
Terminology Associated with Cardiac Pacing

Unipolar	Having one "pole"; in a unipolar pacing system, one electrode is in or on the heart and the other is the pacemaker can itself.
Bipolar	Having two "poles"; in a bipolar pacing system, both electrodes are located on the lead in close proximity to each other.
End of life (EOL)	The point at which the pacemaker battery needs mandatory replacement because the usable energy is nearly exhausted.
Elective replacement indicator (ERI)	An indicator or sign that the pacemaker battery is nearing depletion, allowing time for an "elective" replacement; such indicators include change in pacing rate (magnet and/or nonmagnet), pacing mode, measured values, or telemetry message.
Capture	Depolarization and contraction of a chamber in response to electrical stimulation.
Sensing	The degree to which a pacing system "SEES"; it senses (sees) intrinsic P waves or R waves.
Oversensing	Sensing of events other than those which are desired; for example, R wave noted on the atrial lead, muscle artifact, environmental noise, etc.
Undersensing	Failure of the pacemaker to sense (see) intrinsic cardiac activity.
Sensing threshold	The minimum atrial or ventricular intracardiac signal amplitude required to inhibit or trigger a demand pacemaker.
Pacing threshold	The minimum amount of electricity/energy that is required to consistently depolarize the tissue being paced.
Lower rate	In a dual chamber device, the lowest possible atrial rate; in a rate-adaptive device, the lowest possible rate, either atrial or ventricular, depending on the programmed mode.

(continues)

Table 3
Terminology Associated with Cardiac Pacing (*cont.*)

Upper rate	In DDD mode, the highest rate that the atrium will be tracked by the ventricle in a 1:1 manner; in a rate-adaptive device the highest paced rate, either atrial or ventricular, depending on the programmed mode.
Upper rate limit behavior	In DDD mode, the response of the pacemaker to the upper rate; in most cases, it is Wenckebach behavior, but other responses include fallback, 2:1 block, and rate smoothing.
Telemetry	In pacing, this refers to information received from the pacemaker through an external programmer via radiofrequency signals; this information may include battery status, impedance measurements, intrinsic signals, and event data.
Program	The act of making a noninvasive adjustment of the implanted device.
Pulse width	Also known as pulse duration; the length of time the pacing stimulus is applied; it is expressed in milliseconds.
Pulse amplitude	The magnitude of the pacemaker's output voltage; generally expressed in volts, but is also expressed in milliamperes.
Refractory period	In a pacemaker, the refractory period is a time when the device is unresponsive to all intrinsic signals from the heart.
Impedance	Also known as resistance; total opposition to current flow; expressed in ohms.
Rate-adaptive pacing	Pacing in which the rate changes in response to an internal sensor; this sensor could be body movement or activity and/or minute ventilation.

diograph verifies lead position and can verify such complications as pneumothorax or hemothorax. The ECG will depict pacemaker function, i.e., pacing and/or sensing. The pacemaker testing includes the performance of pacing thresholds, sensing thresholds, and determination of underlying rhythm. Diagnostic data counters are programmed at this time, as well as any other parameters requiring programming or reprogramming. Patients

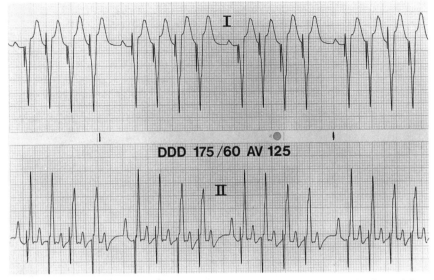

Figure 10. Upper rate limit behavior in a dual chamber pacemaker. As the atrial rate approaches 175 ppm, the atrial sense and ventricular pace interval increases until the P wave falls in the post ventricular refractory period resulting in nonsensing of one P wave. The rhythm resumes after the next P wave and resembles a Wenckebach pattern, typical of desirable upper rate limit behavior.

who have undergone epicardial pacemaker placement may undergo echocardiography to assess for pericardial or pleural effusions as well.

Discharge Planning

Prior to discharge, the dressing is removed from the pacemaker incision. Patients with endocardial pacemakers are instructed to use Polysporin powder, which is applied to the wound twice daily. They are instructed not to remove the steri-strips and to expect a small amount of serosanguinous drainage with increased ambulation. They are also instructed about the signs and symptoms of wound infection, as well as ways to bathe without getting the incision wet. The authors require the use of subacute bacterial endocarditis prophylaxis on all transvenous implants even though the American Heart Association/American Dental Association no longer recommend it. The educational guidelines for home care of the child with a permanent cardiac pacemaker can be found in Table 4.

An outpatient follow-up appointment is scheduled for 6 to 8 weeks post implant. If the wound is thought to be at particular risk, an interim visit is scheduled at 2 to 3 weeks post procedure. Patients with epicardial devices are seen at 2 weeks and again at 6 to 8 weeks. The child's activity level is slowly increased and strenuous physical activity is moderated according to the patients' overall cardiac condition.[72] Pacemaker patients with anatomically normal hearts are allowed to compete at any level of

Table 4
Education Guidelines for Home Care of the Child
with a Permanent Cardiac Pacemaker

Wound care	1. Observe site for redness, swelling, purulent drainage, and tenderness 2. Keep wound dry and allow steri-strips to fall off spontaneously 3. Cover wound with plastic wrap (plastic cling wrap or baggie) for bathing and showering 4. Apply Polysporin antibiotic powder to wound twice daily
Activity allowances/restrictions	1. Specific for each patient 2. No PE or contact sports until wound is completely healed (approximately 6–8 weeks) 3. Carry backpack on shoulder opposite pacemaker pocket site 4. No swimming or water sports activities until wound is completely healed 5. For most patients, limitations are imposed by underlying disease versus pacemaker presence 6. No varsity sports (i.e., full-contact karate, football, boxing, or hockey) for any pacemaker patient; in children with concomitant CHD, individual disease-specific allowances/restrictions are determined by MD
Endocarditis prophylaxis	1. Specified by implanting physician preference 2. Not necessary for epicardial implants unless accompanied by CHD 3. Authors recommend SBE prophylaxis in all transvenous pacemaker patients regardless of concomitant CHD
When to contact the doctor/nurse	1. Any of the following symptoms: dizziness, fatigue, palpitations (fast or extra heartbeats), SOB, "hiccoughing," signs of wound infection (see above), recurrence of any prepacemaker symptoms, muscle stimulation, or injury to the pacemaker
Avoidance of environmental hazards	1. Avoid the following: large magnets, arc welding equipment, high-energy electrical fields, high-output radio transmitters, MRI 2. Use with caution the following: cellular phones

(continues)

Table 4
Education Guidelines for Home Care of the Child
with a Permanent Cardiac Pacemaker (*cont.*)

Follow-up schedule	1. **Transtelephonic:** weekly for 6 weeks, then monthly for 1 year, then every third month until battery depletion or suspected malfunction 2. **Clinic visit:** 2 weeks (interim wound check) and 2 months (for new leads to reprogram output), and then every 6–12 months per physician preference

CHD = congenital heart disease; MRI = magnetic resonance imaging; PE = physical education; SBE = subacute bacterial endocarditis; SOB = shortness of breath.

athletics with the exception of contact sports such as varsity football, hockey, and full-contact karate. Patients with CHD often have restrictions placed more so because of their structural rather than their conduction system disease.

Last, the patient and family are instructed in the use of a transtelephonic monitor as an adjunct to "hands-on" outpatient follow-up. The pacemaker nurse provides verbal and written instructions and each family is required to provide a return demonstration. They are instructed to call weekly for the first 6 weeks or anytime a problem with the child's rhythm or pacemaker is suspected. This component of pacemaker follow-up has proven to be both valuable and cost effective for the pediatric pacemaker population.[73]

Follow-Up Care

Pacing system follow-up should ideally begin at the time the decision is made to implant a permanent cardiac pacemaker. This follow-up is equally important to the implant itself and is crucial in maintaining optimal hemodynamics and battery longevity. Additionally, follow-up provides early recognition of inadequate or even inappropriate pacing system performance. Although it is not always feasible, it is desirable to have the implanting physician also be the follow-up physician. It is not only cost efficient, but provides continuity in the patient's care. This follow-up care should consist of regular "hands-on" outpatient clinic visits, with complimentary transtelephonic monitoring of pacemaker function in between.

Transtelephonic Monitoring

Transtelephonic monitoring can be accomplished by providing an "on-site" service or by utilizing a "centralized" service. The use of a "centralized" service is not optimal when caring for children, but for some pacemaker follow-up centers it is more cost effective. The authors believe that this type of transtelephonic service is not optimal for several reasons.[74] First, the geographical distance between the patient and the service is often very wide with differing time zones, making communication with the service and the following physician more difficult. Second, the service has complete knowledge of the pacing system but does not really "know the patient," which can be problematic in patients with CHD and a malfunctioning pacemaker. Third, once an abnormal ECG is obtained by the service, the following physician must be notified in order to make arrangements for pacemaker adjustment. This procedure is time consuming and could result in occasional unwanted sequelae.

The use of an on-site transtelephonic surveillance system provides a continuum of care unrivaled by the use of the "off-site" method. Several pieces of equipment as well as personnel who are knowledgeable about the patient and pacing system are necessary. Many systems are now computerized, obviating the need for much of the equipment used in the early days of pacemaker follow-up. The ECG receiving center is attached to an answering machine that allows the patient and family to transmit at their convenience, using a toll-free number for the call. Reminder letters are sent to each patient approximately 2 weeks prior to a scheduled transmission. If a transmission is not obtained, pacemaker clinic personnel contact the family to request a transmission.

This system works fairly well, but an adjunct system has been placed in the event that problems occur outside of regular "business hours." A second receiving center is located on the inpatient telemetry unit and is attached to an acoustic coupler. If a problem arises, the physician on call simply transfers the call to the nursing unit for a real-time transmission. Once the ECG has been obtained, the physician reviews it, either by facsimile or direct visualization, and proceeds from there. It is very rare that the use of this secondary method is required, but the few times that it has been used, it has resulted in prompt identification and treatment of pacemaker-related problems.

It is helpful for the individual receiving the transtelephonic ECG to have some knowledge of the various transmitters used for pacemaker surveillance. In the authors' institutions, the nurses who provide the patient education regarding transmitter usage are the same individuals who receive the transtelephonic ECGs. On occasion, patients/parents become flustered when attempting to send an ECG and may place the phone backward on the transmitter or in the phone cradle. Knowledge of the type of transmitter allows the receiver to solve potential problems related to technique in these cases.

The type of transmitter used for transtelephonic follow-up varies from institution to institution. Transmitters with wrist electrodes, finger electrodes, or chest electrodes with leads are not desirable for the pediatric population for several reasons. First, the wrist and finger electrodes, because they are made for adults, are too large for use on small patients. Second, chest electrodes attached to ECG leads are disliked by most children, because they "hurt" when being removed. The use of a transmitter with metal "electrodes" on the back or of one with a phone cradle with chest probe are the transmitters of choice for children.[17,74] The latter allows the operator to hold the chest probe with one hand and soothe the child with the other. Prior to hospital discharge from the pacemaker implant procedure, the patient and family are taught how to use the specific transmitter and are introduced to the transtelephonic service.

Transtelephonic ECGs are received on a routine basis, but the families are told to transmit any time that they perceive a problem with the pacing system or that the child experiences symptoms, e.g., syncope, dizziness, tachycardia, or palpitations. In the authors' institutions, transtelephonic ECGs are received weekly for the first 6 to 8 weeks after initial implantation. At this time, a hands-on follow-up visit will determine the frequency of telephone transmissions. If there is a problem, patients may require more intensive phone follow-up. In most cases, the phone follow-up proceeds to monthly for the first year and then every 3 months after the pacemaker's first birthday. Once the device reaches approximately 5 years of age or shows evidence of battery depletion, transtelephonic surveillance is intensified as determined by the following physician.

The ECG transmission itself consists of a 30-second ECG *without* magnet application and a 30-second ECG *with* magnet application (Fig. 11). It is important that the person receiving the transtelephonic recording has knowledge of each device's response to magnet application and elective re-

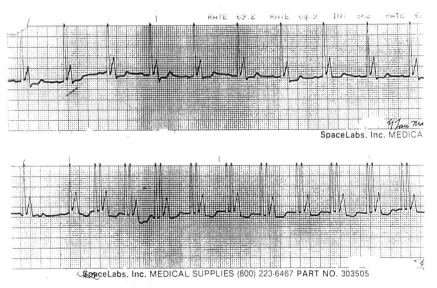

Figure 11. Transtelephonic ECG recording in a patient with a dual chamber pacemaker. The top strip (without magnet) depicts atrial synchronous (VDD) pacing. The second strip (with magnet) depicts magnet application on the third complex resulting in asynchronous (DOO) pacing. The first three beats are at a rate of 100 ppm with output reduction on the third beat, typical of a threshold margin test.

placement indicators. Additionally, many manufacturers include a threshold margin test to allow verification that an adequate safety margin has been programmed. In general, the threshold margin test consists of a specific number of beats at a predetermined rate, with a percent reduction in output on a specified beat. Often, the pulse width is temporarily reduced by 25% to 50%, depending on the device manufacturer (Fig. 12).

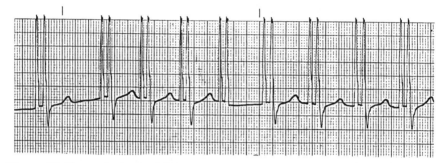

Figure 12. Transtelephonic ECG recording in a patient with a dual chamber pacemaker and magnet application. On the fifth complex, the ventricular pacing spike is not followed by a QRS complex denoting ventricular noncapture.

Hands-On Follow-Up

Outpatient, hands-on follow-up is scheduled on an individual patient basis, depending on underlying rhythm, concomitant structural heart disease, patient and/or device age, and previous pacemaker history (e.g., elevated thresholds, lead fracture). In general, patients younger than 2 years of age, patients with epicardial pacing leads, patients who are considered pacemaker-dependent, patients with complex CHD, and patients with previous threshold problems are seen every 6 months. All others are seen on an annual basis. Once impending battery depletion is noted, the hands-on as well as transtelephonic follow-up schedule is intensified as prescribed by the following physician.

The hands-on follow-up visit may include a multitude of tests, depending on the specific needs of each individual patient. All patients should undergo a complete history and physical examination as well as a complete pacemaker evaluation. The value of obtaining a history cannot be overstated, as it often reveals problems that might otherwise go unidentified. Symptoms such as dizziness, new-onset exercise intolerance, syncope, and generalized fatigue may be indicative of pacemaker malfunction.[17] The physical examination allows the physician to evaluate the patient's overall physical status, but also provides an opportunity to detect problems that may be directly related to the pacing system such as irregular heart rhythms, pacemaker pocket infections, changes in valve function, etc.

Other tests that are important in the follow-up of the pediatric pacemaker patient include chest roentgenogram, exercise stress testing, echocardiography, routine 12- to 15-lead ECG, and 24-hour ambulatory monitoring. Chest roentgenography should be performed at least annually in the growing child (i.e., <17 years of age) to assess lead length and position as well as lead migration/interference with cardiac function (Figs. 13 through 15).

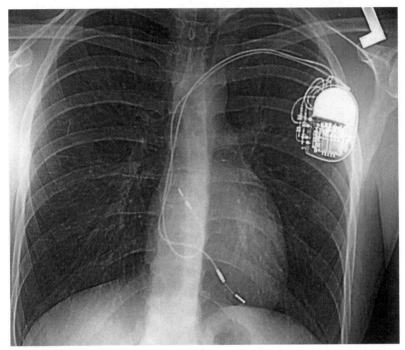

Figure 13. Chest radiograph (posteroanterior view) of typical transvenous lead placement in an adolescent. The ventricular tined bipolar lead is positioned in the right ventricular apex, while the atrial bipolar screw-in lead is positioned in the right atrial appendage. A small amount of excess lead has been left in each chamber for growth.

Echocardiography is generally performed in those patients who have concomitant CHD and is performed at the discretion of the following physician.

Exercise stress testing is an invaluable tool for the pediatric pacemaker patient.[5] A multitude of information can be obtained regarding the pacemaker's performance that may not be evident during pacemaker testing.[75] The problems identified during exercise stress testing can relate to undesirable upper rate limit behavior, inadequate heart rate increase with exercise, variation of pacing thresholds with exercise, and atrial undersensing due to changes in atrial electrogram voltage during exercise.[64,76–79] Many of these problems are easily corrected by parameter reprogramming.

Twenty-four-hour ambulatory monitoring is another invaluable tool in the follow-up of the pediatric pacemaker patient.[80,81] It is especially helpful in younger patients who are unable to perform exercise stress test-

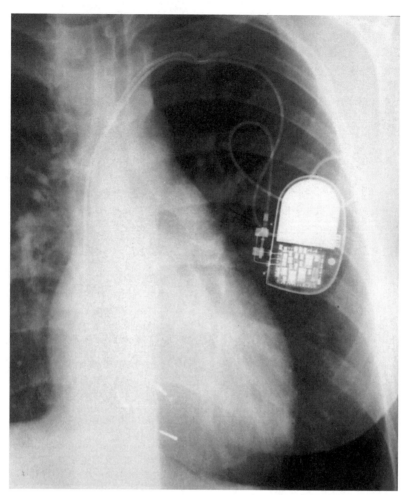

Figure 14. Chest radiograph depicting a patient with subclavian crush syndrome. Two separate ventricular leads have been placed in the left subclavian vein during two separate procedures. The punctures were very medial resulting in an increased likelihood of "subclavian crush." The first lead ceased functioning and was abandoned, and the second lead (also crushed) is beginning to malfunction as well.

ing (Fig. 16). Intermittent problems such as undersensing or oversensing and/or noncapture can be detected by 24-hour ambulatory monitoring. Additionally, competition between the patient's paced and intrinsic rhythm can be identified. Last, any symptomatology that the patient may be experiencing related to the pacing system may be verified in this manner (Fig. 17).

Noninvasive pacemaker evaluation in the child should be performed by qualified personnel who are adept at dealing with children and their families. A calm child is a cooperative child, which allows a complete pacemaker evaluation. Limb leads are attached to the patient for a baseline

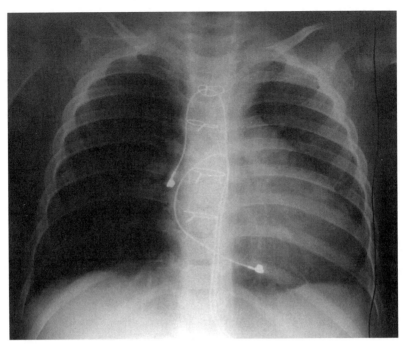

Figure 15. Chest radiograph on a patient with an epicardial pacing system. The leads placed on the right atrium and right ventricle are unipolar, steroid-eluting leads.

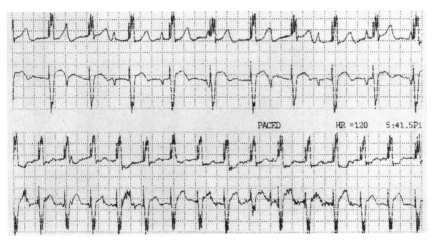

Figure 16. Twenty-four-hour ambulatory monitor recording in a patient with a ventricular rate-adaptive pacemaker. The first two simultaneous leads exhibit a paced rate of approximately 75 ppm followed by an increase in the rate to 120 ppm on the second set of recordings, demonstrating an adequate rate response with activity.

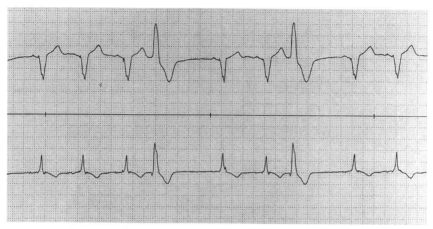

Figure 17. Surface ECG recordings from a patient with a dual chamber pacemaker exhibiting appropriate sensing of premature ventricular contractions.

ECG recording of leads I, II, and III. If available, an ECG cable that hooks into the specific pacemaker programmer is also attached. The pacemaker is then interrogated for programmed settings, measured data, and diagnostic data. Measured data include performance data such as battery voltage, lead impedance, measured pulse width and amplitude, current flow, and energy delivered.

The programmed values should be evaluated and compared with those from the last visit, to ensure that no reprogramming has occurred. Some generators revert to noise reversion modes or elective replacement when exposed to electromagnetic interference (EMI). Although this information is frequently discussed with the patient and parents, exposure to such hazards occasionally occurs.

The measured data are very valuable to the clinician. The pacemaker's battery voltage and cell impedance should be assessed and compared with the previous values in order to estimate battery longevity and determine frequency of follow-up. The cell impedance of most lithium batteries increases as the battery voltage decreases. This does not occur logarithmically and is very hard to predict in devices with very small batteries. Lead impedance is critical, as it is a very good indicator of how the lead is functioning. Normal lead impedance measurements vary according to lead polarity and can range from 200 to 1800 Ω. The measurements should be compared with previous values in order to determine any abrupt or subtle changes. A change in either direction of 200 Ω or greater should arouse suspicion, and in these cases, for consistency, repeat measurements should be taken at the same pulse width and pulse amplitude.[74] In general, an abrupt decrease in the lead impedance is indicative of insulation problems, while an increase is indicative of lead wire fracture, pacemaker header problems, electrode tip erosion, or impending exit block.

The pacemaker's diagnostic data are very helpful, but vary from one device manufacturer to another. Pacemaker usage as well as heart rate ranges can be assessed using the diagnostic counters (Fig. 18). Other use-

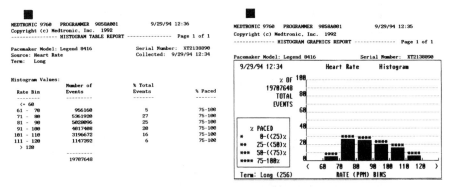

Figure 18. Event counters obtained on a patient with an older model rate-adaptive pacemaker. The heart rate histogram is depicted on the right with the table of rate ranges on the left, both indicating good heart rate variability.

ful information that can be obtained includes incidence of premature beats and/or runs of tachycardia and the number of tachycardia episodes and subsequent modes of termination, the latter being found in atrial antitachycardia devices.

Intracardiac electrograms and annotation markers are available in most commercially available devices. These features can be extremely useful in identifying the source of sensing problems or other unclear problems (Fig. 19). A frequently encountered problem in patients with atrial antitachycardia pacemakers with postoperative IART is the presence of R wave oversensing on the atrial electrogram. On the surface ECG, it appears that the device is malfunctioning because the paced rate is less than that of the programmed rate. On the atrial electrogram, a ventricular intrinsic deflection is present, causing the device to appropriately inhibit. If one were to measure from the atrial pacemaker artifact to the previous QRS complex on the surface ECG, the measured interval should correlate to the programmed pacing rate. Intracardiac electrograms are also helpful in identifying obscure atrial arrhythmias that are difficult to ascertain on the surface ECG.

The actual provocative testing of the device includes pacing thresholds, sensing thresholds, and underlying rhythm. The pacing thresholds are performed in the chamber(s) being paced. Pulse width thresholds are performed at various pulse amplitudes. The threshold is considered to be the lowest pulse width value that produces a cardiac depolarization 100% of the time. For leads that are older than 6 weeks, the programmed output is permanently programmed as follows: for the atrium, the threshold pulse width value is doubled, and for the ventricle, the threshold pulse

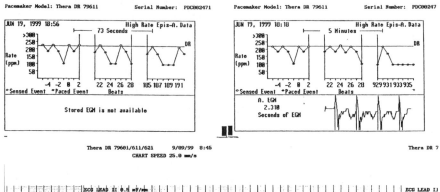

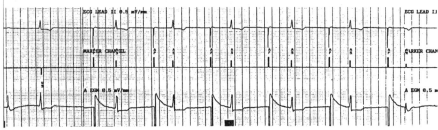

Figure 19. Event counters and ECG with annotation markers and intracardiac electrograms on a patient with a dual chamber pacemaker. The ECG recordings depict atrial pacing with far field R wave on the atrial electrogram that is sensed as if it were an atrial depolarization. This occurs because of its size and the long PR interval, which causes it to be outside of the sensing refractory period. Although this patient has concomitant atrial reentry tachycardia, the number of high-rate episodes may be exaggerated secondary to the R wave oversensing.

width value is tripled. It is also important to evaluate sensing thresholds, which should correlate with the intracardiac electrogram when using bipolar leads.[82] Newer generation devices allow automatic sensitivity measurements and electrogram amplitudes in lieu of performing manual sensitivity testing. Recent research data[83] show the former values to be significantly greater than the manually obtained values, suggesting that clinicians should use the aforementioned with caution and perhaps verify the findings with manual testing. Because the atrial electrogram voltage decreases with exercise,[64] the atrial sensitivity is left at the maximal setting, i.e., 0.5 mV in most devices. In the case of unipolar leads, the atrial sensitivity is programmed to a slightly less sensitive setting because of their propensity to sense skeletal muscle.[84] The ventricular sensitivity is generally programmed to at least two settings more sensitive than where sensing was lost. Again, judgment must be used when programming the sensitivity in a unipolar device.

The determination of the patient's underlying rhythm is important for several reasons. First, it answers the question of pacemaker dependency, which is critical in caring for pacemaker patients of any age. The majority of pediatric pacemaker patients are not pacemaker-dependent. Second, it shows the patient and family that the fact that a person has a pacemaker does not make that person dependent on it. Third, it reassures the cardiovascular caregivers and the patient and family that in the case of pacemaker/lead malfunction, the child will more often than not revert back to the rhythm that initially required the pacemaker. The optimal way to determine underlying rhythm is NOT to suddenly inhibit the pacemaker. This results in a brief (sometimes prolonged) period of asystole and is generally despised by the patient. With slow decreases (in 10-ppm increments) in the programmed pacing rate, the child's underlying rhythm will gradually emerge. In the patient with a DDDCO pacemaker in which the patient is atrial tracking or in patients with rate adaptation, it is first necessary to program the mode to VVICO. Once this has been accomplished, one can then proceed with lowering the rate. Of course, all of the information obtained during pacemaker evaluation should be documented in the patient's record, including any and all changes made in the programmed settings.

The programmed pacing rate in the pediatric patient requires periodic adjustment with increasing age. Once the child reaches the age of 16, the lower rate can be programmed as low as 40 ppm in both rate-adaptive and atrial synchronous modes. In the child with postoperative bradycardia-tachycardia syndrome, a higher than normal lower rate is chosen. In adolescents that rate is usually 80 ppm due to its propensity to prevent tachycardia episodes.[74]

Other parameters that can be adapted to the needs of the individual patient include AV intervals, rate-adaptive parameters, and antitachycardia recognition and termination algorithms. Because the normal PR interval shortens with exercise,[85] a rate-adaptive AV delay is preferable to a fixed AV delay in the majority of pediatric pacemaker patients. This parameter can be programmed to as low as 50 ms without adverse sequelae. Rate-adaptive parameters must be individualized for the type of sensor and to meet each patient's specific needs. In most cases, the various settings must be evaluated with exercise stress testing and/or 24-hour ambulatory monitoring.[86] Antitachycardia recognition and termination algorithms are programmed according to the tachycardia characteristics and are usually patient specific, but should be reassessed if any antiarrhythmic drug therapy is initiated (Fig. 20).

Troubleshooting

Many patients remain quite stable throughout the follow-up period, but some require extra attention. Many of the problems encountered during this time can be alleviated with simple reprogramming of the implanted device. These problems include, but are not limited to, failure to capture, phrenic nerve stimulation, undersensing or oversensing, pacemaker-mediated tachycardia, atrial tachycardia recurrence in the patient with an implanted atrial antitachycardia device, and new-onset atrial tachycardia in a patient with a DDDCO pacemaker.

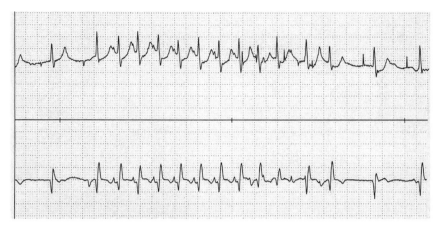

Figure 20. Surface ECG recording from a patient with an automatic atrial antitachycardia pacemaker after the Fontan procedure. The first two beats exhibit atrial pacing followed by an episode of atrial reentry tachycardia. The pacemaker appropriately detects and successfully overdrives the tachycardia resulting in an atrial paced rhythm on the last two beats.

Failure to capture in the immediate postoperative period requires prompt attention. In most cases, programming the output to a higher value will correct the problem. Because this is only palliative and because the pacing threshold normally rises to peak during this time, this could potentially become a bigger problem. In the authors' institutions, if the pacing threshold is ≥0.2 ms at 5.0 V and there is no contraindication to steroid administration, oral prednisone is initiated at a dosage of 60 mg/m²/day. The dose is tapered by 10 mg/day over a 7- to 10-day period. This can be done on an outpatient basis if an adequate safety margin can be attained; otherwise, the patient should be hospitalized for constant rhythm monitoring. Intravenous Decadron can be used for faster results.

Phrenic nerve stimulation, although rare, can present in the followup period. It is characterized by complaints of "jerking or hiccoughing." In the majority of cases, it can be reduced or even eliminated by programming a lower pulse amplitude coupled with a longer pulse width or duration. If it cannot be alleviated, one must, in conjunction with the patient and family, consider the frequency of occurrence and tolerability. If it is intolerable to the patient, lead repositioning/replacement may be necessary.

Sensing abnormalities can generally be corrected, due to the broad range of sensitivity settings currently available in most pulse generators. As previously mentioned, in patients with the bradycardia-tachycardia syndrome and CHD, it may be necessary for the clinician to "allow" the device to R wave oversense in those who have atrial antitachycardia pacemakers. If the R wave oversensing is alleviated, it generally results in undersensing of the IART. A better "effective" rate can be achieved by increasing the lower rate of the device. Undersensing can occur with some bipolar leads due to a decrease in electrogram size; however, this can be corrected by reprogramming the sense configuration to unipolar while allowing the pace configuration to be bipolar.

Pacemaker-mediated tachycardia is rare in the pediatric population because most of the patients who require device placement do not have intact retrograde conduction. It is characterized by a rapidly paced ventricular rhythm that is the result of the loss of AV synchrony in the presence of retrograde (VA) conduction. The most common causes of pacemaker-mediated tachycardia in children are premature ventricular contractions, loss of atrial capture, and/or loss of atrial sensing. When any of these events occurs, a retrograde P wave occurs outside of the atrial refractory period, which in turn will initiate an AV delay and subsequent ventricular pacing setting up an endless loop tachycardia. It does not always occur at the upper rate limit and will persist until the retrograde pathway is blocked or terminated, which can be accomplished by simple magnet application. It can be alleviated by lengthening the PVARP, decreasing the atrial sensitivity, and/or eliminating premature ventricular contractions. In order to determine how long the PVARP should be programmed, one can assess retrograde conduction by pacing the ventricle at varying rates and measuring the VA interval using the atrial electrogram.

Atrial tachycardia recurrence in children with implanted atrial antitachycardia devices may occur in patients who have more than one arrhythmogenic substrate and in whom antiarrhythmic drugs that may have altered the tachycardia characteristics are present. Most recurrences can be treated by reprogramming the tachycardia detection and termination sequences. In rare cases, noninvasive programmed stimulation may offer some insight if the tachycardia is inducible.

Many postoperative patients with pacemakers for acquired AV block will subsequently develop atrial tachycardia in the follow-up period. Because these patients need AV synchrony for optimal hemodynamics, it is best not to reprogram the device to single chamber mode. This lack of AV synchrony will often lead to tachycardia exacerbations. If the mode is programmed to DDICO or DDIRO, the atrium will not sense the tachycardia but will provide back-up ventricular pacing during the tachycardia episode. During periods without tachycardia, the device will pace AV sequentially. A more attractive option is that of mode switching, in which the device senses or averages a specific number of beats and reverts to an alternate mode until the episode has terminated.

Patient and Family Considerations

There are many considerations for patients who must undergo permanent pacemaker implantation and for their families. The individual needs of pediatric pacemaker recipients provide the foundation of the nursing care plan, including assessment, planning, implementation, and evaluation. Since nurses have assumed most of the patient education responsibilities,[87] the success with which this is implemented depends largely on the nurse/family relationship, the nurse's level of expertise/proficiency, and commitment/communication between members of the health care team.[88] The authors recommend a family-centered approach in which the philosophy of care used is one that recognizes and respects the critical role that the family plays in the lives of the children with special care needs. Family-centered care positions parents and health providers/professionals as equal partners who are committed to excellence in all aspects/levels of patient care.[89] This section focuses on the specific needs of the patient and family undergoing permanent pacemaker implantation, with specific emphasis on patient and family education and the psychosocial implications of life with a pacemaker.

Patient and Family Education

Patient and family education should begin as soon as the decision for pacemaker implantation has been made. Shannon[90] states that the assessment phase should include the identification of previous pacemaker knowledge, the identification of myths/misconceptions regarding pacemakers, and the establishment of a level of teaching that is dependent on the patient's age and intellectual abilities. The assessment phase should also include the family's understanding of the upcoming procedure, lifestyle, play habits, previous hospitalizations, and coping mechanisms.[88] All families have strengths and weaknesses[91]; however, if cardiovascular clinicians strive to assess the family's strengths (as opposed to their weaknesses) and use them as a foundation on which to build, the patient and family will be more likely to respond to our interactions. Allowing the patient and family to elaborate on what they already know and tailoring their education in a manner understandable to them will help to decrease fear and anxiety while hopefully establishing/reinforcing a trusting relationship between clinicians and family members.

After the assessment phase is initiated, the nurse can identify problems and establish goals and anticipated outcomes with the patient and family. The goals should be realistic and individualized for each specific patient and family. Implementation of the plan then ensues with care to solicit observations, complaints, and/or requests from the patient and family in order to evaluate whether the set goals and objectives have been met.

Patient education should be carried out in a quiet, relaxed atmosphere with few interruptions. This generally takes place after a discussion with the implanting physician regarding the procedure, risks associated with the procedure, and potential complications. The discussion should begin with the assessment data previously obtained with clarification of any myths regarding pacemakers. A basic explanation of how the pacemaker works is extremely helpful, since many patients believe that the pacemaker will somehow make them dependent on it. The implant technique should be reviewed at this time and any visual aids about the conduction system, pacing system, and implant technique can also assist in the patient/family's understanding. The patient and family should also be given the opportunity to visualize and handle the pacing system at this time, so that the child knows what will be inside of him or her. Any written information that can be provided at this time is also very useful. The use of play during the preoperative education phase is another helpful approach for clinicians. It may be used to help the child understand and feel more comfortable about the upcoming procedure, but it may also be used by clinicians to learn the child's specific fears, interests, and coping mechanisms.[88]

Patients and parents should be told what to expect immediately after the procedure. The best approach is to be honest with both the child and family, especially regarding painful interventions and/or procedures. An explanation of the physician's orders is very helpful, since the family can know what to expect once the child arrives on the postoperative care unit. Any routine tests that will be performed during the hospitalization should be reiterated as well as the anticipated length of stay. If problems are noted during the hospitalization, the clinician should explain them to the patient and family, especially if they are likely to prolong the hospitalization.

Discharge planning is an extremely important component of the patient and family educational process. In addition to the guidelines presented in Table 4, the clinician should give an overview of what is to be expected in the days and weeks following hospital discharge. Receiving telephone numbers of key personnel to contact after discharge can provide comfort to the family as well. It is very important that clinicians be accessible to patients and families for support and to help them support each other after hospital discharge.

Psychosocial Considerations

The psychosocial aspects of having a pacemaker during childhood were studied as early as the late 1960s.[92] This early study was undertaken at a time when devices were large, batteries depleted quickly, and postoperative complications greater. Despite the obstacles that the 18 patients and their families faced, the majority of them (17/18) were found to be functioning normally, with only one patient demonstrating what has become known as "cardiac neuroses."

Twenty years later, Alpern and colleagues[93] compared 30 pediatric patients with two age- and sex-matched control groups. One control group consisted of children with similar heart defects and no pacemaker and the other consisted of physically healthy children. The authors found that the children with pacemakers experienced a decreased sense of personal control and less autonomy, while all groups perceived negative peer reactions toward the children with pacemakers, although the pacemaker recipients themselves did not see themselves as different. The investigators postulated that the pacemaker recipients in this study cope by using denial and intellectualization in a highly adaptive way.

Nearly half a decade later, Andersen and colleagues[94] evaluated the psychosocial aspects and mental health in 15 Danish children after permanent pacemaker implantation. The children underwent psychological as well as intelligence testing and were found to have normal IQs, but all had an abnormal body image. Seven families faced "strained" conditions and sought social and psychiatric therapy.

Zeigler and Corbett[95] used open-ended interviewing techniques to evaluate the meaning of living with a pacemaker in 20 adolescent and young adult pacemaker recipients. Several themes were evident throughout the data analysis, including normalization, parental overprotectiveness, peer integration, consistent caregivers, procedural fear, body image, adjustment period, and the future.

These data support the fact that pacemaker implantation during childhood is a very stressful life event for children and their families. Health care professionals should include an ongoing psychosocial assessment in the overall physical care of the pediatric pacemaker patient. This awareness of the psychosocial issues faced by these patients will aid clinicians in making an early identification and subsequent treatment referral for those patients and families at high risk.

Interventions that might be helpful for these children and their families include meeting other children of similar age who have pacemakers, being treated as normally as possible under the patient-specific circumstances, having consistent caregivers that they know and trust, and hearing an explanation that there is somewhat of an adjustment period after pacemaker placement.

Related Issues

There are several related issues regarding pediatric pacemaker patients that warrant discussion. One pertinent issue is that of EMI with implanted pacemakers. Additionally, special consideration is warranted in certain situations involving the patient with a permanently implanted cardiac pacemaker. The following discussion includes EMI considerations as well as situations that require special attention in patients with implanted pacemakers, including pulse generator replacements for battery depletion, other medical procedures not associated with pacemaker implantation (including radiofrequency catheter ablation), and cardioversion/defibrillation in the patient with a permanent cardiac pacemaker.

Electromagnetic Interference

EMI can occur in the hospital as well as in the nonindustrial and home environment. Although most modern devices are protected from most sources of EMI because of shielding of the device's circuitry by the pacemaker can, the clinician should be knowledgeable about sources of

EMI in all environments so that he or she can educate the patient and the family and, importantly, coordinate care to reduce exposure and/or damage to the permanently implanted device.

The potential responses that a device may have to EMI include pacemaker output inhibition, pacemaker output trigger, asynchronous pacing, inadvertent reprogramming (usually to a back-up mode), and damage to the pacemaker's circuitry.[96] Electrocautery is the most common source of EMI in patients with pacemakers, and is discussed in more detail below. Other sources of EMI in the health care environment include external cardioversion/defibrillation (which is discussed below), catheter ablation, magnetic resonance imaging, lithotripsy, transcutaneous electrical nerve stimulation, some dental equipment, radiation, electroconvulsive therapy, and diathermy.[96]

There are sources of EMI in the nonindustrial and home environments. Importantly, although signs remain in some public places warning patients with pacemakers that microwave ovens are in use, this is no longer a concern. Recently, cellular telephones and antitheft devices have caused concern among pacemaker patients and pacemaker personnel. Antitheft devices may cause inhibition and asynchronous pacing, but this incidence is decreased if the device is bipolar.[96] Patients are instructed not to linger near these devices. Cellular phones, in addition to the aforementioned effects, can cause complete inhibition of the pacemaker.[96] Pacemaker patients who use cellular phones are advised to hold them to the ear opposite the side of the pacemaker and not to place them directly over the device. Clinicians should inform patients and families that if a specific situation evolves concerning the patient and the possibility of EMI, the customer service department of the specific manufacturer can be contacted with any specific concerns.

Pulse Generator Replacements

When replacing a pulse generator that is at elective or imminent replacement, certain factors should be considered in advance. Since many older style leads are still implanted, the compatibility of these leads with the newer pulse generators must be taken into account. In most cases, the various manufacturers provide pulse generators with headers that accept older lead pins, such as the 3.2-mm in-line with a long connector pin. Lead and pulse generator compatibility/availability must be verified prior to the implant procedure.

Pads for emergent temporary pacing should be placed on the patient in the event that the battery-depleted device fails completely. A cardioverter defibrillator with external pacing capabilities can be used in place of the former "stand-alone" external, transcutaneous pacemaker. If this is not available, a temporary venous pacing catheter should be placed in those patients who are considered pacemaker-dependent or hemodynamically vulnerable.

The use of electrocautery should be avoided with pulse generator replacements that are battery depleted because the pacemakers will often cease to function when electrocautery is applied, sometimes permanently. Additionally, the risk of damaging the chronic lead is higher. The use of an ultrasonic scalpel has alleviated some of these problems and is now preferred in "redo" cases for this reason. A review of written reports of previous pacemaker procedures may be helpful in determining where the lead may have been placed, i.e., over or under the implanted pulse generator.

One should also be prepared for inadvertent damage to the lead during opening of the pocket or for previously undetected lead problems that materialize during intraoperative testing. Additional leads, stylets for the chronically implanted lead(s), and a tool used to disconnect the pulse generator from the lead must be readily available.

Other Medical Procedures on the Child with a Pacemaker

Any time the child with a permanent cardiac pacemaker undergoes medical or surgical procedures, the pacemaker team should be made aware. This often does not occur, but it is the most desirable way of treating these patients. The physician performing the procedure should be aware of the patient's underlying rhythm, pacemaker indication, programmed settings of the device, and pocket location. When using electrocautery, care must be taken to avoid use directly over the implanted device. Ideally, it should be kept at least 4 to 6 inches from the pacemaker.[96]

The most common adverse effect of electrocautery is pacemaker inhibition, although other adverse effects can occur including device reprogramming, reversion to a noise or fallback mode, permanent damage to the pulse generator, and thermal damage to the myocardium resulting in myocardial infarction or ventricular fibrillation.[96] It is feasible to program to an asynchronous mode (by programming or magnet application) in adults, but this is not always feasible in children due their ability to track the atrium at much higher rates than the adult. If feasible for a particular patient, this should certainly be undertaken. The use of a bipolar electrocautery system and multiple, short bursts during the procedure may help minimize permanent pacemaker damage. The grounding pad for the electrocautery should be placed as far away from the implanted device as possible and the pacing system evaluated by pacemaker personnel immediately after the procedure.

Patients with permanent pacemakers undergoing radiofrequency catheter ablation are at risk for the same EMI sequelae as those exposed to electrocautery because the frequency current is the same for both. Hayes and Strathmore[96] recommend device interrogation with threshold measurements and reprogramming of rate-adaptive devices to a non-rate-adaptive mode prior to the ablation procedure. Additional recommendations include the availability of a programmer during the procedure and a complete pacemaker evaluation following the procedure.

Cardioversion/Defibrillation in the Pacemaker Patient

Pacemaker patients rarely require cardioversion or defibrillation. If necessary, it can be performed by using defibrillation paddles or self-adhesive electrode pads that attach directly to the patient's skin. It is crucial to be aware of the location of the pulse generator in order to correctly place the pads or paddles, which should be placed as far away from the pulse generator as possible (Table 5). The adverse effects of cardioversion/defibrillation range from no change in pacemaker function to complete device destruction. Pacemaker function should be assessed immediately after cardioversion/defibrillation, including sensing and pacing thresholds and lead impedance assessment. Altamura and colleagues[97] report a significant rise in ventricular pacing threshold, including transient loss of capture in 50% of patients, worsening of sensing function, and generator failure (in 2 cases) after transthoracic direct current shock. The lead impedance measurement(s) may be increased or decreased immediately following cardioversion/defibrillation, but generally return to normal in several hours. It is not unusual after cardioversion/defibrillation for the device to exhibit elective replacement indicators or be in a back-up mode. This can usually be eliminated by simply reprogramming the device.

Table 5
Defibrillation Pad/Paddle Placement in the
Permanent Pacemaker Patient

Pacemaker Pocket Location	Pad/Paddle Placement
Left subpectoral/subcutaneous	left anterior apex (low) and right posterior (clavicular)
Right subpectoral/subcutaneous	front-back on the left side
Left rectus	left anterior (high) and right anterior or posterior
Right rectus	left anterior and right anterior or posterior

From: Gillette PC, Zeigler VL (eds.): Pediatric Cardiac Pacing. Armonk, New York: Futura Publishing Company, Inc.; 1995:239, with permission.

In summary, the care of the pediatric pacemaker recipient is multifaceted and requires that the clinician possess a wealth of knowledge regarding pacing system technology and care of children and their families. The use of this knowledge can help to provide the child and family with a positive pacemaker experience, making this subspecialty rewarding and challenging to the cardiovascular clinician.

References

1. Elmqvist R, Landegren J, Petterson SO, et al: Artificial pacemaker for treatment of Adams-Stokes syndrome and slow heart rate. Am Heart J 1963; 65:731–748.
2. Karpawich PP, Perry BL, Farooki ZQ, et al: Pacing in children and young

adults in non-surgical atrioventricular block: Comparison of single-rate ventricular and dual-chamber modes. Am Heart J 1987; 113:316–321.
3. Kugler JD, Danford DA: Pacemakers in children: An update. Am Heart J 1989; 117:665–679.
4. Yabek SM, Wernly J, Check TW, et al: Rate adaptive cardiac pacing in children using a minute ventilation biosensor. Pacing Clin Electrophysiol 1990; 13:2108–2112.
5. Cabrera ME, Hanisch DG, Cohen MH, et al: Cardiopulmonary responses to exercise in children with activity rate responsive ventricular pacemakers. Pacing Clin Electrophysiol 1993; 16:1386–1393.
6. Celiker A, Alehan D, Oto A, et al: Long-term clinical experience with a steroid-eluting active fixation ventricular electrode in children. Am J Cardiol 1997; 80:355–358.
7. Frye RL, Collins JJ, DeSanctis RW, et al: Guidelines for permanent cardiac pacemaker implantation, May 1984. A report of the Joint American College of Cardiology/American Heart Association Task Force on Assessment of Cardiovascular Procedures (Subcommittee on Pacemaker Implantation). Circulation 1984; 70:331A-339A.
8. Dreifus LS, Fisch C, Griffin JC, et al: Guidelines for implantation of cardiac pacemakers and antiarrhythmia devices. A report of the Joint American College of Cardiology/American Heart Association Task Force on Assessment of Cardiovascular Procedures. J Am Coll Cardiol 1991; 18:1–13.
9. Gregoratos G, Cheitlin MD, Conill A, et al: ACC/AHA guidelines for implantation of cardiac pacemakers and antiarrhythmia devices. J Am Coll Cardiol 1998; 31:1175–1209.
10. Gillette PC: Pacing indications and choosing the most appropriate generator. In Gillette PC, Zeigler VL (eds.): Pediatric Cardiac Pacing. Armonk, New York: Futura Publishing Company, Inc.; 1995:9–22.
11. Shearin RP, Fleming WH: Fourteen years of implanted pacemakers in children. Ann Thorac Surg 1978; 25:144–147.
12. Simon AB, Dick M II, Stern AM, et al: Ventricular pacing in children. Pacing Clin Electrophysiol 1982; 5:836–844.
13. Waelkens JJ: Cardiac pacemakers in infants and children as observed in The Netherlands. Pediatr Cardiol 1982; 3:337–340.
14. Ector H, Dhooghe G, Daenen W, et al: Pacing in children. Br Heart J 1985; 53:541–546.
15. Serwer GA, Mericle JM: Evaluation of pacemaker pulse generator and patient longevity in patients aged 1 day to 20 years. Am J Cardiol 1987; 59:824–827.
16. Walsh CA, McAlister HF, Anders CA, et al: Pacemaker implantation in children: A 21 year experience. Pacing Clin Electrophysiol 1988; 11:1940–1944.
17. Serwer GA, Dorostkar PC, LeRoy SS: Pediatric pacing and defibrillator usage. In Ellenbogen KA, Kay GN, Wilkoff BL (eds.): Clinical Cardiac Pacing and Defibrillation. 2nd ed. Philadelphia: WB Saunders Company; 2000:953–989.
18. Dorostkar P, Serwer GA, LeRoy S, et al: Long-term course of children and young adults with congenital complete heart block. J Am Coll Cardiol 1993; 21:295A.
19. Michaelsson M, Riesenfeld T, Jonzon A: Natural history of congenital complete atrioventricular block. Pacing Clin Electrophysiol 1997; 20:2098–2101.
20. Beder SD, Gillette PC: Non-surgical etiologies of sick sinus syndrome. In Yabek SM, Gillette PC, Kugler JD (eds.): The Sinus Node in Pediatrics. Edinburgh: Churchill Livingstone; 1984:121–132.
21. Gillette PC, Wampler DG, Shannon C, et al: Use of cardiac pacing after the Mustard operation for transposition of the great arteries. J Am Coll Cardiol 1986; 7:138–141.
22. Rishi F, Hulse JE, Auld DO, et al: Effects of dual-chamber pacing for pediatric

patients with hypertrophic obstructive cardiomyopathy. J Am Coll Cardiol 1997; 29:741–743.

23. Karpawich PP, Justice CD, Cavitt DL, et al: Developmental sequelae of fixed-rate ventricular pacing in the immature canine heart: An electrophysiologic, hemodynamic, and histopathologic evaluation. Am Heart J 1990; 199:1077–1083.

24. Fukushige J, Porter CB, Hayes DL, et al: Antitachycardia pacemaker treatment of postoperative arrhythmias in pediatric patients. Pacing Clin Electrophysiol 1991; 14:546–556.

25. Gillette PC, Ross BA, Zeigler VL: Antitachycardia pacing. In Garson A Jr., Bricker JT, McNamara DG (eds.): The Science and Practice of Pediatric Cardiology. Philadelphia: Lea & Febiger; 1990:2156–2161.

26. Gillette PC, Zeigler VL, Case CL, et al: Atrial antitachycardia pacing in children and young adults. Am Heart J 1991; 122:844–849.

27. Celiker A, Tokel K, Lenk MK, et al: Dual sensor pacemakers in children: What is the choice of sensor blending? Pacing Clin Electrophysiol 1997; 20:1301–1304.

28. Serwer GA, Uzark K, Beekman R, et al: Optimal programming of rate altering parameters in children with rate-responsive pacemakers using graded treadmill exercise testing. Pacing Clin Electrophysiol 1990; 13:541. Abstract.

29. Walsh CA, McAlister HF, Anders CA, et al: Pacemaker implantation in children: A 21 year experience. Pacing Clin Electrophysiol 1988; 11:1940–1944.

30. Till JA, Jones S, Rowland E, et al: Endocardial pacing in infants and children 15 kg or less in weight: Medium term follow up. Pacing Clin Electrophysiol 1990; 13:1385–1392.

31. Spotnitz HM: Transvenous pacing in infants and children with congenital heart disease. Ann Thorac Surg 1990; 49:495–496.

32. Esperer HD, Singer H, Riede FT, et al: Permanent epicardial and transvenous single- and dual chamber cardiac pacing in children. Thorac Cardiovasc Surg 1993; 41:21–27.

33. Serwer GA, Mericle JM, Armstrong BE: Epicardial ventricular pacemaker electrode longevity in children. Am J Cardiol 1988; 61:104–106.

34. Serwer GA, Uzark K, Dick M II: Endocardial pacing longevity in children. J Am Coll Cardiol 1990; 15:212A. Abstract.

35. Serwer GA, Dorostkar PC, LeRoy S, et al: Comparison of chronic thresholds between differing endocardial electrode types in children. Circulation 1992; 86:I-43. Abstract.

36. DeLeon SY, Ilbawi MN, Koster N, et al: Comparison of the sutureless and suture-type epicardial electrodes in pediatric cardiac pacing. Ann Thorac Surg 1982; 33:273–276.

37. Michalik RE, Williams H, Zorn-Chelten S, et al: Experience with a new epimyocardial pacing lead in children. Pacing Clin Electrophysiol 1984; 7:831–838.

38. Kugler J, Monsour W, Blodgett C, et al: Comparison of two myoepicardial pacemaker leads: Follow up in 80 children, adolescents, and young adults. Pacing Clin Electrophysiol 1988; 11:2216–2222.

39. DeLeon SY, Ilbawi MN, Backer CL, et al: Exit block in pediatric cardiac pacing. Comparison of the suture-type and fishhook epicardial electrodes. J Thorac Cardiovasc Surg 1991; 102:213–222.

40. Hoyer MH, Beerman LB, Ettedgui JA, et al: Transatrial lead placement for endocardial pacing in children. Ann Thorac Surg 1994; 58:97–101.

41. Hamilton R, Gow R, Bahoric B, et al: Steroid-eluting epicardial leads in pediatrics: Improved epicardial thresholds in the first year. Pacing Clin Electrophysiol 1991; 14:2066–2072.

42. Karpawich PP, Hakimi M, Arciniegas E, et al: Improved chronic epicardial pacing in children: Steroid contribution to porous platinized electrodes. Pacing Clin Electrophysiol 1992; 15:1151–1157.

43. Lau YR: Lead selection. In Gillette PC, Zeigler VL (eds.): Pediatric Cardiac Pacing. Armonk, New York: Futura Publishing Company, Inc.; 1995:23–36.
44. Friedman RA, Moak JP, Garson A Jr.: Active fixation of endocardial pacing leads: The preferred method of pediatric pacing. Pacing Clin Electrophysiol 1991; 14:1213–1216.
45. Seiden HS, Camunas JL, Fishburger SB, et al: Use of single lead VDD pacing in children. Pacing Clin Electrophysiol 1997; 20:1967–1974.
46. Rosenthal E, Bostock J, Qureshi SA, et al: Single pass VDD pacing in children and adolescents. Pacing Clin Electrophysiol 1997; 20:1975–1982.
47. Gillette PC, Shannon C, Blair H, et al: Transvenous pacing in pediatric patients. Am Heart J 1983; 105:843–847.
48. Case CL: Cardiac pacing in the infant and child with postoperative congenital heart disease. In Gillette PC, Zeigler VL (eds.): Pediatric Cardiac Pacing. Armonk, New York: Futura Publishing Company, Inc.; 1995:95–113.
49. Silka MJ, Rice MJ: Paradoxic embolism due to altered hemodynamic sequence following transvenous pacing. Pacing Clin Electrophysiol 1991; 14:499–503.
50. Parsonett V, Furman S, Smyth NPD, et al: Optimal resources for implantable cardiac pacemakers. Circulation 1983; 68:227A–244A.
51. Gillette PC, Edgerton J, Kratz J, et al: The subpectoral pocket: The preferred implant site for pediatric pacemakers. Pacing Clin Electrophysiol 1991; 14:1089–1092.
52. Sharma AD, Guiraudon GM, Klein GJ, et al: Pacemaker implantation techniques. In El-Sherif N, Samet P (eds.): Cardiac Pacing and Electrophysiology. 3rd ed. Philadelphia: WB Saunders Company; 1998:561–567.
53. Brenner JI, Gaines S, Cordier J, et al: Cardiac strangulation: Two-dimensional echo recognition of a rare complication of epicardial pacemaker therapy. Am J Cardiol 1988; 61:654–656.
54. Perry JC, Nihill MR, Ludomirsky A, et al: The pulmonary artery lasso: Epicardial pacing leads causing right ventricular outflow obstruction. Pacing Clin Electrophysiol 1991; 14:1018–1023.
55. Eyskens B, Mertens L, Moerman P, et al: Cardiac strangulation, a rare complication of epicardial pacemaker leads during growth. Heart 1997; 77:288–289.
56. Ott DA, Gillette PC, Cooley DA: Atrial pacing via the subxyphoid approach. Tex Heart Inst J 1982; 9:149–152.
57. Ulicny KS Jr., Detterbeck FC, Starek PJK, et al: Conjoined subrectus pocket for permanent pacemaker placement in the neonate. Ann Thorac Surg 1992; 53:1130–1131.
58. Robertson JM, Laks H: A new technique for permanent pacemaker implantation in infants and children. Ann Thorac Surg 1987; 44:209–211.
59. Shepard RB, Sand ME, Colvin EV: Cardiac pacing in children. In Grillo HC, Austen WG, Wilkins EW Jr., et al. (eds.): Current Therapy in Cardiothoracic Surgery. Philadelphia: BC Decker, Inc.; 1989:564–567.
60. Rees PG: Use of pacemakers in children. In Stark J, deLeval M (eds.): Surgery for Congenital Heart Defects. Philadelphia: WB Saunders Company; 1994: 139–153.
61. Kratz JM, Gillette PC, Crawford FA, et al: Atrioventricular pacing in congenital heart disease. Ann Thorac Surg 1992; 54:485–489.
62. Stokes K, Bornzin G: The electrode-biointerface: Stimulation. In Barold SS (ed.): Modern Cardiac Pacing. Mt. Kisco, New York: Futura Publishing Company, Inc.; 1985:79–95.
63. Irwin M, Carbol B, Senaratne M, et al: Long-term survival of chosen atrial-based pacing modalities. Pacing Clin Electrophysiol 1996; 19:1796–1798.
64. Ross BA, Zeigler V, Zinner A, et al: The effect of exercise on the atrial electrogram voltage in young patients. Pacing Clin Electrophysiol 1991; 14:2092–2097.
65. Zeigler VL: Intraoperative testing. In Gillette PC, Zeigler VL (eds.): Pediatric

Cardiac Pacing. Armonk, New York: Futura Publishing Company, Inc.; 1995: 63–77.

66. Daubert C, Ritter P, Mabo P, et al: Rate modulation to the AV delay in DDD pacing. In Santini M, Pistolese M, Alliegro A (eds.): Proceedings of the International Symposium on Progress in Clinical Pacing. Amsterdam, The Netherlands: Excerpta Medica, Medical Communications BV; 1990:415–430.

67. Ragonese P, Guccione P, Drago F, et al: Efficacy and safety of ventricular rate responsive pacing in children with complete atrioventricular block. Pacing Clin Electrophysiol 1994; 17:603–610.

68. Conway SP: Pediatric pacemakers for patients with complete heart block. Dim Crit Care Nurs 1997; 16:29–39.

69. Association of Operating Room Nurses: Proposed recommended practice: Monitoring the patient receiving IV conscious sedation. AORN J 1992; 56:316–324.

70. Brownlee JR, Serwer GA, Dick M II, et al: Failure of electrocardiographic monitoring to detect cardiac arrest in patients with pacemakers. Am J Dis Child 1989; 143:105-107.

71. Kleinschmidt KM, Stafford MJ: Dual-chamber cardiac pacemakers. J Cardiovasc Nurs 1991; 5:9–20.

72. Gutgesell HP, Gessner IH, Vetter VL, et al: Recreational and occupational recommendations for young patients with heart disease. A statement for physicians by the Committee on Congenital Cardiac Defects of the Council on Cardiovascular Disease in the Young, American Heart Association. Circulation 1986; 74:1195A-1198A.

73. Vincent JA, Cavitt DL, Karpawich PP: Diagnostic and cost effectiveness of telemonitoring the pediatric pacemaker patient. Pediatr Cardiol 1977; 18:86–90.

74. Zeigler VL: Pacing system follow up. In Gillette PC, Zeigler VL (eds.): Pediatric Cardiac Pacing. Armonk, New York: Futura Publishing Company, Inc.; 1995:205–242.

75. Bricker JT, Barison A, Traveek MS, et al: The use of exercise testing in children to evaluate abnormalities of pacemaker function not apparent at rest. Pacing Clin Electrophysiol 1985; 8:656–660.

76. Serwer GA, Dorostkar PC, LeRoy S, et al: Evaluation of rate variable pacemaker function at maximal exercise exertion in children and young adults. Pacing Clin Electrophysiol 1991; 16:899. Abstract.

77. Serwer GA, Kodali R, Eakin B, et al: Changes in pacemaker threshold with exercise in children and young adults. J Am Coll Cardiol 1991; 17:207A. Abstract.

78. Gillette PC, Zinner A, Kratz J, et al: Atrial tracking (synchronous) pacing in a pediatric and young adult population. J Am Coll Cardiol 1987; 9:811–815.

79. Frohlig G, Blank W, Schwerdt H, et al: Atrial sensing performance of AV universal pacemakers during exercise. Pacing Clin Electrophysiol 1988; 11:47–60.

80. Strathmore NF, Mond HG: Noninvasive monitoring and testing of pacemaker function. Pacing Clin Electrophysiol 1987; 10:1359–1370.

81. Janosik DL, Redd RM, Buckingham TA, et al: Utility of ambulatory electrocardiography in detecting pacemaker dysfunction in the early postimplantation period. Am J Cardiol 1987; 60:1030–1035.

82. Brandt J, Attewell R, Fahraeus T, et al: Acute atrial endocardial P wave amplitude and chronic pacemaker sensitivity requirements: Relation to patient age and presence of sinus node disease. Pacing Clin Electrophysiol 1990; 13:417–424.

83. Gura MT, Ching E, Humphrey D, et al: Reliability of pacemaker autosensing and electrograms in comparison to manual programming of sensitivity: A multicenter study. Pacing Clin Electrophysiol 2000; 23:588. Abstract.

84. Chui CC, Gow RM, McCrindle BW, et al: Impact of programmed sensitivity safety factor on atrial sensing in children. Pacing Clin Electrophysiol 1997; 20:2163–2170.

85. Daubert C, Ritter P, Mabo P, et al: Physiological relationship between AV interval and heart rate in healthy subjects: Applications to dual chamber pacing. Pacing Clin Electrophysiol 1986; 9:1032–1039.
86. Zeigler VL, Gillette PC, Kratz J: Is activity sensored pacing in children and young adults a feasible option? Pacing Clin Electrophysiol 1990; 13:2104–2107.
87. Stewart JV, Sheehan AM: Permanent pacemakers: The nurse's role in patient education and follow-up care. J Cardiovasc Nurs 1991; 5:32–43.
88. Winslow AT: Nursing care of the pediatric pacemaker patient. In Gillette PC, Zeigler VL (eds.): Pediatric Cardiac Pacing. Armonk, New York: Futura Publishing Company, Inc.; 1995:149–180.
89. Brewer EJ Jr., McPherson M, Magrab PR, et al: Family-centered, community-based, coordinated care for children with special health care needs. Pediatrics 1989; 83:1055–1060.
90. Shannon C: Care of the pediatric pacemaker patient. In Dreifus L, Breast A, Purcell JA (eds.): Pacemaker Therapy: An Interprofessional Approach. Philadelphia: FA Davis Company; 1986:219–240.
91. Dunst C, Trivette C, Deal A: Enabling and Empowering Families-Principles and Guidelines for Practice. Cambridge, MA: Brookline Books; 1988.
92. Galdston R, Gamble WJ: On borrowed time: Observations on children with implanted cardiac pacemakers and their families. Am J Psychiatry 1969; 126:142–146.
93. Alpern D, Uzark K, Dick M: Psychosocial responses of children to cardiac pacemakers. J Pediatr 1989; 114:494–501.
94. Andersen C, Horder K, Kristensen L, et al: Psychosocial aspects and mental health in children after permanent pacemaker implantation. Acta Cardiol 1994; 49:405–418.
95. Zeigler VL, Corbett KS: Psychosocial aspects of caring for pediatric pacemaker recipients and their families. In Gillette PC, Zeigler VL (eds.): Pediatric Cardiac Pacing. Armonk, New York: Futura Publishing Company, Inc.; 1995:181–203.
96. Hayes DL, Strathmore NF: Electromagnetic interference with implantable devices. In Ellenbogen KA, Kay GN, Wilkoff BL (eds.): Clinical Cardiac Pacing and Defibrillation. 2nd ed. Philadelphia: WB Saunders Company; 2000:939–952.
97. Altamura G, Bianconi L, LoBianco F, et al: Transthoracic DC shock may represent a serious hazard in pacemaker dependent patients. Pacing Clin Electrophysiol 1995; 18:194–198.

Chapter 8

Implantable Cardioverter Defibrillators

Vicki L. Zeigler, RN, MSN, Karen Corbett, PhD, RN, Ann Lewis, RN, BSN, and Paul C. Gillette, MD

The use of implantable cardioverter defibrillators (ICDs) in the pediatric and young adult population has steadily increased since the first human implant more than 20 years ago.[1–7] Pediatric electrophysiologists were originally somewhat hesitant to implant these devices in children due to their large size and technological limitations. Today, the devices are much smaller and the explosion in technology has produced many more features and programming options that are more suitable to the pediatric population. Additionally, the proven efficacy of the ICD in the adult population has helped to establish it as the primary therapy for the treatment of ventricular arrhythmias resulting in sudden cardiac death (SCD) in children and young adults. Common terminology associated with ICDs can be found in Table 1.

This chapter includes a brief historical perspective of ICDs, a discussion of SCD in the young, the indications for ICD implantation, device technology (including hardware and software), implant technique (transvenous and epicardial), implications for clinicians who care for these patients, follow-up care, patient and family considerations, and, finally, related issues.

Historical Perspective

Starting with the first human implant of an ICD in 1980,[8] the US Food and Drug Administration approved these devices for the treatment of re-

The psychosocial data published in this chapter were supported by the Center for Nursing Research, College of Nursing, Medical University of South Carolina, Charleston, SC.

From Zeigler VL, Gillette PC: *Practical Management of Pediatric Cardiac Arrhythmias.* Armonk, NY: Futura Publishing Co., Inc.; ©2001.

Table 1
Common ICD Terminology

Antitachycardia pacing (ATP)	A train of pacing impulses in response to preset pacing criteria; the pacing can be delivered synchronously or asynchronously at a fixed or decreasing cycle length.
Autodecrement	The automatic and progressive shortening of the interval between paced beats in burst pacing.
Automatic gain control	A feedback mechanism in which the gain of an amplifier can be adjusted automatically according to the sensed magnitude of the input or output signal in order to sense both small and large inputs without undersensing or oversensing.
Biphasic shock	The shock delivered by a biphasic waveform.
Biphasic waveform	A waveform in which the polarity of the shock changes at each electrode part way through the defibrillation waveform.
Capacitor reformation	A process in which the capacitors of the ICD are exercised in order to keep them functional and to evaluate charge times of the device.
Charge time	The time required for the capacitors of the ICD to be charged prior to delivering a shock.
Cycle length	The length of time between one event and the next in a repetitive signal; a measurement of rate expressed in milliseconds.
Dedicated bipolar	A lead configuration in which rate sensing occurs between the tip electrode and a ring electrode positioned approximately 1–2 cm proximal to the lead tip.
Defibrillation threshold (DFT)	The minimum amount of energy required to successfully terminate ventricular fibrillation.
Detection algorithm	A criterion or criteria in which sensed intervals are used for tachycardia recognition; such criteria include sudden onset and rate stability.

(continues)

Table 1
Common ICD Terminology (*cont.*)

Detection enhancements	Criteria used to enhance arrhythmia detection, such as sudden onset, rate stability, and arrhythmia duration.
Detection interval	The cycle length required for a device to detect an arrhythmic event.
Integrated bipolar	A lead configuration in which rate sensing occurs between the tip electrode and the RV defibrillation electrode; the difference between integrated and dedicated bipolar is a function of interelectrode distance and size of the proximal anodal electrode.
Monophasic shock	The shock delivered by a monophasic waveform.
Monophasic waveform	A waveform that changes from a zero-potential baseline in either a positive or negative direction, but not both.
Morphology	The shape of the ECG or electrogram waveforms.
Noncommitted shock	A shock that is aborted if the device is allowed to "reconfirm" the arrhythmia after charging.
Probability density function (PDF)	A detection criterion in which the QRS morphology is monitored and the device calculates the amount of time the complex spends on or near the baseline in order to determine if the rhythm requires shocking.
Rate stability	A tachycardia detection criterion in which the variability of the cycle length is assessed in order to determine if tachycardia has occurred.
Redetection interval	The interval after a shock in which redetection of the arrhythmia can occur.
Sudden onset	A tachycardia detection criterion in which the rate of change of rate (or suddenness of onset) is assessed in order to determine if tachycardia has occurred.
Tiered therapy	Treatment modality in which the least aggressive therapy is delivered first, followed by more aggressive therapies, e.g., ATP followed by low-energy cardioversion followed by high-energy shock.

ATP = antitachycardia pacing; ICD = implantable cardioverter defibrillator; RV = right ventricular.

fractory ventricular arrhythmias leading to SCD. The first ICD systems were simple "shock boxes" that depended on probability density function criteria for detection and had batteries that lasted approximately 1 to 2 years. These devices worked well at saving lives, but were technically primitive compared to today's devices. These early systems included a generator, typically sized 145 cc's and 250 g, and a lead/patch system which provided electrodes and insulated wires that connected the ICD to the heart.

In the first decade of ICD use, almost all lead systems were placed epicardially, entailing a thoracotomy or median sternotomy procedure to allow placement of epicardial patches for shocking and screw-in leads for sensing. The ICD was placed in the abdominal area either above or below the rectus muscle, with the lead system tunneled to the device. The implant was performed in the operating room with a surgeon, anesthesiologist, and electrophysiologist present. The procedure took approximately 3 hours. Operative mortality was in the 4% to 5% range and complications were noted in up to 15% of patients.[9] Current ICD systems consist of a generator, which is less than 40 cc's and 77 to 90 g in size, and a lead system. The majority of lead systems are now placed transvenously and can include anywhere from one to three leads. Devices are generally placed in the left pectoral area, either above or below the pectoralis muscle, similar to a permanent pacemaker. Most implants are done by an electrophysiologist in the cardiac catheterization or electrophysiology laboratory, where various levels of sedation and/or anesthesia are used. The procedure takes approximately 60 to 90 minutes and operative mortality is greatly decreased. Transvenous leads and decreased ICD size have reduced implant costs as well as complications, and smaller devices placed subpectorally are more acceptable to most pediatric patients from a comfort and cosmetic standpoint (Fig. 1).

ICD systems have undergone rapid improvements in technology since their inception. Detection algorithms, shock waveforms, and electrogram storage capabilities have improved significantly, resulting in less frequent delivery of inappropriate therapy, more efficacious defibrillation, and improved diagnostic ability. The addition of antitachycardia pacing (ATP) as a therapy for ventricular tachycardia (VT) was a major breakthrough in the therapy arena, providing painless episode termination for many patients with VT.

Until recently, all ICDs were limited to providing single chamber antibradycardia pacing. Presently, dual chamber devices are now available for patients with concomitant bradycardia and/or atrioventricular (AV) node disease. These devices have helped to improve discrimination of supraventricular tachycardia (SVT) from ventricular arrhythmias and contain rate adaptive parameters, mode switching capabilities, a variety of diagnostic features as well as ventricular ATP, cardioversion, and defibrillation algorithms. Therapy delivery by the ICD has seen marked improvement in the last decade as well. Until 1993, the only available ICD therapy was defibrillation and/or cardioversion.

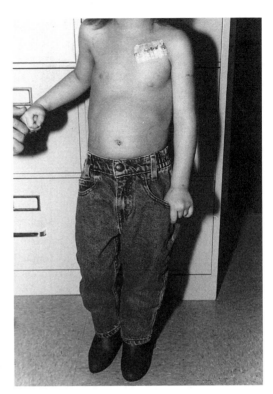

Figure 1. Photograph of a 4-year-old female with long QT syndrome who underwent placement of a single chamber "active can" implantable cardioverter defibrillator in the left subpectoral position.

Hemodynamically stable VT, amenable to ATP, was treated with a painful shock. Bradycardia was either not treated or a concomitant pacemaker was implanted. In 1993, "tiered" therapy was introduced, allowing ATP, low-energy cardioversion, defibrillation, and bradycardia pacing. Multiple tachycardia detection zones can now be programmed, one of which can deliver ATP in an attempt to terminate the VT without a shock, but with shock ability if the tachycardia is not terminated, accelerates, or degenerates into ventricular fibrillation (VF).

Cardioversion and defibrillation methods have also improved. In early devices, all shocks were delivered utilizing a monophasic waveform, i.e., current traveled in only one direction across the heart. In 1993, the biphasic waveform was introduced allowing bidirectional current flow and resulting in improved ability to successfully defibrillate the heart, lower defibrillation thresholds (DFTs),[10] use of simpler lead systems, and decreased overall implant times. An additional feature added around this same time was VF reconfirmation. This feature requires the device to "reconfirm" the arrhythmia after delivering therapy in order for the second shock to be aborted if the arrhythmia has been terminated. In a device with a "noncommitted shock," the device can "reconfirm" the arrhythmia after charging in order to abort the shock if the arrhythmia has terminated; this only applies to the first shock as all subsequent shocks are "committed."

Great strides have been made in the last decade with respect to available diagnostics within the ICD. Stored electrograms (intracardiac electrocardiograms [ECGs] recorded during tachycardia episodes) provide enormous assistance to the clinician in determining the appropriateness of delivered therapies. Many "alerts" have been added that provide notification of certain occurrences such as changes in lead impedance, low battery status, and excessive charge times. These technological advances require that clinicians remain up to date in their knowledge regarding a variety of devices from a variety of manufacturers.

Sudden Cardiac Death in Children

SCD in adults with coronary artery disease and ventricular arrhythmias is a very large public health concern. Unlike in the adult population, in the pediatric population SCD is relatively uncommon, with an estimated incidence of 1 to 13 events per 100,000 patient-years.[11–13] The fundamental difference between children and young adults in the documented arrhythmia mechanism is that in most pediatric patients, asystole versus VF is the most commonly documented terminal arrhythmia.[14] Early reports indicate that children with cardiovascular disease are more likely to have ventricular arrhythmias as a cause of sudden death.[15] More recent data indicate that late sudden death risk in postoperative congenital heart disease (CHD) patients is 25 to 100 times greater than in age-matched controls, with the increased risk occurring primarily in patients with cyanotic or obstructive left heart lesions following the second postoperative decade.[16]

SCD is associated with three principle forms of cardiovascular disease in the pediatric patient: cardiomyopathy, primary electrical disease, and CHD. The relative risk profile for each of these subgroups of pediatric patients varies, as do the associated risk factors and electrophysiologic mechanisms,[17] which are delineated in Table 2.

The most common cause of SCD in young patients is hypertrophic cardiomyopathy.[3] There is a 4% to 6% per year sudden mortality rate in children with hypertrophic cardiomyopathy, a risk that is much higher in children than in adults.[18] Dilated cardiomyopathy has been associated with SCD in children, but the sudden death rate in these patients is more likely associated with congestive heart failure and bradyarrhythmias than ventricular arrhythmias.[19,20] Another form of cardiomyopathy emerging as a role player in SCD in the young is arrhythmogenic right ventricular dysplasia. Studies have reported mixed conclusions regarding the precise cause of sudden death in these patients, ranging from ventricular arrhythmias to acute heart failure.[21,22]

By far, the most expanding category of patients who experience SCD in the pediatric population are those with primary electrical diseases, specifically idiopathic VF and the congenital form of the long QT syndrome (LQTS).[6,23,24] Of 287 young patients with LQTS studied by Garson and colleagues,[24] 9% presented with sudden cardiac arrest as their initial symptom.

The third category of children experiencing SCD are those with CHD.

Table 2
Sudden Cardiac Death in the Young—Relative Risk Profile

	SCD Risk (per year)	Electrophysiologic Mechanism of SCD	Associated Risk Factors
Congenital heart disease			
Tetralogy of Fallot	0.1%–1.5%	VT→VF AV block (??)	RV/LV dysfunction
Aortic stenosis	0.3%–1.0%	Ischemia → VF	LV hypertrophy/fibrosis
Transposition of the great arteries	0.2%–2.0%	Atrial flutter 1:1 conduction VT → VF (?) Bradycardia→ asystole (??)	RV dysfunction
Cardiomyopathies			
Idiopathic dilated	0.4%–1.5%	Bradycardia→ asystole Electromechanical dissociation VT → VF (?)	CHF Sustained VT
Hypertrophic	3.0%–6.0%	VT → VF SVT → VF (??)	Familial SCD Inducible VT
Primary electrical diseases			
Idiopathic VF	1.0%–11.0%	Polymorphic VT → VF	Syncope
Long QT syndromes	4.0%–6.0%	Torsades de pointes → VF	Syncope AV block

AV = atrioventricular; CHF = congestive heart failure; LV = left ventricular; RV = right ventricular; SCD = sudden cardiac death; SVT = supraventricular tachycardia; VF = ventricular fibrillation; VT = ventricular tachycardia.

Reproduced from Silka MJ, Kron J, Gillette PC: Implantable cardioverter-defibrillators in children and adolescents. In Estes NAM, Manolis AS, Wang PJ (eds.): Implantable Cardioverter-Defibrillator: A Comprehensive Textbook. New York: Marcel Dekker Inc.; 1994:206, with permission.

Children with CHD differ from adults with coronary artery disease in three ways: 1) children are more likely than adults to suffer from bradycardia as a terminal event[15]; 2) atrial tachyarrhythmias (specifically postoperative atrial flutter/intraatrial reentry tachycardia) are correlated with SCD in children[24]; and 3) coronary artery abnormalities or diseases are generally not associated with SCD in the young.[25]

The most studied of the congenital heart defects associated with SCD in children and young adults include tetralogy of Fallot, aortic stenosis, transposition of the great arteries,[26–29] and, more recently, coarctation of the aorta.[16] Although the electrophysiologic mechanisms of SCD in these patients may vary, some of them will experience a ventricular arrhythmia as a cause of their sudden cardiac arrest.

Indications

Since pediatric patients comprise less than 2% of the total number of ICD recipients,[3] the guidelines proposed for ICD implantation include both adults and children.[30] These indications can be found in Table 3 and are

Table 3
Indications for ICD Therapy

Class I
1. Cardiac arrest due to VF or VT, not due to a transient or reversible cause. (Level of evidence: A)
2. Spontaneous sustained VT. (Level of evidence: B)
3. Syncope of undetermined origin with clinically relevant, hemodynamically significant sustained VT or VF induced at electrophysiology study when drug therapy is ineffective, not tolerated, or not preferred. (Level of evidence: B)
4. Nonsustained VT with coronary disease, prior MI, LV dysfunction, and inducible VF or sustained VT at electrophysiology study that is not suppressible by a Class I antiarrhythmic drug. (Level of evidence: B)

Class IIa
None

Class IIb
1. Cardiac arrest presumed to be due to VF when electrophysiology testing is precluded by other medical conditions. (Level of evidence: C)
2. Severe symptoms attributable to sustained ventricular tachyarrhythmias while awaiting cardiac transplantation. (Level of evidence: C)
3. Familial or inherited conditions with a high risk for life-threatening ventricular tachyarrhythmias such as long QT syndrome or hypertrophic cardiomyopathy. (Level of evidence: B)
4. Nonsustained VT with coronary artery disease, prior MI, and LV dysfunction, and sustained VT or VF at electrophysiology study. (Level of evidence: B)
5. Recurrent syncope of undetermined etiology in the presence of ventricular dysfunction and inducible ventricular arrhythmias at electrophysiology study when other causes of syncope have been excluded. (Level of evidence: C)

Class III
1. Syncope of undetermined cause in a patient without inducible ventricular tachyarrhythmias. (Level of evidence: C)
2. Incessant VT or VF. (Level of evidence: C)
3. VF or VT resulting from arrhythmias amenable to surgical or catheter ablation; for example, atrial arrhythmias associated with the Wolff-Parkinson-White syndrome, RV outflow tract VT, idiopathic LV tachycardia, or fascicular VT. (Level of evidence: C)
4. Ventricular tachyarrhythmias due to a transient or reversible disorder (e.g., AMI, electrolyte imbalance, drugs, trauma). (Level of evidence: C)
5. Significant psychiatric illnesses that may be aggravated by device implantation or may preclude systematic follow-up. (Level of evidence: C)
6. Terminal illnesses with projected life expectancy ≤6 months. (Level of evidence: C)
7. Patients with coronary artery disease with LV dysfunction and prolonged QRS duration in the absence of spontaneous or inducible sustained or nonsustained VT who are undergoing coronary bypass surgery. (Level of evidence: B)
8. NYHA Class IV drug-refractory congestive heart failure in patients who are not candidates for cardiac transplantation. (Level of evidence: C)

AMI = acute myocardial infarction; ICD = implantable cardioverter defibrillator; LV = left ventricular; MI = myocardial infarction; NYHA = New York Heart Association; RV = right ventricular; VF = ventricular fibrillation; VT = ventricular tachycardia.

Reproduced from Gregatoros G, Cheitlin MD, Conill A, et al: ACC/AHA guidelines for implantation of cardiac pacemakers and antiarrhythmia devices. Circulation 1998; 97:1325–1335, with permission.

expressed in the standard American College of Cardiology/American Heart Association format. Class I indications are those in which there is general agreement and/or evidence that the ICD will be useful, effective, and beneficial; Class II indications are those in which there is divergence of opinion and/or conflicting evidence about the efficacy and/or usefulness of the ICD; and Class III indications are those in which there is general agreement and/or evidence that the ICD is not useful and may even be harmful. Class II is divided as follows: Class IIa indicates that the weight is in favor of the usefulness/efficacy of the device, while in Class IIb, that usefulness/efficacy is less well established. This document contains no Class IIa indications. The "levels of evidence" denoted after each classification are defined as follows: Level A ranking denotes that multiple, randomized clinical trials involving a large number of subjects were used to derive the data's evidence; Level B denotes the data were derived from a limited number of trials with smaller numbers of patients that may have been performed in a nonrandomized or observational manner; and Level C is based on expert consensus among those with years of clinical experience.[30]

Current data suggest that 60% of ICD recipients less than 20 years of age have a form of cardiomyopathy, 25% have primary electrical disease, and only 15% were postoperative for CHD.[3] In addition to the aforementioned subcategories, there have been reports of ICD recipients with the following conditions: double outlet right ventricle,[4] arrhythmogenic right ventricular dysplasia,[4,5] and Marfan syndrome.[7] The ICD has also been used as a "bridge" to transplantation in certain high-risk children. The use of ICDs as a prophylactic treatment in children with genetic diseases such as congenital LQTS may see a surge in the future.

The clinical indications for ICD placement in children vary. Silka and Gillette[31] have identified the three most common clinical scenarios representing the indications for ICD implantation in young patients: 1) the patient who has been resuscitated from a sudden cardiac arrest in whom no arrhythmia can be identified, nor can reliable treatment be established; 2) the patient with recurrent, symptomatic VT who has been identified at high risk for sudden death and who is intolerant of antiarrhythmic treatment; and 3) the patient who is asymptomatic, but who has known cardiovascular disease and a strong family history of SCD.[31] The decision to implant an ICD in a young patient is multifaceted. The clinician must take into account many variables when making this decision, including the patient's relative risk of sudden death, underlying structural heart disease, arrhythmia mechanism, other available treatment options, and the risk/benefit ratio of having an ICD implanted. Genetic diseases and a family history of SCD are also key variables to consider in making this decision.

Device Technology

To appreciate the complexity of ICDs today, it is important to understand the specifics of device technology. This technology can be viewed in two different ways of equal importance: hardware and software, both of which are necessary to detect the low-amplitude, high-frequency signals produced by VF and to deliver the high-energy shocks needed to terminate the arrhythmia. The hardware of the ICD system consists of the device itself and the leads and/or patches that are used along with the device to complete the system. The software, considered the "brain" of the system, includes the various energy waveforms, tachycardia detection capabilities, tachycardia termination therapies, bradycardia pacing parameters, tachycardia discrimination features, and diagnostic capabilities (including event counters and stored electrograms).

Hardware

Devices

The newer devices are similar in size to the average beeper. The device header (made of polyurethane or epoxy) is housed at the top of the device and functions as the lead/patch connection structure. The generator itself is housed in a titanium case with its serial number usually engraved on the anterior surface of the device. Additional radiopaque identifiers are placed on the device to allow visual radiographic identification once the device has been implanted.

The device "can" houses the microcircuitry, a battery, and high-voltage capacitors. The battery of the ICD is slightly different than the battery in a conventional pacemaker and consists of lithium silver vanadium oxide rather than lithium iodide, because the latter source is not able to deliver energy rapidly enough to charge the high-voltage capacitors.[32] The capacitor is the largest component of the device and accounts for its somewhat large size when compared with conventional pacemakers.

Lead Systems

Lead systems vary from manufacturer to manufacturer, but have some similarities. Conventional ICD leads are composed of electrodes, conductors, insulating coating, connectors, and a fixation mechanism. The distal tip of nearly all ICD leads incorporates an electrode that maintains electrical contact with the heart for sensing of cardiac activity. The conductors (coils of wire) conduct the electricity between the electrode(s) and the ICD. The fixation mechanism of the lead is either active or passive (Fig. 2). *Active fixation* leads utilize a mechanism, usually a screw of some sort, that allows penetration into the myocardium. The benefits of active fixation leads are thought to be decreased incidence of dislodgment (when compared with passive fixation leads), easier removal, and physician preference in postoperative CHD patients. *Passive fixation* leads are secured in place with a combination of the use of fins (or tines), which are 2- to 3-mm-

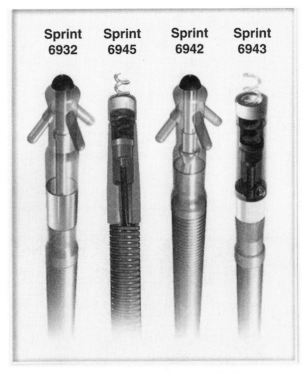

Figure 2. Four endocardial implantable cardioverter defibrillator leads with the two fixation mechanisms. The first (from the left) and third are passive fixation leads, while the second and fourth are active fixation leads.

long extensions of the insulation proximal to the electrode that lodge into fibrous tissue at the lead's tip. The major benefit of passive fixation leads is thought to be superior pacing and sensing thresholds. Both of these types of leads are now available in a steroid-eluting form, in which approximately 1.0 mg of dexamethasone has been added to the tip. This type of lead has almost eliminated the acute peaks in pacing thresholds seen after implantation and has also significantly reduced chronic pacing thresholds. Defibrillation leads range in size from 7 Fr to 12 Fr, are approximately 58 & 65–75 cm in length, and are insulated with silicone or polyurethane.

Defibrillation leads typically incorporate 2 to 4 electrodes that are used for sensing, pacing, and shocking. Endocardial sensing and pacing are accomplished using two electrodes, one at the lead tip and one just proximal to the former, providing a bipolar sensing and pacing configuration. Epicardial sensing leads utilize a small screw on the proximal end that is embedded in the epicardial surface. Epicardial bipolar sensing and pacing can now be accomplished using a bipolar, steroid-eluting epicardial lead or, as in the past, by using two separate unipolar leads attached to a bipolar connector.

Most transvenous ICD lead systems consist of one lead that incorporates a high-output shocking coil and a bipolar sensing pole. In the case of dual chamber application, the atrial sensing and pacing lead is a standard pacemaker lead. In the past, if two shocking coils were insufficient in providing adequate DFTs, a third shocking coil, a subcutaneous patch, or a subcutaneous array was added. The "active" or "hot can" system uses a single, unipolar defibrillation lead with the metallic housing of the device can itself as the second shocking electrode.

Patches/Arrays

Due to advances in technology and decreased device size, epicardial patches are rarely used today. The patches, square or oval in shape and similar in appearance to a fly swatter, are made of titanium or aluminum alloy mesh with a stainless steel and silver composite conductor[33] (Fig. 3).

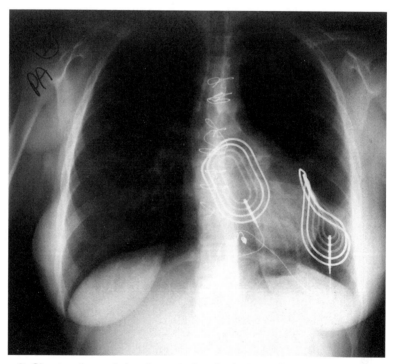

Figure 3. Chest radiograph (posteroanterior view) of a patient with an epicardial implantable cardioverter defibrillator. The two defibrillating patches as well as the two screw-in sensing leads can be seen in this 20-year-old postoperative tetralogy of Fallot patient.

Insulation is accomplished using silicone or polyurethane, and the various shapes and sizes are chosen based on the ventricular access approach and heart size. Larger patches are thought to decrease impedance (resulting in a greater current flow between electrodes) by providing a higher voltage gradient within the shock field over a greater ventricular mass.[34]

The subcutaneous patch is made of conductive mesh that is laminated and sewn between two silicone rubber sheets, one of which contains windows that expose the mesh. These patches can be positioned subcutaneously at the apex or in the prepectoral region and are used primarily to lower monophasic DFTs. The subcutaneous array is also used for this purpose and consists of three flexible defibrillator leads that are joined at a common connector; this is rarely used in children. With advent and success of the nonthoracotomy approach and the long-term problems associated with epicardial patches, manufacturers are no longer producing them.

Software

The ICD software has advanced immensely since the original devices. The ICD sensing circuitry must be able to sense very fine amplitude signals consistent with VF, while at the same time avoiding oversensing that may lead to inappropriate therapy. The older approach to sensing used an algorithm that applied high sensitivity (0.15 to 0.6 mV) prior to each incoming cardiac signal, with a slightly lower sensitivity (0.5 to 3.0 mV) immediately after each signal. This decreased sensitivity prevented T wave sensing that may have resulted in "double counting" leading to an inappropriate shock. Newer technology allows the sensitivity threshold to be adjusted on a "beat-to-beat" basis (known as auto gain or auto sensitivity adjustment), resulting in prompt rhythm recognition change.

Detection algorithms now allow more than one criterion for tachycardia detection, including heart rate, rate stability, and onset. The primary criterion used for tachycardia detection is that of heart rate, but rate stability and onset can be used in conjunction with heart rate in select patients. The *stability* criterion is used to determine if the detected rhythm is variable on a beat-to-beat basis, which may be useful in avoiding detection of atrial tachyarrhythmias that are irregular, e.g., atrial fibrillation. This criterion utilizes a certain percentage that the heart rate is not allowed to change on a beat-to-beat basis. *Onset* criteria are used to determine how fast or how slow the arrhythmia starts. For example, sinus tachycardia slowly accelerates (or gradually warms up) and is not considered to be of sudden onset. These criteria can be used in combinations for arrhythmia detection in order to provide the most appropriate therapy as well as to avoid inappropriate shocks.

Shock waveforms can be delivered in a monophasic or biphasic fashion. Biphasic shocks have been associated with lower defibrillation energy requirements compared with their monophasic counterparts.[10] With a biphasic waveform, most of the energy is delivered with the initial pulse; the polarity then reverses on the second pulse delivering the balance of the available energy.[35–37] On average, when the waveforms are optimized for efficiency, it takes 44% less energy to defibrillate using the biphasic waveform.[35] Although biphasic waveforms are now preferred, most devices have the capability to deliver either a biphasic or monophasic waveform. The microcircuitry in most devices allows the waveform polarity to be noninvasively reprogrammed and provides "noncommitted" shocks that allow the device to "reevaluate" the arrhythmia after charging prior to therapy delivery.

The monitoring capabilities of currently available ICDs have expanded enormously in the past several years, providing the clinician with a somewhat overwhelming amount of data. Arrhythmia episode data are stored, including number of episodes, number of termination attempts (successful and unsuccessful), charge time, and intracardiac electrograms, including prior to, during, and after therapy delivery. Tachyarrhythmia induction capabilities are present in current devices, allowing noninvasive arrhythmia induction using programmed electrical stimulation. Real time telemetry provides measured data obtained from the device, such as lead impedances, battery voltage, and charge times, to name a few. A broad range of bradycardia pacing capabilities also exist, including automatic mode switching and SVT discrimination algorithms in dual chamber devices.

Implant Technique

The first reports of ICD implantation in young patients involved the use of the epicardial technique.[1,2] In Kron and colleagues' report of 40 patients,[2] a lateral thoracotomy was used in 56% of patients, a midline sternotomy in 31% of patients, and a subcostal or subxiphoid in the remaining 13%. The first report of a nonthoracotomy approach was published in 1994 and included 17 young patients,[4] and in a smaller, more recent series comparing the two approaches,[38] the transvenous approach was found to be associated with lower morbidity and decreased length of hospital stay.[38]

Today, the choice of ICD implant technique in children and young adults is determined by several factors including patient size, presence of intracardiac shunts, superior vena cava obstruction, lack of a connection at the atrial level, and structural anatomy that will not allow endocardial lead placement. In patients with CHD, careful consideration to cardiac position, the location of the major ventricular mass, and the presence of prosthetic valves must also be given with respect to implant technique. The endocardial approach is preferred over the epicardial approach due to the presumption that endocardial sensing with ICD leads is superior to epicardial sensing based on previous experience with sensing and pacing in the pacemaker population.[39]

Select noninvasive data should be reviewed by the clinician prior to ICD implantation, including but not limited to 12-lead ECG, 24-hour ambulatory monitor, exercise stress test, previous operative reports, previous catheterization/electrophysiology study reports, current medications, and, importantly, an echocardiogram. Since the incidence of embolic events is increased in children with intracardiac shunts,[40] all efforts to document their presence must be undertaken in patients about to undergo the transvenous approach. This can be accomplished in most cases with simple transthoracic echocardiography, but in some cases may require contrast or even transesophageal echocardiography. The following discussion includes ICD system selection, a description of the transvenous and epicardial placement techniques, and intraoperative testing.

Implantable Cardioverter Defibrillator System Selection

Once the decision to implant an ICD has been made, the clinician must determine the system that will be best suited for the individual patient's needs. Determining factors include the patient's size, the specific arrhythmia mechanism, concomitant arrhythmias, and the patient's overall cardiac condition. Due to the complexity of currently available devices, the clinician must consider the overall risk/benefit ratio for a particular system for each individual patient. For example, a small child with LQTS may benefit more from a simple single lead system that serves to defibrillate in the event of a sustained episode of VT/fibrillation. The teenager with ventricular arrhythmias after repair of tetralogy of Fallot with concomitant third-degree AV block may benefit more from a dual chamber device capable of providing atrial synchronous pacing as well as tiered therapy.

An important factor in determining which ICD system is best suited for a particular patient is whether the system will be implanted transvenously or epicardially. Once the specific implant technique has been determined, the clinician must decide whether to implant a single chamber system or a dual chamber system. The authors prefer a single chamber system that uses an active can configuration in very small patients, i.e., less than 30 kg.

A dual chamber system is generally reserved for those patients with conduction system disease as well as ventricular arrhythmias, in particular patients who have undergone previous surgery for CHD. These devices, capable of providing AV synchrony and rate-adaptive bradycardia pacing, also have other desirable features. They allow shorter AV intervals for sensing and pacing, the latter of which is especially important in patients with hypertrophic cardiomyopathy. They are equipped with algorithms that can provide discrimination between supraventricular and VTs, and can provide overdrive pacing for reentrant VTs as well as back-up cardioversion or defibrillation.

There are a multitude of electrode systems from which to choose, including epicardial, endocardial, and subcutaneous varieties. Each type is needed to care for patients with CHD. In order to be most effective, the defibrillation shock must pass through the heart's major ventricular mass; thus, in patients with normal hearts or a hypertrophic left ventricle, defibrillation from the right ventricle to an active can in the left shoulder is often very effective. On the other hand, this would not be a good arrangement for a patient with dextrocardia where a right shoulder implant of an active can should be more effective in providing the optimal shocking vector. Many variations are possible and each patient must be considered individually (Fig. 4). Although patients who have had a Mustard or Senning operation

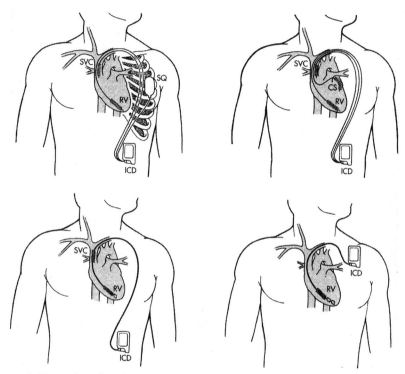

Figure 4. Examples of various placements for nonthoracotomy lead systems. Clockwise from upper left-hand corner: A three-lead system with shocks delivered from the right ventricular (RV) electrode to the superior vena cava (SVC) electrode and also to the subcutaneous patch (SQ) electrode; a three-lead system with shocks delivered from the RV to SVC electrodes and also to the coronary sinus; a single lead system with shocks delivered from the RV to SVC electrodes; and a single lead system with shocks delivered from the RV electrode to the pulse generator can. Reproduced from Stephenson N, Combs WJ: Artificial cardiac pacemakers and implantable cardioverter-defibrillators. In Kinney MR, Packa DR (eds.): Andreoli's Comprehensive Cardiac Care. 8th ed. St. Louis: Mosby-Year Book, Inc.; 1996:248, with permission.

for transposition of the great arteries possess ventricles in the normal position, the ventricular mass is reversed due to the right ventricular hypertrophy and left ventricular atrophy. This may require a subcutaneous patch in the right upper abdominal quadrant or a coil placed in the inferior vena cava with the main defibrillating electrode in the left (blue) ventricle.

Transvenous Technique

Transvenous implantation of an ICD in a pediatric patient is best carried out by a pediatric electrophysiologist in a pediatric electrophysiology/catheterization laboratory with a team consisting of clinicians who routinely care for children and who have a working knowledge of CHD. As previously mentioned, angiography and even interventional procedures are often needed in children with CHD, and the procedure room should be readily equipped for any and all patient scenarios. As with permanent pacemaker implantation outside of the operating room environment, sterility and air handling/filtration standards in the catheterization/electrophysiology laboratory should be consistent with those of the operating room, with the staff remaining cognizant of maintaining strict sterile technique.

Transvenous ICD implantation may be carried out in very small children. Reported implantation weights range from 32 kg[4] to 27 kg[7] to 20 kg.[41] In the authors' experience, the smallest recipient of a transvenous system weighed 15 kg. The endocardial approach is very similar in technique to that of transvenous pacemaker implantation. Once adequate anesthesia has been obtained, the authors place an indwelling femoral artery catheter for invasive blood pressure monitoring and blood gas analysis throughout the procedure. Additionally, a venous catheter is placed via the femoral vein all the way into the left subclavian vein for contrast analysis of venous anatomy. Preapplied self-adhesive pacing/defibrillation pads are placed prior to the procedure for back-up defibrillation and/or bradycardia pacing.

In most children and young adults, the device is placed in a left subpectoral position, with a single coil electrode and the device itself functioning as the second electrode (Fig. 5). In most cases the subclavian vein is used for lead placement, although the cephalic vein can also be used. The ICD lead is placed using the same technique described in chapter 7 for permanent pacemakers, using a 10.5 Fr introducer. Pacing and sensing thresholds are evaluated in the same manner as one would utilize with permanent pacing leads.

As previously mentioned, the ICD generator can be placed subpectorally or abdominally by tunneling the lead from the subclavicular area to the abdominal pocket, which may be above or under the rectus muscle. Serwer and colleagues[41] report that the use of a single coil, bipolar pacing, steroid-eluting lead placed into the subclavian vein and tunneled to an upper left quadrant abdominal pocket has yielded DFTs less than 10 J in all cases, has not required an additional electrode in any patient, and has been performed in patients weighing as little as 20 kg.

Once the stylets and sheaths are removed and the leads affixed to the ICD, the device is placed in its pocket for tachycardia induction and detection and termination algorithm testing using the device itself (this is discussed below in the section on intraoperative testing). After adequate pacing, sensing, and DFTs are obtained, the lead or leads are sutured to the chest wall using 2.0 Dexon®. The subpectoral pocket is closed using absorbable 2–0 suture as is the subcutaneous tissue. A 4–0 running absorbable skin suture completes the three-layer closure. Steri-strips are applied over benzoin and the incision lightly dressed. The arterial and ve-

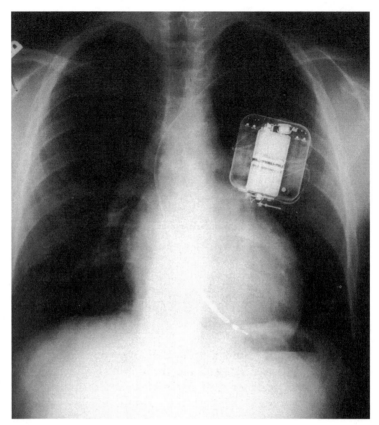

Figure 5. Chest radiograph (posteroanterior view) in patient with a single chamber ICD implanted by the transvenous approach. The lead has a single defibrillating coil and dedicated bipolar sense/pace configuration.

nous sheaths are removed and the patient is awakened, extubated, and transported to the postanesthesia recovery unit.

Epicardial Technique

As previously discussed, the preferred implant technique for ICDs in most children and young adults is the endocardial or transvenous technique; however, some pediatric patients require the use of the epicardial technique. These patients include those with right-to-left or left-to-right intracardiac shunts, very small children (<20 kg), patients without a venous connection at the atrial level (such as patients who have undergone the Fontan repair), and patients with prosthetic tricuspid valves.

The epicardium can be approached using several techniques, including a median sternotomy, a thoracotomy, or a subcostal or substernal approach. These various approaches are discussed in detail in chapter 7. The specific epicardial approach used is determined by the individual patient characteristics such as cardiovascular anatomy, previous operations, size, and ventricular anatomy, as well as by surgeon preference.

In the past, two unipolar screw-in leads were placed no farther apart than 1 cm on the epicardium to be used for bipolar sensing. Historically, the epicardial rate-sensing lead was commonly placed on the left ventricle due to its greater ventricular mass and the increased amplitude of the bipolar electrogram in adult ICD recipients.[42] Currently, either ventricle may be used for the rate-sensing electrodes, with one patch typically placed on the right ventricle.

Epicardial patches are placed either inside or outside the pericardium, with one over the posterolateral wall or the left ventricular apex and the other onto the right ventricle or right atrium in order to position the maximum ventricular mass between the two electrodes. Serwer and colleagues[41] recommend suturing the patches to the pericardium rather than the epicardial surface to minimize the effect of growth and to decrease the incidence of patch distortion. The patches should be placed so that maximum and equal amounts of cardiac mass are between them. The patches should not overlap and the electrodes should not come in contact with each other. More than two patches may be used if necessary due to increased DFTs. Care must be taken to avoid the coronary arteries in small children, as well as the phrenic nerve, when placing epicardial leads and patches. Epicardial patch placement is virtually the same regardless of the congenital heart defect.

Intraoperative Testing

The pacing and sensing parameters are tested for each lead in the manner described in chapter 7. Once these measurements are completed, the impedance of the defibrillating electrode is tested with a low-output shock. An acceptable range for this value is 10 to 40 Ω.[43] Prior to device placement, most manufacturers recommend an initial interrogation while the device is still within its sterile packaging. A manual capacitor formation is performed by dumping any charge on the capacitors then charging to the highest stored energy. By not dumping this stored charge, the capacitors are reformed. Any pertinent patient data, as well as the bradycardia pacing parameters, can be programmed into the device at this time.

The device is then attached to the lead and placed in the device pocket for DFT testing. External defibrillation capabilities must be confirmed at this time. Induction can be performed using programmed electrical stimulation (including burst pacing), T wave shock, or 50-Hz shock (Figs. 6 and 7). Prior to VF induction, the VF detection parameters should be optimized for sensing and quick therapy delivery, including the detection interval itself as well as the number of intervals required for detection. The energy and pathway of the shock should also be programmed at this time. The initial shock is programmed to deliver 20 J and the second is programmed at the maximum output. If 20 J is successful in terminating the arrhythmia, the permanent settings used are set for 30 or 35 J. A DFT of at least 10 J less than

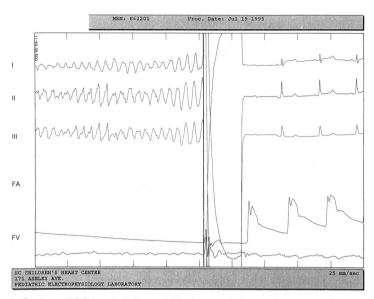

Figure 6. Surface ECG leads I, II, and III along with femoral artery and venous pressure tracings during an episode of ventricular fibrillation that was successfully terminated with a 20-J shock during transvenous defibrillation threshold testing.

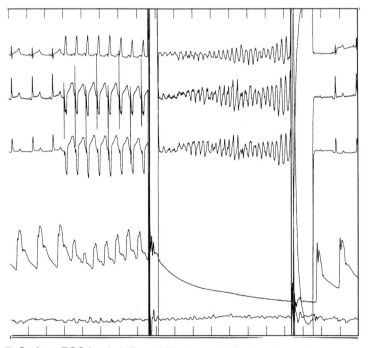

Figure 7. Surface ECG leads I, II, and III along with femoral artery and venous pressure tracings during induction of torsades de pointes using ventricular pacing followed by a T wave shock during implant defibrillation threshold testing. The 20-J shock is successful in restoring normal sinus rhythm.

the device's maximum output is considered an acceptable DFT by most implanting physicians.[44] After tachycardia induction and termination, the clinician can evaluate the appropriateness of the recognition and termination algorithms by recording ECGs with annotation markers during device testing as well as obtaining measured data from the device after an appropriate postshock interval.

If 20 J does not successfully terminate the arrhythmia, the polarity is reversed and DFTs are performed again. If the DFT continues to be greater than 20 J, the lead is repositioned. If high DFTs persist, a second coil or subcutaneous patch is added. The first choice for coil placement is the innominate vein in most patients, the superior vena cava in larger patients, and the inferior vena cava in patients with transposition of the great arteries. A subcutaneous patch is also used if the veins are too small, stenosed, or thrombosed.

Once acceptable DFTs have been obtained, the tachycardia recognition and termination algorithms can be permanently programmed (Fig. 8). If ATP is to be used as a termination algorithm, the arrhythmia should be induced and the algorithm tested for efficacy. The bradycardia pacing parameters should be patient specific and are discussed in detail in chapter 7. The remainder of this discussion pertains to the parameters specific to optimum ICD functioning. Most manufacturers recommend a ventricular sensitivity setting of 0.3 mV in order to maximize VF detection.

An issue specific to young ICD recipients is that of inappropriate shocks.[4,6,7] Inappropriate shocks in children are associated with SVT, non-sustained VT, and high sinus rates (when compared with adults). Several developments in tachycardia detection have alleviated some of these problems, but this issue continues to remain a concern among pediatric electrophysiologists. In most cases, a detection interval of 272 ms/220 beats per minute will be sufficient, but exercise stress testing may elucidate the need to reconsider this interval in some patients. The number of intervals to detect is an important criterion that must be patient specific. Patients with LQTS may experience nonsustained episodes of VT or torsades de pointes. By using a ratio of beats for detection, e.g., 18/24 or 24/32, unnecessary shocks may be avoided. The redetection interval programmed should be relatively short for therapy to be delivered in a timely manner.

The termination algorithms must be patient specific. In most cases, the devices are programmed for a VF zone with a lower output on the first shock and maximum outputs on the remainder of shocks. The energy pathway should be programmed in conjunction with the implant DFTs and, if the clinician desires, the device can be programmed to "reconfirm" the arrhythmia after charging but just before energy is delivered. In the case of documented and tested VT, the termination algorithm can be programmed in a tiered fashion going from least aggressive therapy (ATP) to more aggressive (low-energy cardioversion) to most aggressive (high-energy defibrillation). Several termination algorithms can be used for ATP, including fixed rate, burst pacing, ramp pacing, or a combination. *Burst*

ICD Model: Gem DR 7271

Sep 28, 2000 14:08:27
9960 Software Version 3.0
Copyright (c) Medtronic, Inc. 1997

Parameter Settings Report   Page 2

VF Therapies	Rx1	Rx2	Rx3	Rx4	Rx5	Rx6
VF Therapy Status	On	On	On	On	On	On
Energy	35 J	35 J	35 J	35 J	35 J	35 J
Pathway	AX>B	AX>B	AX>B	AX>B	AX>B	AX>B
Reconfirm VF after initial charge?	Yes					

FVT Therapies	Rx1	Rx2	Rx3	Rx4	Rx5	Rx6
FVT Therapy Status						
Therapy Type	None	None	None	None	None	None
Initial # Pulses						
R-S1 Interval=(%RR)						
S1S2(Ramp+)=(%RR)						
S2SN(Ramp+)=(%RR)						
Interval Dec						
# Sequences						
Smart Mode						
Energy						
Pathway						
Anti-Tachy Pacing Minimum Interval	200 ms					

ICD Model: Gem DR 7271

Sep 28, 2000 14:08:38
9960 Software Version 3.0
Copyright (c) Medtronic, Inc. 1997

Parameter Settings Report   Page 3

VT Therapies	Rx1	Rx2	Rx3	Rx4	Rx5	Rx6
VT Therapy Status						
Therapy Type	None	None	None	None	None	None
Initial # Pulses						
R-S1 Interval=(%RR)						
S1S2(Ramp+)=(%RR)						
S2SN(Ramp+)=(%RR)						
Interval Dec						
# Sequences						
Smart Mode						
Energy						
Pathway						
Anti-Tachy Pacing Minimum Interval	200 ms					

Shared Anti-Tachy Pacing Therapy

V. Amplitude	8 V
V. Pulse Width	1.6 ms
V. Pace Blanking	240 ms

Shared VF, FVT, and VT Therapy

Progressive Episode Therapies	Off

A

Figure 8A. Programmed parameter settings report from an implanted dual chamber implantable cardioverter defibrillator after successful implant defibrillation threshold testing. There are no therapies programmed for VT, and all six ventricular fibrillation therapies are set at maximum energy output. *Continues.*

pacing is when a percentage of the tachycardia cycle length is used to calculate the ATP interval, which is then delivered at that cycle length for a programmed number of intervals. *Ramp pacing* is similar, but allows a beat-to-beat decrement in the ATP cycle length for a predetermined number of cycles. In general, ATP is chosen as an initial therapy, but all subsequent therapies use cardioversion and/or defibrillation.

An important parameter to be programmed at this time is the automatic capacitor reformation interval, which in most cases is programmed for every 3 or 6 months. If mode switching is necessary, the associated parameters should be programmed at this time. Data collection set-up can be programmed at this point or just prior to hospital discharge. If the de-

ICD Model: Gem DR 7271

9960 Software Version 3.0
Copyright (c) Medtronic, Inc. 1997

Parameter Settings Report — Page 4

Modes/Rates

Mode	DDD
Mode Switch	Off
Lower Rate	50 ppm
Upper Tracking Rate	120 ppm

A-V Intervals

Paced AV	180 ms
Sensed AV	180 ms
Rate Adaptive AV	Off

Rate Therapy Features

V. Rate Stabilization	Off

Post Shock Pacing

A. Amplitude	4 V
A. Pulse Width	1.6 ms
A. Pace Blanking	240 ms
V. Amplitude	6 V
V. Pulse Width	1.6 ms
V. Pace Blanking	240 ms

Atrial Lead

Amplitude	2 V
Pulse Width	0.4 ms
Sensitivity	0.3 mV
Pace Blanking	240 ms

Ventricular Lead

Amplitude	2 V
Pulse Width	0.4 ms
Sensitivity	0.3 mV
Pace Blanking	240 ms

Refractory

PVARP	250 ms
PVAB	150 ms

Refractory Features

PMT Intervention	Off
PVC Response	On
V. Safety Pacing	On

Sep 28, 2000 14:09:06
9960 Software Version 3.0
Copyright (c) Medtronic, Inc. 1997

ICD Model: Gem DR 7271

Parameter Settings Report — Page 5

Telemetered and Stored EGM

	EGM 1 (A or V)	EGM 2 (V)
EGM Source	Atip to Aring	Vtip to Vring
EGM Range	+/- 8 mV	+/- 8 mV
Store this channel?	Yes	Yes

Store EGM during charging?	Yes
Store EGM before tachycardia starts?	No

Additional Setup

Device Date/Time	Sep 28, 2000 14:22
Holter Telemetry	Off
Premature Event Threshold	69 %

Auto Cap Formation

Minimum Auto Cap Formation Interval	2 month

B

Figure 8B. Continuation of programmed parameters from Figure 8A with bradycardia pacing parameters. The lower report indicates how the telemetered and stored electrograms have been set up for tachycardia events and the automatic capacitor reformation has been set for 2-month intervals.

vice has the capability of providing patient notification of certain events, those parameters can be programmed on as well.

Implications for Clinicians

Clinicians caring for children and young adults with ICDs have a multitude of responsibilities regarding both the patient and the family. Children are inherently different from their adult counterparts who receive ICDs, and a family-centered approach should be taken when assessing, planning, implementing, and evaluating their care.[45] Their needs are specific before, during, and after ICD implantation, and therefore it is necessary that the clinician remain abreast of current technology and possess updated knowledge regarding the indications, available devices, and, importantly, follow-up care. Patient and family education, a pivotal component of caring for children and their families, is discussed in the section on patient and family considerations, which also includes a discussion of the psychosocial issues faced by these children and their families. The following discussion addresses knowledge that the clinician must possess in order to care for these children and their families, as well as issues to consider when planning care before, during, and after the ICD implantation.

Baseline Knowledge for the Clinician

All clinicians caring for children with ICDs must possess baseline knowledge regarding specific aspects of the overall ICD experience. The clinician should be knowledgeable regarding the individual child's specific ICD indication and able to share that knowledge with the patient and family. Although it is fairly easy for some patients and families to understand the need for ICD placement (e.g., the child with LQTS and cardiac arrest), other families may need further clarification from the clinician.

The clinician, regardless of where he or she comes into contact with the ICD patient, must also understand and be able to identify the components of the ICD system. In most of the ICDs currently being used, the device houses a pulse generator, battery, capacitors, microcircuitry, and header. The can itself is similar to a pacemaker and, internally, consists of a lithium silver battery coupled with high-voltage capacitors for storing the energy used to defibrillate. The capacitor is the largest component of the ICD and is necessary because the battery alone cannot deliver the energy rapidly enough, nor does it have a high enough voltage to defibrillate the heart. Before the capacitor can deliver the energy required for cardioversion or defibrillation, it must first "store" the energy, a process known as "charging." Once the charge process has been completed, the capacitor is able to deliver the energy.

The microcircuitry or brain of the ICD is similar to a computer that is intelligent enough to provide a multitude of tasks as well as a wealth of information to aid the clinician. The tiered therapy devices are capable of providing ATP as an initial option, followed by low-energy cardioversion, and, finally, back-up defibrillation. Additionally, these devices can provide back-up single or dual chamber bradycardia pacing. The clinician can obtain specific information from the device, such as pacing lead impedance, charge time, battery voltage, electrograms, and a variety of episode counters. The longevity of the ICD is difficult to predict and is dependent on the number of times that the capacitors are charged, pacemaker usage, auto capacitor reformation interval, and the type and number of therapies delivered. A typical ICD capacitor charges approximately 100 times before the battery is depleted.[42] Similar to permanent pacemakers, the longevity of the ICD is dependent on the aforementioned factors, making it nearly impossible for the clinician to predict exactly when the battery will become depleted. Typically, an ICD lasts approximately 3 to 5 years.

The device header is housed at the top of the ICD and functions as the lead/patch connection structure. The number of leads depends on the type of system used, i.e., single or dual chamber, or problems associated with obtaining acceptable DFTs at implant. Unlike permanent pacing leads, the ICD leads not only have the functions of pacing and sensing but are also capable of delivering the high-voltage shocks necessary for defibrillation. The ICD leads consist of electrodes, conductors, insulating coating, connectors, and a specific fixation mechanism. The distal tip electrode of nearly all ICD leads is used for sensing, with the defibrillation coils (usually positioned at the right ventricular apex and superior vena cava) used for cardioversion and defibrillation.

Defibrillation patches can be used in specific circumstances, although their production is on the decline and future availability is questionable. They are commonly used for epicardial implants along with epicardial pacing leads to complete the system. The epicardial patches are placed onto the epicardium in such a way that the maximum ventricular mass is between the two patch electrodes. An additional use for the patch is its placement into a subcutaneous pocket. The subcutaneous patch is used in part to control the direction of the shock pulses given through the lead system; it is needed less often with the development of biphasic shocking waveforms.

Last, the clinician should be able to differentiate between the endocardial and epicardial implant techniques. Since the transvenous approach is now preferred over the epicardial approach in most cases, the clinician should be able to explain to the patient and family the reason that one approach was chosen over the other. In most cases, the epicardial approach is used for anatomic reasons, e.g., patient size, presence of intracardiac shunts, lack of venous access (Fontan patients), prosthetic tricuspid valves, unsuccessful attempts to balloon or stent the superior vena cava to right atrium junction, and/or stenosed or thrombosed veins commonly used for transvenous lead placement.

Prior to the Procedure

The team of clinicians caring for children and young adults undergoing ICD implantation has a wide array of responsibilities. This care begins at the moment the decision has been made to implant the ICD and includes not only physical care but emotional and psychological care as well. The tasks necessary to ensure a safe and uncomplicated procedure involve those concerning the patient as well as those regarding the catheterization/electrophysiology laboratory or operating room. The following preprocedural tasks are discussed relative to the patient and family considerations (excluding patient and family education and psychosocial considerations) and the laboratory considerations.

Patient Considerations

Since the majority of ICD recipients are admitted on the day of the procedure, most will be required to come in the day before for a preprocedural work-up and evaluation. This evaluation generally includes specific tests ordered by the implanting physician as well as a history and physical examination. In the physician author's center, the work-up is coordinated by a nurse clinician who also provides the patient and family education and follow-up care.

The clinician should ensure that the patient and family know where to report for the work-up and that they are given an approximate idea of how long the testing will take and what to expect in regard to the tests the child may undergo. If the child is receiving antiarrhythmic medications, the decision to withhold these medications should be made by the implanting physician based on relative risk to the patient. Diagnostic tests that may be ordered by the implanting physician prior to the procedure include blood work, urinalysis, chest radiograph, 12-lead ECG, 24-hour ambulatory monitor, exercise stress test, and echocardiogram. It is the policy in the physician author's institution that all females aged 12 years and older undergo pregnancy testing prior to the procedure. Blood work may include a complete blood count, clotting studies, and a type and cross-match for 1 to 2 units of packed red blood cells. Some of the aforementioned tests may not be necessary for all patients and should be ordered by the implanting physician on an individual patient basis. An exercise stress test may be performed in order to assist the clinician in determining tachycardia detection rates as well as the type and mode of bradycardia pacing, if applicable. An echocardiogram is nearly always performed to obtain a final disposition regarding the presence of intracardiac shunts in patients scheduled for transvenous placement. In patients with complex CHD or those who may have been lost to follow-up, a diagnostic cardiac catheterization may be performed to define structural anatomy in order to determine the most feasible implant technique or to delineate problems that may be amenable to interventional procedures ultimately allowing a transvenous implant.

Patients should also be evaluated for the type of anesthesia to be used, and special consideration given to previous sedation/anesthesia experience. The authors prefer the use of general anesthesia for ICD implantation. It is important that the patient and family meet with anesthesia personnel prior to the procedure to discuss the type of sedation agents that will be used for the child's procedure and when to withhold food and fluids in preparation for the implant procedure. The coordinating clinician should provide anesthesia personnel with any records from the child's previous hospitalizations, procedures, and/or surgeries, especially in children with cardiovascular or other congenital anomalies and in those with a history of airway problems.

The coordinating clinician should ensure that the patient and family meet with the implanting physician to answer any additional questions about the procedure, recovery period, and ICD itself. At this time, consent is obtained and a history and physical examination performed. After all diagnostic tests have been completed, sedation issues discussed with anesthesia personnel, and a patient and family education session completed, the clinician should review the plans for implant day with the patient and family. The family should be instructed on where to report on the day of the procedure and what to bring to the hospital on the day of the procedure. They should also be given a review of the child's NPO (nothing by mouth) instructions and an overview of the events that will take place on the day of the procedure. This overview should include where the family is expected to wait during the procedure, where the child will go after the procedure, and how the family will get messages regarding their child during the procedure.

Once the preprocedural work-up is completed, the clinician should ensure the availability of any and all necessary supplies that may be needed during the implant procedure. If the procedure is for device placement only, the clinician must have previous implant records available and be knowledgeable enough (or have someone available who is) regarding lead connector and ICD compatibilities in order to have the correct supplies available. All equipment necessary for permanent pacemaker implantation should be readily available and is listed in chapter 7. Additional ICD-specific equipment includes devices, ICD leads, lead adaptors, lead adaptor sleeves and caps, patches, arrays, guidewires, tunneling tools, extra rate-sensing leads, high-voltage cables, external/AC fibrillator, programmable stimulator, and two external defibrillators. To quote Drs. Belott and Reynolds, "one cannot have too many supplies and spare parts."[46] Collaboration and communication between the implanting physician and the clinician or manufacturer's representative responsible for the technical aspects of the procedure are critical.

Laboratory Considerations

Clinicians involved in the ICD implant itself have ongoing responsibilities regarding room as well as patient preparation. Maintaining a safe environment for both the patient and the staff is critical, and all electrical equipment should be properly grounded with efficient performance as evidenced by frequent evaluations by the institution's biomedical department. The clinician working in the procedure room should have an adequately stocked supply of pacing system equipment in addition to diagnostic and interventional catheters for a variety of patient sizes and clinical situations. Equipment specific for pacemaker and ICD implantation, such as those previously mentioned, should be readily available. Both external defibrillators should be tested prior to the procedure as well.

Once the child arrives in the procedure room, clinicians must obtain adequate surface ECG recordings by assessing electrode placement and replacing any that may inhibit high-quality ECGs. The grounding pad for the electrocautery is generally placed on the patient's thigh and preapplied self-adhesive defibrillation pads placed for external rescue defibrillation. Pulse oximetry is measured throughout the procedure and adequate body temperature should be maintained as well. Strict sterile technique should be used and radiation safety precautions taken at all times.

During the Procedure

During the implant procedure, the clinician must constantly assess the child's overall hemodynamic condition and also be prepared to assist with any urgent or emergent procedures if necessary. Nurses and other cardiovascular clinicians directly involved in ICD implantation must remain cognizant of pediatric drug dosages and should constantly monitor the patient for any signs or symptoms of ICD- or procedural-related complications. The complications associated with ICD implantation are listed in Table 4.

Table 4
Potential Complications Associated with ICD Implantation

Hemorrhage
Infection
Arrhythmia exacerbation
Embolism
Pleural/pericardial effusion
Cardiac perforation/tamponade
Stroke
Pericarditis (epicardial implant)
Pneumothorax
Hemothorax
Death

ICD = implantable cardioverter defibrillator.

Immediately After the Procedure

Once the procedure has been completed, the patient is transferred to the postanesthesia care unit or cardiovascular telemetry unit. The clinician assuming care for the child with an ICD must obtain specifics of the procedure from implant personnel, including the type of ICD implanted, the ICD pocket location, the type and amount of sedation/anesthesia used, any problems or complications encountered during the procedure, the presence of any drainage tubes, condition of any dressings, and the following ICD parameters: bradycardia pacing parameters (including pacing mode, pacing rate, output settings, sensitivity settings, refractory periods, rate-adaptive parameters [if applicable], and sleep rate [if applicable]), arrhythmia detection rates, tachycardia termination algorithms, and number of termination attempts.

An overall clinical assessment of the patient should be performed by the clinician assuming the child's care immediately upon the patient's arrival on the unit. If venous and/or arterial catheters were used, their puncture sites should be inspected for the presence of hemorrhage, swelling, or hematoma, and the affected extremity evaluated for warmth, color, capillary refill, and palpable pulses. The child's level of consciousness and airway patency should be assessed and documented, as should his or her heart rate and rhythm, blood pressure, respiratory rate, and temperature. Telemetry should be placed upon arrival to the telemetry unit and a baseline recording obtained. The bradycardia pacing parameters should be compared with the baseline recording and ECG recordings obtained at a minimum of every 8 hours or when abnormalities are noted (Fig. 9). Care should be taken not to place any electrodes on or near the ICD pocket, due to the increased risk of infection if skin integrity is altered with electrode removal or irritation.

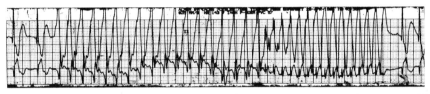

Figure 9. Surface ECG leads II and V$_1$ recorded during an episode of monomorphic ventricular tachycardia (VT) in a 14-year-old postoperative tetralogy of Fallot patient. The VT is appropriately sensed and successfully overdriven using a 16-beat burst into normal sinus rhythm with right bundle branch block.

The postoperative orders should include frequent assessment of vital signs in the immediate postoperative period. An intravenous line is generally left in place for hydration and medication administration. Oral fluids are allowed when the patient is fully awake and alert. Ambulation is permitted the next day, and in transvenous implants a shoulder immobilizer is placed on the affected extremity to decrease the possibility of early lead dislodgment. All patients are monitored on telemetry until discharge. Medications include any previous medications taken prior to ICD implantation, prophylactic antibiotics, pain medication, antipyretics, antiemetics, and occasionally Decadron or prednisone for acute elevated pacing thresholds.

The dressing over the ICD pocket should be inspected with each vital sign assessment and any drainage noted on the bandage. If excessive drainage or hemorrhage is noted, the clinician should immediately notify the responsible physician. The intravenous site should be inspected each shift for signs of infiltration and/or infection. Parents should be informed of the necessity to ask for their child's pain medication rather than it being given at routine intervals. Pediatric and young adult ICD recipients will remain hospitalized for 24 to 48 hours or 2 to 4 days, depending on the implant technique used and any early complications or problems.

Implantable Cardioverter Defibrillator Rhythm Analysis

Clinicians caring for young ICD recipients must have advanced knowledge of pacemaker function. The basics of pacemaker function are discussed in chapter 7 and the remainder of this discussion is limited to the tachycardia aspects of the device. Most young ICD recipients will have an uneventful postoperative course in regard to device discharge. The clinician should remain cognizant of each child's reason for ICD implantation. If frequent ventricular ectopy or nonsustained episodes of VT is noted during the monitoring period or nonsustained episodes of VT, the clinician should obtain a recording, assess the patient's response to the arrhythmia, and notify the responsible physician. If the device should discharge, the physician should be informed immediately. Additionally, some patients may be prone to supraventricular arrhythmias as well as ventricular arrhythmias. The clinician should be aware of this predisposition and remain cognizant of the device's role in these concomitant arrhythmias.

Magnet Application

On many units, a pacemaker magnet is available for ICD patients. The clinician must be aware of each manufacturer's ICD magnet mode because these modes can vary among manufacturers. In general, placement of a magnet over the ICD results in temporary suspension of arrhythmia detection and subsequent therapy delivery. In some devices, the magnet can permanently program the device off if left over the ICD long enough, until it can be turned back on with the specific device programmer. Some devices even allow the magnet mode to be programmed on or off; therefore, clinicians caring for patients with ICDs must remain cognizant of each manufacturer's specific magnet mode prior to magnet application.

Prior to discharge, all ICD recipients undergo the following tests: 12-lead ECG, chest radiograph, echocardiogram, and noninvasive device testing. Device testing includes evaluation of pacemaker sensing and pacing functions, including the performance of pacing thresholds and sensing thresholds, and determination of underlying rhythm. Diagnostic counters are programmed or cleared at this time, as well as any other parameters that require change or initial programming. The defibrillation lead is evaluated by assessing high-voltage impedance in addition to pacing lead impedance. Tachycardia induction with device testing is not routinely performed in most patients prior to discharge, although it may be indicated in specific patients. Some centers require that the patient return 1 week after discharge for device testing,[41] but this practice varies among pediatric electrophysiologists. The tachycardia recognition and termination algorithms are assessed and changes made if necessary.

Discharge Planning

Prior to discharge, the dressing (if transvenous implant) is removed from the ICD site. Patients and families with this type of incision in the physician author's institution are instructed in the application of Polysporin powder to the wound twice daily. They are asked to allow the steri-strips to fall off spontaneously and to expect a small amount of drainage (serosanguinous) with increased ambulation. They are also instructed as to the signs and symptoms of wound infection to report to their physician or nurse, as well as techniques used for bathing without immersing the incision. The authors require subacute bacterial endocarditis prophylaxis on all transvenous implants, in contrast with the current recommendations of the American Heart Association/American Dental Association. Educational guidelines for home care of children with ICDs can be found in Table 5.

Table 5
Education Guidelines for Home Care of the Child with an ICD

Wound care	1. Observe site for redness, swelling, purulent drainage, and tenderness 2. Keep wound dry and allow steri-strips to fall off spontaneously 3. Cover wound with plastic cling wrap or baggie for bathing and showering 4. Apply Polysporin powder to wound twice daily
Activity allowances/restrictions	1. Specific for each patient 2. No PE or contact sports until wound is completely healed (approximately 6–8 weeks) 3. Carry backpack on shoulder opposite ICD site 4. Avoid restrictive clothing over device pocket, e.g., bras or tight-wasted pants 5. No swimming or water sports activities until wound is completely healed 6. For most patients, limitations dependent on underlying disease 7. No varsity sports (i.e., football, full-contact karate, boxing, or hockey)—ask MD for allowable sports once wound has healed
Endocarditis prophylaxis	1. Specified by implanting physician preference 2. Recommend for all transvenous systems

(continues)

Table 5
Education Guidelines for Home Care of the Child with an ICD (*cont.*)

When to contact doctor/nurse	1. Any of the following symptoms: signs of wound infection (see above), temperature greater than 101°F, device discharge, dizziness, palpitations, shortness of breath, muscle stimulation, injury to the device, or device protrusion 2. Notify nurse or MD of any surgeries child may be scheduled for
Avoidance of environmental hazards	1. Avoid the following: large magnets, arc welding equipment, high-voltage electrical fields, and MRI 2. Take precautions with the following: **Cellular phones:** Use on opposite side of ICD pocket, keep 6 inches from ICD when in use **Antitheft devices:** Walk through quickly, do not linger **Airport metal detectors:** May walk through without device malfunction; device may make metal detector go off; show ID card to avoid passing through **Airport wands:** Avoid, due to magnet mode response
Follow-up schedule	Outpatient Visits: 1. Per physician preference 2. Generally 6–8 weeks post implant but may be seen at 1–2 weeks as well 3. Every 6 months for device interrogation per physician preference 4. As needed for device discharge

ICD = implantable cardioverter defibrillator; MRI = magnetic resonance imaging; PE = physical education.

An outpatient follow-up appointment is scheduled for 6 weeks post implant. If the wound is thought to be at particular risk or if an echocardiogram is warranted, an interim visit is scheduled at 1 to 2 weeks. The child's activity level is slowly increased and strenuous physical activity is moderated based on the child's overall cardiac condition[47] and the associated arrhythmia substrate. Children with ICDs and anatomically normal hearts are allowed no contact sports, such as football, hockey, or full-contact karate; however, children with associated LQTS are not allowed to participate in any competitive athletics and may have more individualized restrictions as well. Patients with CHD and ICDs often already have imposed restrictions that are secondary to their structural diseases.

Patients with ICDs are not routinely prescribed transtelephonic monitors; however, in some cases, this diagnostic tool may be very helpful. If parents have not had in-hospital cardiopulmonary resuscitation training, a community course should be arranged for a time as close to discharge as possible. Verbal and written home care instructions are discussed with the patient and family, and are discussed in more depth in the section on patient and family considerations.

Follow-Up Care

Follow-up of the ICD recipient should begin at the time that the decision to implant the device has been made. This follow-up provides recognition of inadequate or inappropriate system performance and consists of regularly scheduled follow-up visits. Follow-up should not only include the child and young adult's physical and device care, but should address psychosocial issues as well. These issues are discussed below in the section on patient and family considerations. The authors require a follow-up visit any time the device discharges, which others require as a part of their follow-up as well.[41] The goals of ICD follow-up as published by Crossley[48] include: 1) assessment of overall cardiovascular status; 2) identification and recording of both the nature and frequency of arrhythmias as well as device activity; 3) assessment of pacing and sensing functions; 4) battery status assessment; 5) pulse generator longevity enhancement; 6) optimization of therapeutic parameters based on device history; and 7) optimization of diagnostic enhancements and other ancillary parameters.[48]

Hands-on follow-up is scheduled for every 6 months or more frequently, depending on concomitant structural heart disease, patient and/or device age, and history of problems or complications. This visit may include a variety of tests, some of which are patient specific. All patients should undergo a complete history and physical examination as well as a complete ICD evaluation. The history may reveal problems that may have occurred in the interim, such as dizziness, syncope, new-onset exercise intolerance, and generalized fatigue, any of which could be indicative of bradycardia pacing system malfunction.[41] Additionally, the patient should be asked to provide a description of any and all device-related issues and/or experiences, including any shocks, since the last hospital or clinic visit. The physical examination may be used to identify problems directly related to the ICD system, such as irregular heartbeats, pocket infection/erosion, or changes in valve function.

Additional tests include a chest roentgenogram to assess lead length, lead position, and migration/interference with cardiac function (Figs. 10 and 11). Echocardiography is performed at the discretion of the following physician. The authors recommend echocardiography at the initial follow-up after ICD implantation, as pericardial effusions can occur up to 2 months following implant.[5]

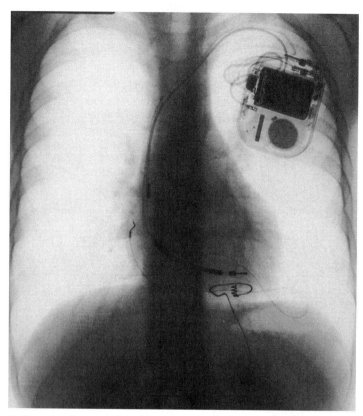

Figure 10. Chest radiograph (posteroanterior view) of a patient with a dual chamber "active can" implantable cardioverter defibrillator implanted by a transvenous approach in an 8-year-old male with long QT syndrome. The old epicardial pacing leads can be seen as well.

Exercise stress testing can be used to evaluate dual chamber pacing performance as well as peak heart rate obtained during exercise. The latter is very useful in programming tachycardia detection intervals, since a major problem for pediatric ICD recipients is the incidence of inappropriate shocks.[4,6,7] Twenty-four-hour ambulatory monitoring is a helpful adjunct for ICD recipients and can assist the clinician in identifying intermittent problems such as under- or oversensing, noncapture, increasing frequency of ectopy, nonsustained tachycardia episodes, and any new-onset arrhythmias.

Noninvasive ICD evaluation should be performed by qualified personnel who are highly trained and knowledgeable about ICDs and their functions and who routinely work with children and their families. When dealing with children, calm equals cooperative, so efforts to make the child feel comfortable and nonthreatened are priority goals. The follow-up should be performed at regular intervals in an organized and systematic manner. The authors use a separate ECG machine for limb lead attach-

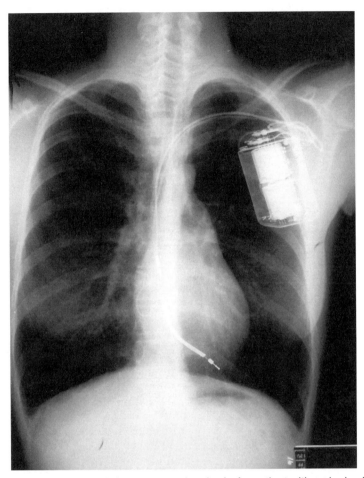

Figure 11. Chest radiograph (posteroanterior view) of a patient with a single chamber "active can" implanted by transvenous approach in a 4-year-old female. The two sensing electrodes can be seen at the distal end of the lead, while the shocking electrode is more proximal.

ment and recording of leads I, II, and III in addition to the patient cable that inserts into the device-specific programmer.

After an assessment of the patient's overall clinical status is obtained, the device is interrogated for currently programmed parameters, measured data, and diagnostic data (Fig. 12). The programmed values are compared with previous settings and correlated with what is seen on the surface ECG (Fig. 13). The battery status should be evaluated and compared with individual manufacturer parameters. It is recommended that this measurement be obtained 30 minutes or more after device discharge or capacitor formation.[49] Once the device reaches elective replacement, it should be replaced, as charge times become increasingly prolonged between elective replacement and end-of-service. With the advent of automatic capacitor re-

Episodes Last Interrogated: Oct 26, 2000 09:07:41

| Since Last Session: Jul 27, 2000 | Current Data |

Episodes

VF	0
FVT	0
VT	0
SVT/NST	0
Mode Switch	0

% Pacing

AS-VS	48 %
AS-VP	0 %
AP-VS	51 %
AP-VP	0 %

Battery Voltage

(ERI=2.55 V, EOL=2.40 V)
Oct 26, 2000   3.14 V

Last Full Energy Charge

Jun 10, 2000   6.96 sec

Last Capacitor Formation

Jun 10, 2000

Lead Impedance

Oct 26, 2000
A. Pacing	611 ohms
V. Pacing	444 ohms
Defibrillation (HVB)	20 ohms

Observations (1)

- The VF Detection Interval (FDI) is < 300 ms. May result in delayed detection of VF.

Figure 12. Data summary episodes obtained noninvasively depicting number of episodes, percentage of pacing, battery voltage, last charge time, last capacitor reformation, and lead impedances of the pacing as well as defibrillation leads.

ICD Model: Gem II DR 7273

Sep 14, 2000 10:29:13
9964 Software Version 1.0
Copyright Medtronic, Inc 1998

Parameter Settings Report   **Page 1**

Detection

	Enable	Interval (Rate)
VF	On	250 ms (240 bpm)
FVT	Off	ms (bpm)
VT	Off	290 ms (207 bpm)

Number of Intervals to Detect

	Initial NID	Redetect NID
VF	12/16	6/8
VT	12	8

Sensitivity

Atrial	0.3 mV
Ventricular	0.3 mV

Dual Chamber SVT Criteria

AFib/AFlutter	On
Sinus Tach	On
Other 1:1 SVTs	On
SVT Limit	240 ms

Ventricular SVT Criteria

VT Stability	Off

Parameter Settings Report   **Page 2**

VF Therapies	Rx1	Rx2	Rx3	Rx4	Rx5	Rx6
VF Therapy Status	On	On	On	On	On	On
Energy	30 J	30 J	30 J	30 J	30 J	30 J
Pathway	AX>B	AX>B	AX>B	AX>B	AX>B	AX>B
Reconfirm VF after initial charge?	Yes					

FVT Therapies	Rx1	Rx2	Rx3	Rx4	Rx5	Rx6
FVT Therapy Status						
Therapy Type	None	None	None	None	None	None
Initial # Pulses						
R-S1 Interval=(%RR)						
S1S2(Ramp+)=(%RR)						
S2SN(Ramp+)=(%RR)						
Interval Dec						
# Sequences						
Smart Mode						
Energy						
Pathway						
Anti-Tachy Pacing Minimum Interval	200 ms					

A

Figure 13A. Parameter settings report obtained noninvasively during a routine follow-up visit. The supraventricular tachycardia discrimination criteria have been programmed, as well as 30-J shocks for all six ventricular fibrillation therapies. *Continues.*

ICD Model: Gem II DR 7273

Sep 14, 2000 10:29:29
9964 Software Version 1.0
Copyright Medtronic, Inc. 1998

Parameter Settings Report

Page 3

VT Therapies	Rx1	Rx2	Rx3	Rx4	Rx5	Rx6
VT Therapy Status	On	On	On	On	On	On
Therapy Type	Burst	Burst	CV	CV	CV	CV
Initial # Pulses	8	8				
R-S1 Interval=(%RR)	72 %	69 %				
S1S2(Ramp+)=(%RR)						
S2SN(Ramp+)=(%RR)						
Interval Dec	10 ms	10 ms				
# Sequences	2	2				
Smart Mode	On	On				
Energy			4 J	30 J	30 J	30 J
Pathway			AX>B	AX>B	AX>B	B>AX
Anti-Tachy Pacing Minimum Interval		200 ms				

Shared Anti-Tachy Pacing Therapy

V. Amplitude	8 V
V. Pulse Width	1.6 ms
V. Pace Blanking	240 ms

Shared VF, FVT, and VT Therapy

Progressive Episode Therapies	Off

Parameter Settings Report

Page 4

Modes/Rates

Mode	DDDR
Mode Switch	Off
Lower Rate	60 ppm
Upper Tracking Rate	150 ppm
Upper Sensor Rate	130 ppm

A-V Intervals

Paced AV	200 ms
Sensed AV	200 ms
Rate Adaptive AV	On
Start Rate	90 bpm
Stop Rate	150 bpm
Minimum Paced AV	140 ms
Minimum Sensed AV	110 ms

Rate Therapy Features

Non-Competitive Atrial Pacing	On
V. Rate Stabilization	Off

Atrial Lead

Amplitude	2 V
Pulse Width	0.2 ms
Sensitivity	0.3 mV
Pace Blanking	240 ms

Ventricular Lead

Amplitude	2 V
Pulse Width	0.2 ms
Sensitivity	0.3 mV
Pace Blanking	180 ms

Refractory

PVARP	310 ms
PVAB	150 ms

Rate Response

Rate Response	7
Activity Threshold	Medium
Activity Acceleration	30 sec
Activity Deceleration	5 min

B

Figure 13B. Continuation of parameters obtained in the patient in Figure 13A. Note that the ventricular tachycardia therapies start with two antitachycardia pacing modalities, followed by a low-joule (4 J) cardioversion then followed by three attempts of 30 J each, which were tested extensively at device implantation. This postoperative congenital heart disease patient has a bradycardia pacing mode of DDDR.

formation, the assessment of the ICD's high-voltage capacitors is determined by evaluating the device's last charge time. Although specific charge times vary among manufacturers, in general, a capacitor's charge time should not exceed 15 to 20 seconds.[50] Excessive charge times may delay shock delivery and must be scrutinized at each clinic visit (Fig. 14).

Event counters contain a vast amount of information in today's devices. Spontaneous episode and therapy data should be reviewed and compared with previous episodes for inconsistencies or increased episode occurrence. In patients in whom multiple tachycardia zones have been programmed, the clinician should evaluate each sequentially, noting how the detection criteria were met and the appropriateness of therapies. Electrograms can be analyzed to assist the clinician in evaluating therapy efficacy (Fig. 15). They can also be used to elucidate SVT as well. With high-energy shocks, it

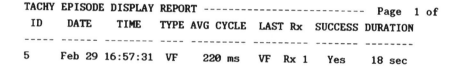

```
STATUS REPORT -------------------------------------------- Page  1 of ¹

DEVICE STATUS INDICATORS:          MOST RECENT CHARGE:
MEMORY RETENTION OK                 Feb 29, 2000  16:57:47
CHARGE CIRCUIT OK                   Energy(J):    0.0 - 30.0
                                    Charge Time(sec):  14.92


BATTERY VOLTAGE:                   LAST CAPACITOR FORMATION:
Mar 01, 2000  11:47:47              Feb 19, 2000  16:47:10
Last Measured (V):  5.67            Energy(J):    0.0 - 30.0
                                    Charge Time(sec):  19.25


MIN. BATTERY VOLTAGE DURING CHARGE: MOST RECENT H.V. LEAD IMPEDANCE:
Feb 19, 2000  16:47:10              Feb 29, 2000  16:57:48
Minimum Measured (V):  4.40         Waveform:                BIPH
                                    Pathway:                 AX>B
                                    Delivered Energy (J): 28.6
MOST RECENT PACING LEAD IMPEDANCE:  Impedance(ohms):         49
Feb 27, 2000  04:34:58
Impedance(ohms):    601
```

Figure 14. Noninvasive interrogation of device data in a 15-year-old patient with an implantable cardioverter defibrillator. Note the prolonged charge time from the last capacitor formation of 19.25 ms.

```
TACHY EPISODE DISPLAY REPORT ------------------------- Page  1 of

ID    DATE    TIME    TYPE AVG CYCLE  LAST Rx  SUCCESS DURATION
----- ------ -------- ---- --------- --------- ------- --------

5    Feb 29 16:57:31  VF    220 ms    VF Rx 1   Yes    18 sec
```

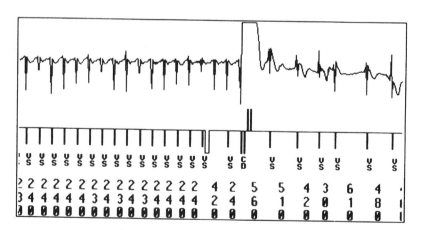

Figure 15. Noninvasively obtained intracardiac electrograms and annotation markers in an implantable cardioverter defibrillator patient during an episode of ventricular tachycardia/ventricular fibrillation. The arrhythmia was successfully converted 18 seconds after being detected by the device.

is important for the clinician to review the lead impedance. A significant decrease in this lead impedance could be indicative of insulation problems, while a significant increase may be indicative of conductor problems.

The provocative testing of the device includes the routine pacing parameter assessment of pacing thresholds, sensing thresholds, and underlying rhythm as discussed in chapter 7. Adequate sensing in the ICD patient is a priority. Electrograms should be used to evaluate sensing (Fig. 16), specifi-

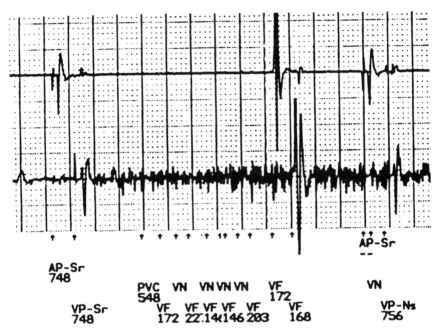

Figure 16. Atrial and ventricular electrograms with annotation markers obtained noninvasively from a dual chamber implantable cardioverter defibrillator during an episode of electromagnetic interference. The device is pacing the atrium (AP) and ventricle (VP), but is sensing far field R wave on the atrial channel (Sr) and noise on the ventricular channel. The noise is interpreted by the device as premature ventricular contractions and ventricular fibrillation with refractory sensing (Sr) on the ventricular channel.

cally T wave oversensing. There are two ways to alleviate T wave oversensing: 1) decrease the sensitivity, or 2) adjust the postpacing ventricular refractory period. The former is not recommended because the new sensitivity setting may not allow the sensing of the low-amplitude signals associated with VF. The refractory period adjustment should be reprogrammed modestly in order to decrease the incidence of compromised sensing.

With epicardial systems, the clinician must be aware of the high lead failure rates and the fact that some epicardial patches will fail at approximately 4 years' follow-up.[50] Brady and colleagues[51] report that 58% of patients with epicardial lead malfunction were asymptomatic, with diagnoses including failed defibrillation, lack of pacing output, lead abnormalities discovered at routine device replacement, or fractures noted on radiography.

Since a large majority of fractures (62% to 68%) were found by radiography, the authors of this study recommend radiographs every 6 months in patients with epicardial patch systems.[51] Due to similarities in design of epicardial and subcutaneous patches, close follow-up of patients with the latter is recommended as well.[50]

At the end of the follow-up session, the device should be interrogated again and the values compared with the values obtained initially. It is critical that the clinician ensure that the tachyarrhythmia recognition and termination sequences have not been turned off inadvertently. The episode data counters can be cleared and pertinent data shared with the child's other health care providers. In addition to computerized records, the authors print a final report indicating the programmed parameters, the pacing and sensing thresholds, the patient's underlying rhythm, the battery voltage, the last charge time, the episode data, and any changes that were made. This report is placed in the ICD chart in addition to the patient's outpatient record.

Troubleshooting

Patients with ICDs can encounter a variety of problems throughout the follow-up period. Troubleshooting issues associated with the bradycardia pacing and sensing functions of the ICD are discussed in chapter 7. Many ICD problems can be discovered using adjunct diagnostic tools generally used in follow-up, including radiography, exercise stress testing, 24-hour ambulatory monitors, and event monitors. The problem should be identified and possible causes of the problem delineated. Nisam and Fogoros[52] have categorized most ICD problems into the following four categories: 1) suspected inappropriate therapy (shocks or ATP); 2) failure to deliver therapy; 3) ineffective therapy (shocks or ATP); and 4) a deactivated device. The following discussion addresses each of these issues regarding possible causes of ICD malfunction and subsequent ways to identify the source of the problem as delineated by Nisam and Fogoros.[52]

Inappropriate therapy can occur as a result of any of the following: sinus tachycardia, SVT, nonsustained VT, T wave or P wave oversensing, lead problems (such as fracture, insulation breaks, dislodgment, or loose set screws), electromagnetic interference (EMI), device-induced proarrhythmia, or inappropriate detection algorithms. The clinician should begin by assessing the events that led up to the therapy delivery, including the therapy history and intracardiac electrograms. If sinus tachycardia is suspected, an exercise stress test may be helpful in identifying this problem. In the case of SVT, most dual chamber devices now have SVT discrimination algorithms to assist the clinician in delineating and treating the problem. Nonsustained VT can be problematic, especially in patients with LQTS. This problem has decreased with newer devices that use detection delays as well as with noncommitted devices that "reconfirm" the arrhythmia after charging. If there are no identifiable problems noted on x-ray, suspected lead abnormalities can often be discerned by having the patient perform upper body exercises or by device/device header manipulation.

Failure to deliver therapy can occur in the presence of lead problems, sensitivity problems, inappropriate detection algorithms, EMI, inadvertent device reprogramming associated with magnet application, or antiarrhythmic medications that may have altered the arrhythmogenic substrate. Once again, the clinician can gain valuable information by evaluating the therapy history, sensitivity settings, intracardiac electrograms, and ECG with annotation markers. Detection criteria could be inhibiting therapy delivery if the detection enhancements (e.g., rate stability or sudden onset) are too sensitive.

Ineffective therapy delivery can result from inadequate output energy, rise in DFTs, lead problems, and increased pacing output necessary for ATP. A chronic rise in DFTs may be a result of changes in impedance or antiarrhythmic drugs and is associated with epicardial patches, congestive heart failure, and decreased left ventricular function. If DFTs are elevated and the device is not programmed to maximum output, the clinician should immediately program the energy to its highest value. If the device is programmed to maximum output, invasive lead testing and subsequent system enhancement or replacement might be necessary. Certain antiarrhythmic drugs can increase DFTs, and patients who begin antiarrhythmic drug therapy after device placement should undergo DFT testing after adequate serum concentrations are reached (if applicable) or when the physician deems the drug has had an appropriate clinical effect. If ATP was previously successful, steps should be taken to ascertain if the pacing threshold has increased, and if so, the output should be increased.

A deactivated device can result from EMI, battery depletion, or, as previously mentioned, magnet application. Device interrogation should provide information regarding the device's functional status as well as specifics regarding the battery status. The clinician should question the patient about potential sources of EMI and if concerns exist, an ambulatory monitor such as a Holter or event recorder can be prescribed to assist in determining if the patient is coming in contact with an EMI source while engaged in his or her activities of daily living.

Troubleshooting of ICDs can usually be traced back to any four of the previously discussed problems. The clinician should use a systematic approach, as well as the diagnostic tools that are available within the device itself, to determine the etiology of these problems. In most cases, the problem can be identified and proper steps can be taken to alleviate or repair it.

Patient and Family Considerations

The many issues involved in caring for patients and families with ICDs can be quite challenging for the clinician. The individual needs of each patient and family should be considered when developing a family-centered plan of care. The following discussion focuses on the specific educational needs of the child and family as well as some of the psychosocial implications associated with having an ICD in childhood.

Patient and Family Education

Patient and family education should begin when the decision for ICD implantation has been made. The components of the assessment phase include identification of any previous ICD knowledge, the identification of myths/misconceptions regarding ICDs, and the establishment of a teaching level that is consistent with the patient's age and intellectual abilities. The family's understanding of the upcoming procedure, their lifestyle, the child's play or young adult's work habits, previous hospitalizations, and coping mechanisms should be included in the assessment phase as well. Clinicians should use this information to identify the family's strengths to tailor a patient- and family-specific educational session. Once the assessment is complete, problems, goals, and anticipated outcomes can be identified with the patient and family. While implementing the plan, the clinician should be cognizant of any observations, complaints, and/or requests from the patient and family in order to evaluate specific goals and objectives.

Patient and family education should be carried out in a quiet, relaxed atmosphere with as few interruptions as possible. This generally occurs after the patient and family have met with the implanting physician regarding procedural issues such as the risks and potential complications associated with ICD implantation. The discussion should begin with the data gained from the assessment phase, including the clarification of any myths associated with the ICD system itself. A basic explanation of how the device works, a cardiac conduction system review, and the implant technique should be included. It is important for patients and families to understand that the device will not prevent the arrhythmia from occurring; it only serves to terminate the arrhythmia, and despite the fact that it may not "shock" right away after being implanted, it is constantly monitoring the heart rhythm.[53] Patients and families are very interested in what a "shock" will feel like. Since most cardiovascular clinicians have never experienced a shock, anecdotal information gathered from other patients is used to describe device discharges. It is important to stress that each patient may experience device discharges differently. Some may experience a shock while awake, while others may pass out and feel only the after effects, some of which are described below in the section on psychosocial considerations.

Any visual aids and/or written information can assist with the patient's/family's understanding and should be used whenever possible. The patient and family should be given the opportunity to visualize and handle the device and leads (or patches) at this time, so that they know what will be "inside." Therapeutic play can be used with some children at this time in order for the clinician to determine specific fears, interests, and coping mechanisms that the child may have.

Patients and parents should be instructed on what to expect immediately after the procedure. The best approach is to be honest with both the child and the family, especially regarding painful interventions and/or procedures. An explanation of the postoperative orders is very helpful in assisting the family to know what to expect once the procedure has been completed. Any routine tests or procedures that will be performed during the recovery period should be reiterated. The anticipated length of stay should be verbalized with special emphasis on the fact that unexpected problems may arise necessitating a longer hospital stay. Once unforeseen problems are identified, the clinician should explain them to the patient and family to promote understanding and cooperation.

Discharge planning is a key component of the overall plan of care of the young ICD recipient. In addition to the guidelines presented in Table 4, the clinician should provide an overview of what to expect in the days and weeks to come. Discharge instructions should include the following: wound care, when to notify the physician or nurse, activity allowances/restrictions, precautions regarding electrical hazards, and follow-up care. Information regarding medical alert bracelets should be provided to patients and families and an action plan delineated for emergencies. Telephone numbers of key personnel for contact after discharge will hopefully provide comfort and decrease anxiety for the patient and family. It is extremely important that cardiovascular clinicians not only remain accessible to patients and families after hospital discharge, but to others who come in contact with the patient as well, e.g., school personnel, family practitioners, pediatricians, etc.

Psychosocial Considerations

Literature regarding the psychosocial impact of having an ICD implanted in childhood is virtually nonexistent. Many studies, including quality of life studies, have been conducted in the adult population[54–57] with several implications that may apply to the young ICD patient as well. Adult ICD recipients have reported feelings of isolation, concerns regarding fear of being shocked in public, discomfort of shocks, fear of device failure, role changes, travel restrictions, financial concerns, body image disturbances, disturbances in sexual relations, ability to return to a functional lifestyle, and loss of control associated with dependence on an electrical device.[58–60] Other issues expressed by adults with ICDs include difficulty sleeping (56%), memory problems (64%), depression (54%), overprotective family members (50%), fear of death (38%), and significant anxiety (38%).[61]

A pilot study published in 1995 by Vitale and Funk[62] included two teenagers in its quality of life analysis of nine young ICD recipients. The information obtained from the two adolescents is consistent with most anecdotal experience shared by clinicians who routinely care for pediatric and young adult ICD recipients. Concern that the device "might blow up," fear regarding the future, and concerns about peer rejection were issues identified by these two teenagers.[62]

The issues and concerns of young ICD recipients are similar to those identified in a descriptive study on adolescent pacemaker recipients published in 1995,[63] and include normalization, parental overprotectiveness, peer integration, consistent caregivers, procedural fear, body image, an adjustment period, and concerns regarding the future.[63] This study was repeated by the authors in patients with ICDs followed in a pediatric cardiovascular outpatient clinic in 1995. Six patients were interviewed at a time when few pediatric patients had ICDs. The children ranged in age from 12 to 19 years, with one adult 35 years of age. Three of the patients had previous surgery for CHD (including the adult patient), while the remaining three had LQTS without structural heart disease. All of the devices were placed epicardially.

Open-ended interview techniques were used to obtain data regarding patient descriptions of life with an ICD, including what it felt like to be shocked, peer relationships, activity limitations, and overall general feelings of life with an ICD. The majority of the patients reported initial anxiety, sadness (why me?), and fear of pain when told that an ICD implant was necessary. Many of them reported that an adjustment period of a few months was necessary after implantation, and compared it to being on a roller coaster at first, which is consistent with data obtained from adults.[64] The one adolescent male in the study had the most difficulty accepting the device and exhibited early signs of depression. He reported that "I didn't want the ICD" and "I don't like to talk about it."

Half of the patients had told their peers that they had an ICD, while the remaining three had not. The ones who had told their peers expressed that nothing had changed, "I'm still the same old person." One female asked her friends not to treat her special and told them that she just "wants to be treated like everyone else," while another reported that "belonging is important" and "different is bad," both of which are consistent with other children with chronic disease who want to remain "normal."[65] Many of the patients put unnecessary activity restrictions upon themselves because of the ICD, in part because of fear that certain activities may precipitate a shock. Body image was not expressed as an overwhelming concern in these six patients, which was probably secondary to the fact that the devices were placed in the abdomen and were not clearly visible or protuberant. The various responses to what a shock feels like ranged from "never felt it, I always pass out first," to "feels like a kick in the chest and is sore afterwards," to "it feels like you're fried," to "it feels like being hit by lightening." Some of the patients reported fear of getting shocked with no correlation to fear and previous device discharges.

Serwer and colleagues[41] report severe anxiety in two of their ICD recipients who experienced conscious shocks. Both developed school phobias and one also developed posttraumatic stress disorder. The early identification of problems in this patient population should incite psychological referral in order to avoid catastrophic outcomes. In addition to psychological counseling, these patients may benefit from relaxation methods, biofeedback, support groups, and medication. These reports validate the need for more research in children, adolescents, and young adults with ICDs.

The goal for cardiovascular clinicians in caring for pediatric, adolescent, and young adult ICD recipients should be to facilitate a positive adjustment for both the child and the family while trying to prevent avoidable negative psychosocial outcomes. This involves a psychosocial assessment of the child at each and every follow-up visit. If problems are identified at any visit, the clinician should refer that patient for psychological counseling. Some of these patients will require antidepressant therapy in order to cope with having an ICD.

Returning to school after ICD implantation can be very stressful for both the child and the family as well as for school staff members. The clinician can play a pivotal role in assisting to decrease this anxiety by educating the school personnel about the child's cardiac condition. Serwer and colleagues[41] routinely meet with school personnel (after obtaining parental permission and with the parents present) after ICD implantation to discuss the child's arrhythmia, how the ICD works, and what to do if therapy is delivered, and to develop a plan for emergencies.

Driving is a major concern for adolescent and young adult ICD recipients, and no formal consensus among pediatric electrophysiologists exists regarding this issue. Since each state regulates its own driving restrictions, the recommendation regarding driving should be made based on state regulations and individual, patient-specific circumstances. The authors use their state recommendations for patients with syncope or seizures and allow driving if there have been no episodes in the past 3 months.

Support groups in young ICD recipients have not achieved the success of adult ICD support groups in part because of the small number of young ICD recipients followed at any one center and the geographic distance between this small number of patients.

Patient-to-patient support (i.e., introducing one ICD patient to another of similar age) can be extremely helpful to these patients. Serwer and colleagues[41] report great success with an annual "Youth and Young Adult Support Seminar" aimed at education and interaction between patients and families for ICD patients 30 years of age and younger. Support via the Internet is an option, but health care professionals must warn patients and families about the wealth of misinformation identified and correct any misconceptions they may have as a result.

Cardiovascular clinicians can have a positive impact on the child, adolescent, and young adult's response to life with an ICD. By providing honest and factual information regarding the ICD's function, implant-specific issues, and follow-up care, they can help patients and their families begin to assimilate this technology into their lives. Clinicians can provide support by listening, introducing ICD families to each other, providing support groups and/or networks, and especially by using their clinical observation skills to identify those patients at particular risk for negative outcomes in order to refer them to the appropriate resources.

Related Issues

There are several issues related to caring for ICD recipients that warrant additional discussion. These issues include surgical procedures that use electrocautery, other sources of EMI, device replacements, and external cardioversion/defibrillation.

Surgical Procedures Using Electrocautery

The use of electrocautery with patients with permanent pacemakers is discussed in detail in chapter 7. The issues concerning electrocautery and ICDs are somewhat different in that the electrocautery output can be sensed by the ICD as VF and lead to an inappropriate shock. Pacing output can also be inhibited, which is problematic in pacemaker-dependent patients. Additional concerns include the fact that the electrocautery can cause transient or permanent device reprogramming or that the stimulation threshold can be increased if current from the device is transmitted down the sensing/pacing lead.

In order to avoid erroneous sensing of VF, most manufacturers recommend deactivating the detection and termination algorithms for the duration of the surgical procedure. In this case, external defibrillation should be readily available in the event that the tachyarrhythmia occurs. Others use the magnet to temporarily suspend tachycardia detection if feasible,[48] but this can be problematic if the device is permanently programmed off with magnet application. Pacing output inhibition in pacemaker-dependent patients (rare in the pediatric population) can be minimized by using bipolar cautery in short bursts and by keeping it as far away from the device as possible. External pacing patches/pads can be placed prior to the procedure to be used in emergency situations. The increase in stimulation threshold is not within the clinician's control, but can be evaluated after the surgical procedure and compared with previous results. The use of an ultrasonic scalpel completely obviates the issues regarding EMI with ICDs and pacemakers in most surgical situations.

Collaboration among health care professionals caring for children and young adults with ICDs is critical in maintaining optimal patient and device outcomes. The ICD follow-up team should be notified of impending surgical procedures in order to determine the best options for preventing problems during the surgical procedure. The authors generally program the tachycardia recognition and termination algorithms off for the duration of the procedure and are available for emergencies throughout the procedure. The device is routinely interrogated and reprogrammed immediately following the procedure. If an increase in pacing thresholds is noted, an interim follow-up visit, from 1 to 2 weeks, is scheduled for reevaluation.

Other Sources of Electromagnetic Interference

There are other sources of EMI that ICD recipients may encounter. Cardiovascular clinicians must take the time to educate patients and families about these and provide them with recommendations. Strong magnetic fields, metal detectors at airports, airport wands, antitheft devices, and cellular phones are associated with EMI, but their effects can be minimized with appropriate precautions. Patients should be encouraged to stay away from very strong magnetic fields because of the probability of magnet mode initiation. Airport metal detectors rarely interfere with pacing function, but may "go off" while the ICD patient is passing through. Patients with ICDs can avoid going through them by simply showing their ICD identification card. Airport wands are a little more concerning because they contain a magnet. The potential for activating the magnet mode exists in this situation as well, ranging from momentary to permanent tachycardia detection suspension. Once again patients should show airport personnel their ICD identification card. Antitheft devices, also known as electronic article surveillance equipment, can affect ICD function[66,67] if patients linger while passing through them. Patients should be instructed not to lean on or stand near antitheft devices and to pass through them quickly.[68] The interaction of cellular telephones and ICDs has been studied,[69] with recommendations for use similar to those associated with pacemakers. Patients are instructed not to place the phone over the ICD (such as in shirt pocket in the "on" position), to use the phone with the ear on the opposite side of the ICD pocket, and to keep the phone 8 to 10 cm from the ICD.[68]

Device Replacements

Device replacements are generally performed secondary to battery depletion, device or lead malfunction, or to upgrade the system. Device upgrades may include a new device capable of tiered therapy and/or multiple therapy zones, a device with a higher energy output, or a device capable of providing dual chamber bradycardia pacing. Some replacement procedures include the implantation of additional hardware for inadequate DFTs. Regardless of the reason the device or system is being replaced, the clinician must remain cognizant of the responsibilities associated with ICD replacement.

Similar to pacemaker replacement procedures, the clinician should be familiar with the existing system in order to assess lead connections and compatibilities. Once the device has been removed, the clinician should perform the following tasks: 1) evaluate pacing and sensing functions of the implanted lead; 2) evaluate the integrity of the shocking electrode; 3) measure the impedance of the high-energy electrode; 4) perform DFTs; 5) evaluate intracardiac electrograms; and 6) perform a visual inspection of the lead or leads. These data will provide information regarding the chronic system and will allow changes in the overall system to be made at this time if necessary.

External Cardioversion/Defibrillation

Occasionally, patients with ICDs will require external cardioversion or defibrillation. Similar to permanent pacemakers, the effects can be minimized by taking certain precautions. Hayes[68] recommends the following: 1) if possible, place the paddles/pads in an anterior/posterior position; 2) attempt to keep the paddles/pads at least 4 inches from the device; 3) have the device-specific programmer readily available; and 4) interrogate the device after the procedure.

In summary, caring for children, adolescents, and young adults with ICDs is somewhat different than caring for adults due to the fact that children are in a constant stage of psychosocial, intellectual, and behavioral development. Cardiovascular clinicians must not only understand these developmental issues but also remain abreast of ICD technology and disease etiologies in the pediatric age group. Caring for these children can be challenging, but the rewards far outweigh any difficulties encountered in this patient population.

References

1. Kral MA, Spotnitz HM, Hordof A, et al: Automatic implantable cardioverter defibrillator implantation for malignant ventricular arrhythmias associated with congenital heart disease. Am J Cardiol 1989; 63:118–119.
2. Kron J, Oliver RP, Norsted S, et al: The automatic implantable cardioverter-defibrillator in young patients. J Am Coll Cardiol 1990; 16:896–902.
3. Silka MJ, Kron J, Dunnigan A, et al: Sudden cardiac death and the use of implantable cardioverter-defibrillators in pediatric patients. Circulation 1993; 87:800–807.
4. Kron J, Silka MJ, Ohm OJ, et al: Preliminary experience with nonthoracotomy implantable cardioverter-defibrillators in young patients. Pacing Clin Electrophysiol 1994; 17:26–30.
5. Sokoloski MC, O'Connor BK, Taylor SJ, et al: Pacemaker cardioverter defibrillators in young patients. J Am Coll Cardiol 1995; 25:53A. Abstract.
6. Groh WJ, Silka MJ, Oliver RP, et al: Use of implantable cardioverter-defibrillators in the congenital long QT syndrome. Am J Cardiol 1996; 78:703–706.
7. Hamilton RM, Dorian P, Gow RM, et al: Five-year experience with implantable defibrillators in children. Am J Cardiol 1996; 77:524–526.
8. Mirowski M, Reid PR, Mower MM, et al: Termination of malignant ventricular arrhythmias with an implanted automatic defibrillator in human beings. N Engl J Med 1980; 303:322–324.
9. Holmes DR: The implantable cardioverter-defibrillator. In Furman S, Hayes DL, Holmes DR Jr. (eds.): A Practice of Cardiac Pacing. 3rd ed. Mount Kisco, NY: Futura Publishing Company, Inc.; 1993:465–508.
10. Bardy GH, Ivey TD, Allen MD, et al: A prospective, randomized evaluation of biphasic versus monophasic waveform pulses of defibrillation efficacy in humans. J Am Coll Cardiol 1989; 14:728–733.
11. Molander N: Sudden natural death in later childhood and adolescence. Arch Dis Child 1982; 57:572–576.
12. Neuspiel DR, Killer LH: Sudden and unexpected death in childhood and adolescence. JAMA 1985; 254:1321–1325.
13. Driscoll DJ, Edwards JE: Sudden unexpected death in children and adolescents. J Am Coll Cardiol 1985; 5:118B-121B.
14. Eisenberg M, Bergner L, Hallstrom A: Epidemiology of cardiac arrest and resuscitation in children. Ann Emerg Med 1983; 12:672–674.
15. Walsh CK, Krongrad E: Terminal cardiac electrical activity in pediatric patients. Am J Cardiol 1983; 51:557–561.

16. Silka MJ, Hardy BG, Menashe VD, et al: A population-based prospective evaluation of risk of sudden cardiac death after operation for common congenital heart defects. J Am Coll Cardiol 1998; 32:245–251.
17. Silka MJ, Kron J, Gillette PC: Implantable cardioverter-defibrillators in children and adolescents. In Estes NAM, Manolis AS, Wang PJ (eds.): Implantable Cardioverter-Defibrillators: A Comprehensive Textbook. New York: Marcel Dekker, Inc.; 1994:205–227.
18. Mckenna WJ, Franklin RCG, Nihoyannopoulos P, et al: Arrhythmia and prognosis in infants, children, and adolescents with hypertrophic cardiomyopathy. J Am Coll Cardiol 1988; 11:147–153.
19. Friedman R, Moak JP, Garson A Jr.: Clinical course of idiopathic dilated cardiomyopathy in children. J Am Coll Cardiol 1991; 18:152–156.
20. Burch M, Siddan SA, Celemaier DS, et al: Dilated cardiomyopathy in children: Determinants of outcome. Br Heart J 1994; 72:246–250.
21. Breithardt G, Wichter T, Haverkamp W, et al: Implantable cardioverter defibrillator therapy in patients with arrhythmogenic right ventricular dysplasia, long QT syndrome, or no structural heart disease. Am Heart J 1994; 127:1151–1158.
22. Theine G, Nava A, Corrado D, et al: Right ventricular cardiomyopathy and sudden death in young people. N Engl J Med 1988; 318:129–133.
23. Priori S, Borgreffe M, Camm AJ, et al: Role of the implantable defibrillator in patients with idiopathic ventricular fibrillation. Pacing Clin Electrophysiol 1995; 18:799. Abstract.
24. Garson A Jr., Bink-Boelkens M, Hesslein PS, et al: Atrial flutter in the young: A collaborative study of 380 cases. J Am Coll Cardiol 1985; 6:871–878.
25. Lambert EC, Menon VA, Wagner HR, et al: Sudden unexpected death from cardiovascular disease in children. Am J Cardiol 1974; 34:89–96.
26. Garson A, Randall DC, Gillette PC, et al: Prevention of sudden death after repair of tetralogy of Fallot: Treatment of ventricular arrhythmias. J Am Coll Cardiol 1985; 6:221–227.
27. Campbell M: Natural history of congenital aortic stenosis. Br Heart J 1968; 30:514–526.
28. Flynn CJ, Wolff GS, Dick M II, et al: Cardiac rhythm after Mustard operation for complete transposition of the great arteries. N Engl J Med 1984; 310:1635–1638.
29. Morris CD, Menashe VD: 25 year mortality after surgical repair of congenital heart defect in childhood. JAMA 1991; 266:3447–3452.
30. Gregatoros G, Cheitlin MD, Conill A, et al: ACC/AHA guidelines for implantation of cardiac pacemakers and antiarrhythmia devices: A report of the American College of Cardiology/American Heart Association Task Force on Practice Guidelines. Circulation 1998; 97:1325–1335.
31. Silka MJ, Gillette PC: Advanced electrical management of atrial and ventricular tachyarrhythmias. In Gillette PC, Garson A Jr. (eds.): Clinical Pediatric Arrhythmias. 2nd ed. Philadelphia: WB Saunders Company; 1999:221–230.
32. Stephenson N, Combs WJ: Artificial cardiac pacemakers and implantable cardioverter defibrillators. In Kinney MR, Packa DR (eds.): Andreoli's Comprehensive Cardiac Care. 8th ed. St. Louis: Mosby-Year Book, Inc.; 1996:220–255.
33. Kantharia BK, Callans DJ, Hessen SE, et al: Engineering and clinical aspects of defibrillation leads. In Ellenbogen KA, Kay GN, Wilkoff BL (eds.): Clinical Cardiac Pacing and Defibrillation. 2nd ed. Philadelphia: WB Saunders Company; 2000:151–165.
34. Mehra R, DeGroot PJ, Norenberg MS: Energy waveforms and lead systems for implantable defibrillators. In Luderitz B, Saksena S (eds.): Interventional Electrophysiology. Mount Kisco, NY: Futura Publishing Company, Inc.; 1991: 377–394.

35. Neuzner J, Pitschner HF, Huth C, et al: Effect of biphasic waveform pulse on endocardial defibrillation efficacy in humans. Pacing Clin Electrophysiol 1994; 17:207–212.
36. Block M, Hammel D, Bocker D, et al: A prospective randomized cross-over comparison of mono- and biphasic defibrillation using nonthoracotomy lead configuration in humans. J Cardiovasc Electrophysiol 1994; 5:581–590.
37. Natale S, Sra J, Axtell K, et al: Preliminary experience with a hybrid nonthoracotomy defibrillating system that includes a biphasic device: Comparison with standard monophasic device using the same lead system. J Am Coll Cardiol 1994; 24:406–412.
38. Wilson WR, Greer GE, Grubb BP: Implantable cardioverter-defibrillators in children: A single-institutional experience. Ann Thorac Surg 1998; 65:775–778.
39. Gold MR, Shorofsky SR: Transvenous defibrillation lead systems. J Cardiovasc Electrophysiol 1996; 7:570–580.
40. Silka MJ, Rice MJ: Paradoxic embolism due to altered hemodynamic sequence following transvenous pacing. Pacing Clin Electrophysiol 1991; 14:499–503.
41. Serwer GA, Dorostkar PC, LeRoy SS: Pediatric pacing and defibrillator usage. In Ellenbogen KA, Kay GN, Wilkoff BL (eds.): Clinical Cardiac Pacing and Defibrillation. 2nd ed. Philadelphia: WB Saunders Company; 2000:953–989.
42. Untereker DF, Shepard RB, Schmidt CL, et al: Power systems for implantable pacemakers, cardioverters, and defibrillators. In Ellenbogen KA, Kay GN, Wilkoff BL (eds.): Clinical Cardiac Pacing and Defibrillation. 2nd ed. Philadelphia: WB Saunders Company; 2000:167–193.
43. Medtronic Incorporated: Gem II DR™ Product Information Manual. Minneapolis, MN: Medtronic Inc.; 1999.
44. Hummel JD, Kalbfleisch SJ, Dillon JM: Pocket Guide for Cardiac Electrophysiology. Philadelphia: WB Saunders Company; 2000:266–281.
45. Dunst C, Trivette C, Deal A: Enabling and Empowering Families—Principles and Guidelines for Practice. Cambridge, MA: Brookline Books; 1988.
46. Belott PH, Reynolds DW: Permanent pacemaker and implantable cardioverter-defibrillator implantation. In Ellenbogen KA, Kay GN, Wilkoff BL (eds.): Clinical Cardiac Pacing and Defibrillation. 2nd ed. Philadelphia: WB Saunders Company; 2000:573–644.
47. Kaminer SJ, Hixon RL, Strong WB: Evaluation and recommendations for participation in athletics for children with heart disease. Curr Opin Pediatr 1995; 7:595–600.
48. Crossley GH III: Follow-up of the patient with a defibrillator. In Ellenbogen KA, Kay GN, Wilkoff BL (eds.): Clinical Cardiac Pacing and Defibrillation. 2nd ed. Philadelphia: WB Saunders Company; 2000:931–938.
49. Adams TP: Patient follow up systems. In Kroll MW, Lehmann MH (eds.): Implantable Cardioverter Defibrillator Therapy: The Engineering-Clinical Interface. Norwell, MA: Kluwer Academic Publishers; 1996:421–434.
50. Hayes DL, Friedman PA: Follow-up. In Hayes DL, Lloyd MA, Friedman PA (eds.): Cardiac Pacing and Defibrillation: A Clinical Approach. Armonk, NY: Futura Publishing Company, Inc.; 2000:541–585.
51. Brady PA, Friedman PA, Trusty JM, et al: High failure rate for an epicardial implantable cardioverter-defibrillator lead: Implications for long-term follow up of patients with an implantable cardioverter-defibrillator. J Am Coll Cardiol 1998; 31:616–622.
52. Nisam S, Fogoros RN: Troubleshooting of patients with implantable cardioverter-defibrillators. In Singer I (ed.): Implantable Cardioverter-Defibrillator. Armonk, NY: Futura Publishing Company, Inc.; 1994:433–455.
53. Knight L, Livingston NA, Gawlinski A, et al: Caring for patients with third-generation implantable cardioverter defibrillators: From decision to implant to patient's return home. Crit Care Nurs 1997; 17:46–63.

54. May CD, Smith PR, Murdock CJ, et al: The impact of the implantable cardioverter defibrillator on quality-of-life. Pacing Clin Electrophysiol 1995; 18:1411–1418.
55. Bainger EM, Fernsler JI: Perceived quality of life before and after implantation of an internal cardioverter defibrillator. Am J Crit Care 1995; 4:36–43.
56. Dubin AM, Batsford WP, Lewis RJ, et al: Quality-of-life in patients receiving implantable cardioverter defibrillators at or before age 40. Pacing Clin Electrophysiol 1996; 19:1555–1559.
57. Gallagher RD, McKinley S, Mangan B, et al: The impact of the implantable cardioverter defibrillator on quality of life. Am J Crit Care 1997; 6:16–24.
58. Veseth-Rogers J: A practical approach to teaching the automatic implantable cardioverter-defibrillator patient. Cardiovasc Nurs 1990; 4:7–19.
59. DeBorde R, Aarons D, Biggs M: The automatic implantable cardioverter-defibrillator. AACN Clin Issues Crit Care Nurs 1991; 2:170–177.
60. Teplitz L, Egenes K, Brask L: Life after sudden death: The development of a support group for automatic implantable cardioverter-defibrillator patients. J Cardiovasc Nurs 1990; 4:20–32.
61. Schuster PM, Phillips S, Dillon DL, et al: The psychosocial and physiological experiences of patients with an implantable cardioverter defibrillator. Rehab Nurs 1998; 23:30–37.
62. Vitale MB, Funk M: Quality of life in younger persons with implantable cardioverter defibrillator. Dimen Crit Care Nurs 1995; 14:100–111.
63. Zeigler VL, Corbett KS: Psychosocial aspects of caring for pediatric pacemaker recipients and their families. In Gillette PC, Zeigler VL (eds.): Pediatric Cardiac Pacing. Armonk, New York: Futura Publishing Company, Inc; 1995:181–203.
64. Burke LJ: Securing life through technology acceptance: The first six months after transvenous internal cardioverter defibrillator implantation. Heart Lung 1996; 25:352–366.
65. Wong DL: Impact of chronic illness, disability, or death on the child and family. In Wong DL (ed.): Whaley and Wong's Essentials of Pediatric Nursing. 4th ed. St. Louis: Mosby-Yearbook, Inc., 1993:504–548.
66. Groh WJ, Boschee SA, Engelstein ED, et al: Interactions between electronic article surveillance systems and implantable cardioverter-defibrillators. Circulation 1999; 100:387–392.
67. Santucci PA, Haw J, Trohman RG, et al: Interference with an implantable defibrillator by an electronic antitheft-surveillance device. N Engl J Med 1998; 339:1371–1374.
68. Hayes DL: Electromagnetic interference and implantable devices. In Hayes DL, Lloyd MA, Friedman PA (eds.): Cardiac Pacing and Defibrillation: A Clinical Approach. Armonk, NY: Futura Publishing Company, Inc.; 2000:519–539.
69. Fetter JG, Ivans V, Benditt DG, et al: Digital cellular telephone interaction with implantable cardioverter-defibrillators. J Am Coll Cardiol 1998; 31:623–628.

Index

Page numbers in italics indicate a figure.